# Reflux Aspiration and Lung Disease

Alyn H. Morice • Peter W. Dettmar
Editors

# Reflux Aspiration and Lung Disease

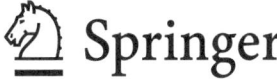
Springer

*Editors*
Alyn H. Morice
University of Hull
Hull York Medical School
Cottingham
East Yorkshire
United Kingdom

Peter W. Dettmar
Castle Hill Hospital
RD Biomed Limited
Cottingham
East Yorkshire
United Kingdom

ISBN 978-3-030-08035-8      ISBN 978-3-319-90525-9   (eBook)
https://doi.org/10.1007/978-3-319-90525-9

© Springer International Publishing AG, part of Springer Nature 2018
Softcover re-print of the Hardcover 1st edition 2018
This work is subject to copyright. All rights are reserved by the Publisher, whether the whole or part of the material is concerned, specifically the rights of translation, reprinting, reuse of illustrations, recitation, broadcasting, reproduction on microfilms or in any other physical way, and transmission or information storage and retrieval, electronic adaptation, computer software, or by similar or dissimilar methodology now known or hereafter developed.
The use of general descriptive names, registered names, trademarks, service marks, etc. in this publication does not imply, even in the absence of a specific statement, that such names are exempt from the relevant protective laws and regulations and therefore free for general use.
The publisher, the authors, and the editors are safe to assume that the advice and information in this book are believed to be true and accurate at the date of publication. Neither the publisher nor the authors or the editors give a warranty, express or implied, with respect to the material contained herein or for any errors or omissions that may have been made. The publisher remains neutral with regard to jurisdictional claims in published maps and institutional affiliations.

This Springer imprint is published by Springer Nature, under the registered company Springer International Publishing AG
The registered company address is: Gewerbestrasse 11, 6330 Cham, Switzerland

# Foreword

Anatomically, the GI track and the respiratory system briefly share common space on their journey to their respective end organs. The clinical relevance of this relationship was emphasised over a century ago in 1892 by Sir William Osler in his elegant medicine textbook when he observed that asthma patients frequently have their largest meal in the middle of the day to avoid an asthma attack. Today we are reminded that "the devil is in the details" as we explore the depths of this relationship in the enclosed international multi-authored, multi-specialty text.

As a clinically active gastroenterologist with a career-long interest in gastroesophageal reflux and its relation to all manner of associated pulmonary disorders, this book is a most welcome addition to this field. Doctors Dettmar and Morice have approached this topic with a most welcome intensity by enlisting input for individual chapters from the correct experts. This text belongs in the personal library of all of us who see patients who likely suffer from a lung disease likely related to aspiration of refluxed gastric contents.

Donald O. Castell
Professor of Medicine, Director,
Esophageal Disorders Program,
Medical University of South Carolina,
Charleston, SC, USA

# Preface

Reflux and aspiration is the Cinderella of medicine. The conjunction of the aerodigestive tract has devolved to three specialities: respiratory medicine, gastroenterology and otolaryngology. Whilst each speciality brings its own expertise to the table, a synthesis is urgently required. Our ambition in this book has been to bring together a disparate collection of world renowned experts to provide the reader with a comprehensive overview in areas which they may not have previously considered in dealing with the patient. Indeed, this dichotomy or rather 'trichotomy' is a source of much frustration with patients bouncing between individual specialities, each denying that the patient's symptoms lie within their area of expertise. Holistic medicine is absent from this paradigm.

The pathological basis of inflammation in the upper and lower airways has moved on from purely acidic damage to a greater understanding of the aggressive factors which are causative factors.

Modern diagnostic techniques have revealed previously unrecognised aetiological mechanisms and are pointing to targeted therapy.

The conventional paradigm of individual lung disease, such as asthma and pulmonary fibrosis, becomes blurred when the aetiological role of aspiration in the pathogenesis of these syndromes is considered. Indeed, we operate a Joint Airways clinic where individual patients are not pigeonholed but have personalised therapy related to the pathological processes determined by the specific investigations. Perhaps the most important innovations have occurred in the area of therapeutics. The realisation that aspiration was not treated by proton pump inhibitors (however effective they are in classical peptic symptoms) has led to an exploration of alternative therapeutic strategies based on the amelioration of reflux rather than acid.

We hope that the reader will dip into this text and find gems which are relevant to them from other specialities.

| | |
|---|---|
| Cottingham, UK | Alyn H. Morice |
| Cottingham, UK | Peter Dettmar |

# Acknowledgement

The editors would like to acknowledge the exceptional contribution of Mrs Julie Crawford to the production of this book. Without her skills in the marshalling the many cats (not least the editors) to produce a cogent whole this volume would have foundered at its inception. She has our grateful thanks.

# Contents

**Part I  Pathology**

1. **Diagnostic Confusion Through the Ages** .................... 3
   Alyn H. Morice

2. **An Overview of Gastroesophageal Reflux Disease** ............ 9
   Serhat Bor

3. **Chemical Composition of Refluxate** ......................... 29
   Iain A. Brownlee

4. **Pathological Processes** .................................... 41
   Jeffrey P. Pearson, Adil Aldhahrani, Peter I. Chater,
   and Matthew D. Wilcox

5. **Pathophysiology in the Lung** ............................... 55
   Chris Ward, Rhys Jones, Mellissa Friel, Eoin Hunt, and Des Murphy

6. **Effect of Reflux on Cough Sensitivity
   and Bronchial Responsiveness** ............................... 71
   Peter V. Dicpinigaitis

**Part II  Diagnosis**

7. **Questionnaire Diagnosis of Airways Reflux** ................. 81
   Shoaib Faruqi

8. **Pepsin Detection as a Diagnostic Test for Reflux Disease** .. 91
   Peter W. Dettmar, Rhianna K. Lenham, Adrian J. Parkinson, and
   Andrew D. Woodcock

9. **Imaging Reflux** ............................................ 105
   Luca Marciani

10. **High Resolution Oesophageal Manometry in the Investigation
    of Unexplained Cough** ...................................... 115
    Jennifer Burke and Warren Jackson

11. **Cough Monitoring in Reflux Lung Disease** .................. 125
    Aakash K. Pandya, Joanne E. Kavanagh, and Surinder S. Birring

## Part III Reflux Aspiration in Specific Lung Diseases

12 **The Relationship Between Asthma and Gastro-Esophageal Reflux** .............................. 137
Adalberto Pacheco

13 **Gastroesophageal Reflux Disease (GERD) and COPD** ............ 165
Nabid Zaer and John R. Hurst

14 **Gastro Oesophageal Reflux and Bronchiectasis** ................. 175
Kirsty L. Hett and Ben Hope-Gill

15 **Reflux Aspiration and Cystic Fibrosis** ........................ 187
Ans Pauwels

16 **Gastroesophageal Reflux and Idiopathic Pulmonary Fibrosis** ...... 195
Lawrence A. Ho and Ganesh Raghu

17 **Gastro-Oesophageal Reflux Disease (GORD) and Chronic Cough** ........................................ 205
Lorcan McGarvey and Kian Fan Chung

18 **Reflux and Aspiration: Their Presumed Role in Chronic Cough and the Development of End-Stage Lung Disease** ................ 213
Jacob A. Klapper, Brian Gulack, and Matthew G. Hartwig

## Part IV Reflux Aspiration in Specific Circumstances

19 **Reflux and Aspiration in the Intensive Care Unit** ................ 227
Peter V. Dicpinigaitis

20 **Incidence and Risk of Aspiration in Mechanically Ventilated Patients** .......................................... 235
Miles J. Klimara, Rahul Nanchal, and Nikki Johnston

21 **Reflux in Pediatrics**.......................................... 245
Nina Gluchowski and Rachel Rosen

22 **Aspiration in the Elderly** .................................... 261
Midori Miyagi and Satoru Ebihara

## Part V Therapy of Airway Reflux

23 **Acid Suppression for Management of Gastroesophageal Reflux Disease: Benefits and Risks** ........................... 269
Carmelo Scarpignato and Luigi Gatta

24 **Reflux Inhibitors and Prokinetics** ............................ 293
Woo-Jung Song

| | | |
|---|---|---|
| **25** | **Macrolides, Reflux and Respiratory Disease** .................... 303 Michael G. Crooks and Tamsin Nash | |
| **26** | **Inhaled, Nebulised and Oral Bronchodilators in Reflux Disease** .... 333 K. Suresh Babu and Jaymin B. Morjaria | |
| **27** | **Speech Pathology: Reflux Aspiration and Lung Diseases** .......... 343 Anne E. Vertigan | |
| **28** | **Anti Reflux Surgery** ........................................... 357 Zainab Rai, Alyn H. Morice, and Peter Sedman | |

**Index** ......................................................... 365

# Abbreviations[1]

| | |
|---|---|
| α-SMA | α-Smooth muscle actin |
| ACE | Angiotensin-converting enzyme |
| ACG | American College of Gastroenterology |
| ADL | Activities of daily living |
| AGA | American Gastroenterological Association |
| AHR | Airway hyper-responsiveness |
| ALI | Acute lung injury |
| AMs | Alveolar macrophages |
| AR | Anti-regurgitation |
| ARS | Anti-reflux surgery |
| ATP | Adenosine triphosphate |
| AUC | Area under curve |
| b.i.d. | Twice daily |
| BAL | Broncho-alveolar lavage |
| BALF | Broncho-alveolar lavage fluid |
| BHR | Bronchial hyper-responsiveness |
| BMI | Body mass index |
| BO | Barrett's oesophagus |
| BOS | Bronchiolitis obliterans syndrome |
| BSG | British Society of Gastroenterology |
| CC | Chronic cough |
| CDCA | Chenodeoxycholic acid |
| CF | Cystic fibrosis |
| CFTR | Cystic fibrosis transmembrane conductance regulator |
| COPD | Chronic obstructive pulmonary disease |

---

[1]Churchill said Britain and the USA were two peoples divided by a common language. This was never truer than in the field of (o)esophageal disease. It would have been nice to agree a common language for this volume; however the literature extensively reviewed by our authors uses both UK and US spelling. To change these and the extensive list of abbreviations to fit a common schema would make location of these references difficult if not impossible. We have decided therefore to leave the choice of GORD or GERD, LOS or LES, etc. to the individual contributor and apologise here to the reader for any confusion that arises.

| | |
|---|---|
| CPAP | Continuous positive airway pressure |
| CPG | Central pattern generator |
| CQLQ | Cough-specific quality of life questionnaire |
| CReSS | Comprehensive Reflux Symptom Scale |
| CV | Cardiovascular |
| CYP | Cytochrome $P_{450}$ |
| DDIs | Drug to drug interactions |
| DIOS | Distal intestinal obstruction syndrome |
| DNase | Deoxyribonuclease |
| EBC | Exhaled breath condensate |
| ECL | Enterochromaffin-like cells |
| ECLIPSE | Evaluation of COPD longitudinally to identify predictive surrogate endpoints |
| EER | Extra-esophageal reflux |
| EGD | Esophagogastroduodenoscopy |
| ELISA | Enzyme-linked immunosorbent assay |
| ENT | Ear, nose and throat |
| ESLD | End-stage lung disease |
| FAK | Focal adhesion kinase |
| FDA | Food and Drug Administration |
| FDG | 18F-Fluorodeoxyglucose |
| FEES | Fibreoptic endoscopic evaluation of swallowing |
| FEV-1 | Forced expiratory volume in 1 second |
| FH | Functional heartburn |
| FVC | Forced vital capacity |
| GABA | γ-aminobutyric acid |
| GABAB | GABA type B receptor |
| GER | Gastroesophageal reflux |
| GERD | Gastroesophageal reflux disease |
| GI | Gastrointestinal |
| GJ | Gastro-jejunal |
| GMP | Guanosine monophosphate |
| GOLD | Global Initiative for Chronic Obstructive Lung Disease |
| GOPG | Gastro-oesophageal pressure gradient |
| GOR | Gastro-oesophageal reflux |
| GORD | Gastro-oesophageal reflux disease |
| GSAS | Gastroesophageal Symptoms Assessment Scale |
| H2 | Histamine2 |
| H2RAs | Histamine2-receptor antagonists |
| HARQ | Hull airways reflux questionnaire |
| HCl | Hydrochloric acid |
| HE | Hypersensitive esophagus |
| HH | Hiatal hernia |
| HOB | Head of bed |
| HP | Helicobacter pylori |

| | |
|---|---|
| HR | Hazards ratio |
| HRCT | High-resolution computed tomography |
| HRIM | High-resolution oesophageal manometry combined with impedance |
| HRM | High-resolution oesophageal manometry |
| HRQL | Health-related quality of life questionnaire |
| HSCT | Haematopoietic stem cell transplant |
| 5-HTR4 | 5-Hydroxytryptamine receptor 4 |
| ICS | Inhaled corticosteroids |
| ICU | Intensive care unit |
| IIP | Idiopathic interstitial pneumonia |
| IL-8 | Interleukin 8 |
| IPF | Idiopathic pulmonary fibrosis |
| IV | Intravenous |
| LARS | Laparoscopic anti-reflux surgery |
| LBP | Lipopolysaccharide binding protein |
| LCM | Leicester Cough Monitor |
| LCQ | Leicester cough questionnaire |
| LDH | Lactic dehydrogenase |
| LES | Lower esophageal sphincter |
| LFD | Lateral flow device |
| LLM | Lipid-laden alveolar macrophages |
| LOS | Lower oesophageal sphincter |
| LPR | Laryngopharyngeal reflux |
| LPR-HRQL | Laryngopharyngeal reflux health related quality of life questionnaire |
| LPS | Lipopolysaccharide |
| LRTI | Lower respiratory tract infection |
| LTRAs | Leukotriene antagonists |
| MAC | Mycobacterium avium complex |
| MCC | Mucociliary clearance |
| MCP | Monocyte chemoattractant protein |
| MDT | Multi-disciplinary team |
| mGluR5 | Metabotropic glutamate receptor 5 |
| MII | Multiple intraluminal impedance |
| MMP | Matrix metalloproteinases |
| MPO | Myeloperoxidase |
| MRI | Magnetic resonance imaging |
| mRNA | Messenger ribonucleic acid |
| MRSA | Methicillin-resistant *Staphylococcus aureus* |
| MTT | An assay |
| NAB | Nocturnal acid breakthrough |
| NAC | N-acetylcysteine |
| NASPGHAN | North American Society of Gastroenterology, Hepatology and Nutrition |

| | |
|---|---|
| NCCP | Non-cardiac chest pain |
| NCFB | Non-cystic fibrosis bronchiectasis |
| NERD | Non-erosive reflux disease |
| nGERD | Nocturnal GERD |
| NNT | Number needed to treat |
| NNTB | Number needed to treat for an additional beneficial outcome |
| NO | Nitric oxide |
| NPV | Negative predictive value |
| NSAIDs | Non-steroidal anti-inflammatory drug |
| NTM | Non-tuberculous mycobacteria |
| OB | Obliterative bronchiolitis |
| OR | Odds ratio |
| OSA | Obstructive sleep apnea |
| OTC | Over-the-counter |
| OVA | Ovalbumin |
| PAR | Protease-activated receptor |
| P-CABs | Potassium-competitive acid blockers |
| PCR | Polymerase chain reaction |
| PDE | Phospho-di-esterases |
| PET | Positron emission tomography |
| PGE2 | Prostaglandin E2 |
| PHD | Prolylhydroxylase domain proteins |
| pH-MII | Multiple intraluminal impedance with pH |
| PP | Post-prandial |
| PPI | Proton pump inhibitor |
| PPV | Positive predictive value |
| PRSQ | Pharyngeal reflux symptom questionnaire |
| PVFM | Paradoxical vocal fold movement |
| QoL | Quality of life |
| QT | Electrocardiogram QT interval |
| RCTs | Randomized control trials |
| RESULT | Reflux Surgery in Lung Transplantation |
| RFS | Reflux finding score |
| rhDNase | Recombinant human DNase |
| RI | Reflux index |
| RNA | Ribonucleic acid |
| ROC | Receiver operating characteristic |
| RSI | Reflux symptom index |
| RSS | Reflux symptom score |
| SAP | Symptom association probability |
| SD | Standard deviation |
| SER | Supraesophageal reflux |
| SERQ | Supraesophageal reflux questionnaire |
| SF-36 | Short form 36-item questionnaire |
| SGRQ | St Georges respiratory questionnaire |

| | |
|---|---|
| SI | Symptom index |
| SIDS | Sudden infant death syndrome |
| SLP | Speech-language pathologists |
| SMC | Smooth muscle cells |
| SPECT | Single photon emission computed tomography |
| SRMD | Stress-related mucosal damage |
| SSI | Symptom sensitivity index |
| TER | Transepithelial resistance |
| TLESR | Transient lower esophageal sphincter relaxation |
| TLOSR | Transient lower oesophageal sphincter relaxation |
| TLOSRs | Transient LOS relaxations |
| TLR | Toll-like receptor |
| TNF | Tumour necrosis factor |
| TNFα | Tumour necrosis factorα |
| TRP | Transient receptor potential |
| TRPV-1 | Transient receptor potential vanilloid-1 |
| UCSF | University of California, San Francisco |
| UES | Upper esophageal sphincter |
| UK | United Kingdom |
| UOS | Upper oesophageal sphincter |
| VAEs | Ventilator-associated events |
| VAP | Ventilator-associated pneumonia |
| VAS | Visual Analogue Scale |
| VATS | Video-assisted thoracoscopic surgery |
| VCD | Vocal cord dysfunction |
| VFSS | Video Fluoroscopic Swallow Study |
| WRAP-IPF | Weighing Risks and Benefits of Laparoscopic Anti-reflux Surgery in Patients with Idiopathic Pulmonary Fibrosis |
| ZO-1 | Zonula occludens-1 |

# Part I
# Pathology

# Diagnostic Confusion Through the Ages

Alyn H. Morice

> There's a sign on the wall
> But she wants to be sure
> 'cause you know sometimes words have two meanings
> Led Zeppelin 'Stairway to heaven'

## Introduction

Medicine is increasingly compartmentalised. Specialism has its advantages, but it occurs at the cost of a holistic approach to the patient. Respiratory and ENT symptoms are ascribed to known diseases with little consideration of other organ systems. In this chapter, I have attempted to illustrate that earlier physicians, not constrained by rigid diagnostic and pathological straitjackets were easily able to see and understand the intimate relationship between reflux, aspiration, and lung disease.

An English psychiatrist is visiting an Italian colleague and sits in on a consultation. The patient enters shaking and explains that he has been unable to settle himself down without his usual morning drink. At the end of the consultation the Englishman suggests that he is a classic alcoholic, but the Italian demurs "he is just a neurotic who drinks too much". This diagnostic confusion has characterised the history of reflux and aspiration throughout the ages. Today if you present in later life with a history of cough and or wheeze and are seen in an asthma clinic you will be diagnosed as having severe possibly neutrophilic asthma. As is admitted in the British Thoracic Society asthma guidelines, there is no agreed definition of asthma. "The diagnosis of asthma is a clinical one; there is no standardised definition of the type, severity or frequency of symptoms, nor the findings on investigation. The absence of a gold standard definition means that it is not possible to make clear evidence

---

A. H. Morice
Respiratory Medicine, HYMS, University of Hull, Castle Hill Hospital, Cottingham, East Yorkshire, UK
e-mail: a.h.morice@hull.ac.uk

© Springer International Publishing AG, part of Springer Nature 2018
A. H. Morice, P. W. Dettmar (eds.), *Reflux Aspiration and Lung Disease*,
https://doi.org/10.1007/978-3-319-90525-9_1

based recommendations on how to make a diagnosis of asthma." Asthma is thus in the eye of the beholder.

Similarly, if you are referred to the COPD service then you will be labelled as COPD probably of the chronic bronchitis phenotype. The recent GOLD guidelines promote a "grade 1" phenotype who have respiratory symptoms but have a percent predicted FEV1 within the normal range. COPD without airflow obstruction! Such foolishness is not restricted to the respiratory community. In chronic upper airways disease dysphonia is common and pseudo-diagnoses such as laryngeal dysfunction abound. Unfortunately the likelihood of the patient achieving the most likely correct diagnosis—that of recurrent reflux and aspiration—is small. Doctors, whether ENT, gastro, or respiratory have been trained to view airway reflux and aspiration as a rarity, when in fact it is probably one of the common cause of airway symptoms. Reflux is an everyday phenomenon, we all experience tasting food which is regurgitated. The intellectual leap required to translate this into a pathological process has proven difficult throughout the ages. The following essay is not meant as a comprehensive history of reflux, aspiration and the airways but is intended to illustrate that we are by no means the first to recognise the connection between the gut and lung.

## True Flatulent Asthma

Sir John Floyer in his "Treatise of the asthma" provides us with beautifully written clinical description of what he calls flatulent asthma [1]. He himself was a sufferer. I have quoted from his third edition (1726) and modified the typography; 's' was written as 'f' in those days which causes confusion when he is talking of the chest sucking the air (Fig. 1.1).

## Page X

Asthma is a Defluxion … and allow the Nerves to be Instruments of the Defluxion (Collins English Dictionary: a flow of bodily humours accompanying a disease—obsolete).

## Page XXVIII

A flatulent slimy *Cacochymia,* which is bred in the Stomach, and creates Inflations there, and givers an Effervescence in the Blood, and an Inflation in the Membranes of the Lungs, and this is the true Periodic Flatulent Asthma.

## Page 5

The main body of text is divided into four sections. In the first there is a detailed and well observed description of what is clearly reflux and aspiration.

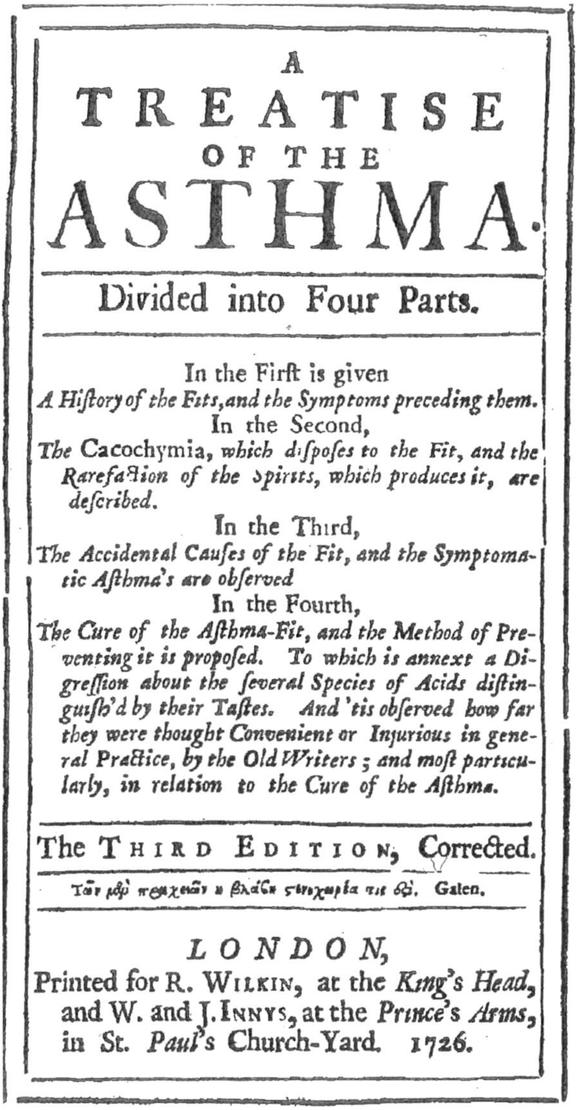

**Fig. 1.1** Frontispiece of Floyer's Treatise on the Asthma, 3rd edition

> A
> TREATISE
> OF THE
> ASTHMA.
>
> Divided into Four Parts.
>
> In the First is given
> A History of the Fits, and the Symptoms preceding them.
> In the Second,
> The Cacochymia, which difpofes to the Fit, and the Rarefaction of the Spirits, which produces it, are defcribed.
> In the Third,
> The Accidental Caufes of the Fit, and the Symptomatic Afthma's are obferved
> In the Fourth,
> The Cure of the Afthma-Fit, and the Method of Preventing it is propofed. To which is annext a Digreffion about the feveral Species of Acids diftinguifh'd by their Taftes. And 'tis obferved how far they were thought Convenient or Injurious in general Practice, by the Old Writers; and moft particularly, in relation to the Cure of the Afthma.
>
> The THIRD EDITION, Corrected.
>
> Τῶν μὲν πραχέων ἡ βλάβη ςυγχωρία τις ᾖ. Galen.
>
> LONDON,
> Printed for R. WILKIN, at the King's Head, and W. and J. INNYS, at the Prince's Arms, in St. Paul's Church-Yard. 1726.

In the afternoon which precedes the Fit of the *Flatulent Asthma* (which is commonly called the *Humid*, or *Spitting Asthma*) about 2 or 3 h after Meat, most Asthmatics are sensible of a great Straightness, or Fulness about the Pit of the Stomach, which is then oppressed with Wind, and an insipid Ructus rises from it, and this Fulness of the Stomach is the first Sign of the ensuing Fit; it appears before any Cough or Straightness Happens in the Lungs. This Fullness in the Stomach Seems to Me to Depend Partly on the Windy Rarefaction of the Digesting Meat Contained in Its Cavity; and Also on the Inflation of the Nervous Fibres of the Skins of the Stomach.

## Page 6

Floyer is the first to observe the characteristic afferent hypersensitivity, recently described as Cough Hypersensitivity Syndrome by the European Respiratory Society task force, 300 years later:

All hot Things disorder them more, as sitting by the Fire, Wine, Tobacco; all cool Liquors, as Water relieve the Fulness at the Stomach … frequent great Retchings.

## Page 9

I must observe, that the Fit of the Asthma happens after Purging, Vomiting, or Fasting, when none or few Contents are in the Stomach, and then this Flattuosity must be a Nervous Affectation of the Membranes.

## Page 10

In the paragraph below Floyer suggests the intimate relationship of nervous control via the vagus nerve. A connection, which is still debated today!

For the *Par Vagum* sends Branches both the Heart and the Lungs, and the Orifice of the Stomach, where the First Nervous effects, or Inflations begin, and that by the same Nerves is communicated to the Heart, and Lungs, and Membranes of the Breast.

## Page 23

Here Floyer points out gaseous nature of the reflux and its origin from the chyle.

That the Preternatural State of the Chyle in the Asthma is a Flatulent Crudity, appears, because all flatulent things, as new Beer, Turnips, Cabbage, … very much disagree with the Asthmatic, by irritating the Spirits, and creating a Windiness in the Stomach, and they also affect the Nerves.

Chapter 3 is devoted to the triggers for asthma. The quality of air is thought to be a crucial precipitant "any kind of smoak offends the Spirits of the Asthmatic; and for that reason many of them cannot bear the Air of *London*". Diet is also seen as an important factor. Strong wine is to be avoided. "But Brandy, above all Liquors, is most pernicious to the Asthma, it rarefies the Windy spirits most of all …". Both exercise and "passions" are described as harmful and he quotes Hippocrates as advising "all Asthmatics to abstain from Anger and Shouting".

The fourth chapter deals with the cure for asthma. It opens with "*First*, To abate the Quantity of the Windy Chyle in the Belly …" But despite cataloguing numerous cures and remedies Floyer is quite frank in that most of them are ineffective. He is particularly dismissive of bleeding and "I have tried Vomiting, Purging, Sweating over Night, and the Cortex to prevent the Fit I apprehended was coming, but all in vain; for the fit was frequently worse for it."

The final section of this marvellous book, full of excellent clinical observation and deduction deals with case reports. Given low level of physiological knowledge at the time (for example the circulation of the blood as described as a newly discovered by Harvey) Floyer's perception is astonishing. I had thought that I was first to describe oesophageal dysmotility as a cause of respiratory symptoms, however....

## Page 176

I remember an old Asthmatic, who was troubled with difficulty of swallowing, upon which his asthma left him; he seemed to me to have some Tumour, or Palsie in the Oesophagus, but no Methods would relieve it; but since that he has continu'd 7 or 8 years without the Asthma who formerly had the Fits periodically for 14 years, and they were occasion'd, as he tells me, by drinking stale beer.

In the Victorian era another perceptive physician, George Congreve, wrote in his text "On Consumption of the Lungs" 1881 [2] that:

There is also a dry or nervous asthma, with the little or no expectoration, accompanied with flatulence, headache, restlessness, dryness of the throat, and intense anxiety. In most cases of this class, *dyspepsia* is an accompanying evil, and perhaps the exciting cause. In addition to the medicinal agents above named, the proper regulation of diet is of vast importance. Nothing that can generate flatulence should be taken. The food should be light and nourishing—no pastry, salt meat, veal, pork, hashes, soups, or stews—but mutton, tender beef (underdone), stale bread, very little vegetable, and light puddings. A very small quantity of the best brandy, well diluted and without sugar, or with half a tumble for of Schweppes Potass or Seltzer Water, may be sipped at dinner. During intervals of attack, course of bitter tonics, such as cascarilla, columba, or quassia, to give tone to the stomach, may be of much advantage.

More recently, but still forgotten, is the review and case series by J. R. Belcher (a better example of nominative determinism would be difficult to find) in Thorax 1946 [3]. "This paper is concerned with the pulmonary aspiration phenomena associated with mechanical dysphagia, and the term "dysphagia pneumonitis" is used for the syndrome". In the discussion Belcher notes "the frequency with which pathological conditions of the oesophagus associated with abnormalities of the lungs is difficult to assess; there is little doubt that it is considerably greater than the number of cases recorded in the literature suggests … AETIOLOGY—the pulmonary changes associated with dysphagia are due to aspiration of oesophageal contents into the bronchial tree. The mechanism of aspiration varies with different oesophageal lesions. During normal deglutition the arrival of a bolus of food in the pharynx sets up a reflex mechanism, part of which is concerned with the onward transmission of the food, and part of which prevents its ingress through the glottis. A lesion which interferes with this protective reflex makes aspiration almost inevitable. When deglutition is not taking place the cough reflex protects the bronchial tree from contamination by liquid in the pharynx or oesophagus. Any lesion which may cause the retention of liquid in this area, in the presence of factors which tend to dull the cough reflex, render the patient liable to "dysphagia pneumonitis". He points out that patients may frequently present without obvious dysphagia, or only admit to the symptom following a close questioning. For the first time he uses the phrase "silent" to describe this phenomenon, but also comments "A long-standing cough in association with the dysphagia has been a frequent feature".

The above is by no means a comprehensive review of the extensive literature stretching back many hundreds of years describing the clinical syndromes associated with reflux and aspiration. What is surprising is that the lessons handed down to us from past generations are largely ignored in modern medical practice. An inpatient with a sudden onset of a cough, breathlessness, and consolidation revealed on the chest x-ray will acquire a diagnosis of HAP—hospital-acquired pneumonia and of course be given intravenous antibiotics. An obese young patient with episodes of wheezing precipitated by lying down and laughing will be diagnosed as acute asthma and be given high dose parenteral corticosteroids. An elderly patient with unilateral pulmonary fibrosis, a large hiatus hernia and a habit of sleeping on their right side will receive a diagnosis of idiopathic pulmonary fibrosis. All of the above examples have occurred in my clinical practice in the last few months. The subsequent chapters in this volume will, I hope, act as a reminder of what our forefathers recognised.

## References

1. Floyer J. A treatise on the asthma. London: Printed for Richard Wilkin; 1698.
2. Congreve GT. On consumption of the lungs, or, decline and its successful treatment: showing that formidable disease to be curable in all its stages: with observations on coughs, colds, asthma, chronic bronchitis etc. 2nd ed. London: Author and Eliot Stock; 1881.
3. Belcher JR. The pulmonary complications of dysphagia. Thorax. 1949;4:44–56.

# An Overview of Gastroesophageal Reflux Disease

## 2

Serhat Bor

## Definition and Clinical Manifestations

Gastroesophageal reflux disease (GORD) is a chronic disorder that is caused by abnormal reflux. It is associated with prolonged exposure of the distal oesophagus and extra oesophageal airways to gastric contents and leads to cardinal symptoms and/or findings, which affect patient quality of life [1]. Typical GORD symptoms include heartburn (usually defined as a rising retrosternal burning discomfort) and/or regurgitation, and atypical symptoms include laryngopharyngeal and pulmonary symptoms, such as cough and non-cardiac chest pain (Fig. 2.1) [2].

From a physician's point of view, the classic GORD patient has typical symptoms, with a satisfactory proton pump inhibitor (PPI) response and/or erosive oesophagitis. Many clinicians believe that the diagnosis of GORD should be primarily based on the presence of these typical symptoms. The specificities of heartburn and acid regurgitation for GORD were found very high in early studies such as 89% and 95%, respectively [3]. However, latest studies concluded that it is not possible to identify reflux disease reliably with symptom questionnaires alone.

In the disease spectrum, there are more caveats rather than a clear-cut diagnosis, particularly in three clinical conditions or in a combination of these conditions:

1. patients with normal endoscopy,
2. PPI unresponsiveness, and
3. the presence of extraoesophageal symptoms, without typical symptoms.

GORD affects not only the oesophagus but also the upper airway, and it is associated with a wide range of extraoesophageal symptoms; therefore,

S. Bor
Ege Reflux Group, Division of Gastroenterology, School of Medicine, Ege University, Izmir, Turkey
e-mail: serhat.bor@ege.edu.tr

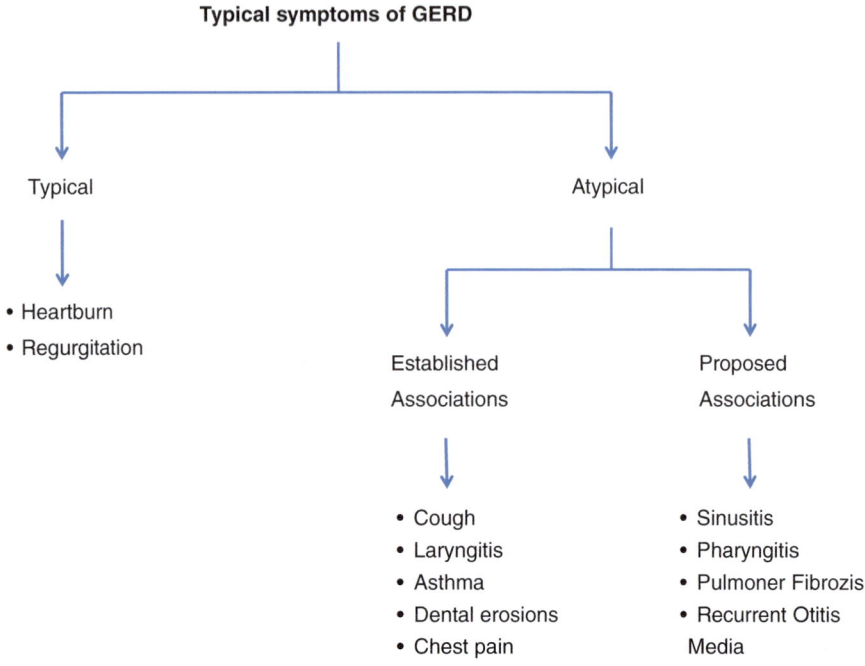

**Fig. 2.1** Typical symptoms of GERD [2]

treating the disease requires collaboration between different disciplines, including gastroenterology, ENT, pulmonary medicine, general surgery, paediatrics, internists and GPs. Thus, a GORD diagnosis might be more difficult because typical symptoms cannot be observed in most patients with extraoesophageal symptoms.

## Epidemiology

Gastroesophageal reflux disease (GORD) is one of the most common chronic diseases in adults in developed countries. If all studies from Western countries were evaluated cumulatively, the prevalence of heartburn and acid regurgitation would be 23% and 16%, respectively [4]. High-quality prevalence studies from Western countries have been performed since the 1990s; such studies have been performed only since the 2000s in Eastern countries. The majority of studies from Eastern countries have been performed in South-East and East Asian populations, and the prevalence of GORD in these populations is 2.5–8.2%, which is markedly lower than that in Western studies (Table 2.1) [1, 4].

According to epidemiological studies, one major difference between Western and Eastern countries is the prevalence of typical GORD symptoms. Patients in Western countries primarily exhibit heartburn, whereas patients in most other

## 2 An Overview of Gastroesophageal Reflux Disease

**Table 2.1** The prevalence of GERD and typical symptoms in studies performed using the Mayo Questionnaire [1]

| Place | Author | No of subjects | Heartburn | Regurgitation | GERD |
|---|---|---|---|---|---|
| Olmsted (USA) | Locke | 1511 | 17.8 | 6.3 | 19.8 |
| Moscow (Russia) | Bor, Lazebnik | 1065 | 17.6 | 17.5 | 23.6 |
| Turkey | Bor | 3214 | 9.3 | 16.6 | 22.8 |
| Argentina | Chiocca | 839 | 16.9 | 16.5 | 23 |
| Eastern Iran | Vossoughinia | 1637 | NA | 25.7 | 25.7 |
| Olmsted (USA) | Jung | 2273 | NA | NA | 18 |
| Philadelphia (USA) | Yuen | 1172 | NA | NA | 26.2 |
| Madrid (Spain) | Rey | 709 | NA | NA | 8.5 |
| Spain | Diaz-Rubio | 2500 | NA | NA | 9.8 |
| China | Wong | 2209 | NA | NA | 2.5 |

**Table 2.2** The prevalence of additional symptoms in studies performed using both the same questionnaire and the same diagnostic criteria [6]

|  | Olmsted (USA) | Moscow (Russia) | Izmir (Turkey) | Argentina | NW China |
|---|---|---|---|---|---|
| NCCP | 23.1 | 15.5 | 37.3 | 37.6 | 34.7 |
| Dysphagia | 13.5 | 25.5 | 35.7 | 26.8 | 6.5 |
| Odynophagia | – | 34.4 | 35.7 | – | 10.7 |
| Globus | 7.0 | 25.5 | 23.8 | 26.3 | 15.2 |
| Dyspepsia | 10.6 | 60.2 | 42.1 | 38.7 | 29.3 |
| Belching | – | 43.0 | 24.6 | – | – |
| Nausea | – | 53.8 | 60.3 |  | – |
| Vomiting | – | 29.1 | 38.1 | – | – |
| Hiccup | – | 6.8 | 9.5 | – | – |
| Cough | – | 36.7 | 19.8 | – | 8.9 |
| Asthma | 9.3 | – | 0.8 | 6.7 | 4.2 |
| Pharyngeal symptoms and hoarseness | 14.3 | 10.4 | 28.6 | 21.8 | 9.4 |

countries predominantly show acid regurgitation [5, 6]. These differences are likely underestimated; however, it is important because regurgitation itself represents a different therapeutic profile compared to heartburn. For example, proton pump inhibitors are less effective compared to heartburn and other medications; motility agents, alginate or other modalities (surgery) might be more effective.

No study has directly compared the atypical symptoms found in different countries, but studies using the same questionnaire have yielded different results. For example, the prevalence of asthma among GORD patients ranges from 0.8% to 9.3%. The prevalence of other symptoms, such as dyspepsia, also differs (range, 10.6–60.2%) (Table 2.2) [6]. There is a strong need for more studies addressing the incidence of the disease, as well as patient quality of life.

## Diagnosis

Currently, different GORD features are measured with different tests, and there is no gold standard used to diagnose the full spectrum of the disease. Some tests have been nearly abandoned, such as radionuclide scintigraphy and the Bernstein test. Others might lose their practicality because of further developments, such as catheter-based 24 h intraoesophageal pH monitoring, barium swallow radiology, and 24 h intraoesophageal bilirubin detection (Bilitec). New and exciting tests are replacing some of these modalities, such as catheter-based intraoesophageal 24 h intraoesophageal pH/impedance monitoring, high resolution manometry, etc. [7]. Some diagnostic tests are under evaluation, with different expectation levels, such as pepsin detection in the saliva (Peptest), mucosal impedance measurements, and laryngeal pH monitoring (Restech). The advantages and disadvantages of different tests are summarized in the Table 2.3.

**Table 2.3** Summary of diagnostic tests in gastroesophageal reflux disease

| Test | Pros | Cons |
| --- | --- | --- |
| 24 h intraesophageal pH monitoring | Quantifies refluxed acid, allows for determination of acid and symptom correlation | Normal even in 30% of erosive esophagitis patients, catheter base, patient discomfort effects the quality of the measurement, acid reflux does not mean the mucosal damage, inter/intra observer variabilities are too high |
| 24 h intraesophageal pH/impedance monitoring | Allows to measure weak or nonacid refluxes. Basal mucosal impedance is a new promising metric. More sensitive determination of all types of reflux and symptom correlation | Catheter base, patient discomfort effects the quality of the measurement. More expensive, less experience. Needs manual analysis especially for research. |
| Wireless pH monitoring | Better tolerance. Allows longer measurements (days), if off-PPI measurement shows pathologic reflux, PPI therapy can be initialized and allows to on-PPI measurement | Needs endoscopy, more expensive |
| Conventional manometry | LES localization for catheter-based monitoring systems, exclude esophageal motility disorders | Catheter base, measures lower esophageal sphincter pressure but the role for GERD is unclear |
| High resolution manometry | Very sensitive to detect HH, motility disorders, esophagogastric junction outflow obstructions. New metrics to detect GERD and combination with other technologies (impedance, ultrasound) are promising | Catheter base. Still needs improvements for the criteria and metrics |

## Proton Pump Inhibitor Trial

Many centres worldwide lack sophisticated diagnostic modalities; therefore, they rely on patient symptoms and upper gastrointestinal endoscopy. The PPI response to typical symptoms is a primary diagnostic tool [8]. However, the PPI response of patients with typical symptoms is approximately 60–65% for heartburn and <50% for regurgitation, and this low response rate decreases the value of the therapeutic trial approach. Recently, all PPI trial studies have been evaluated by the Turkish GORD consensus group [9], which found 16 studies (seven omeprazole, five lansoprazole, two esomeprazole, two rabeprazole). As shown in the table, most of these studies used a high dose (double) of PPI, and the median time was 14 days. There was no consensus for the dose, time of the trial or definition of the "response" (Table 2.4). Despite the heterogeneous design of these studies, the following observations can be asserted;

- The cumulative sensitivity of the PPI trial is 82.3%, and the specificity is 51.5%. The positive predictive value is 79%, and the negative predictive value is 56.9%. These figures indicate that most GORD patients responded well to the PPI trial; however, a negative test does not exclude the possibility of disease. Indeed, the RCT evidence suggests that the effect of PPI is similar to placebo for airway symptoms.
- Patients with erosive oesophagitis and pathologic acid reflux have a greater chance of response, although these groups do not need a PPI trial.

**Table 2.4** PPI trial studies [9]

| Study | PPI | Dose | Time (days) | n= |
|---|---|---|---|---|
| 1. Fass (1998) | Omeprazole | 40 mg AM and 20 mg PM | 7 | 37 |
| 2. Pandak (2002) | Omeprazole | 20 mg AM and PM | 14 | 38 |
| 3. Xia (2003) | Lansoprazole | 30 mg AM | 28 | 36 |
| 4. Bautista (2004) | Lansoprazole | 60 mg AM and 30 mg PM | 7 | 40 |
| 5. Pace (2010) | Omeprazole | 20 mg AM and PM | 15 | 544 |
| 6. Dent (2010) | Esameprazole | 40 mg AM | 14 | 296 |
| 7. Cho (2010) | Lansoprazole | 30 mg AM and 30 mg PM | 14 | 73 |
| 8. Kim (2009) | Rabeprazole | 20 mg Am and 20 mg PM | 14 | 42 |
| 9. Aanen (2006) | Esameprazole | 40 mg AM | 13 | 67 |
| 10. Dekel (2004) | Rabeprazole | 20 mg AM and PM | 14 | 14 |
| 11. Bate (1999) | Omeprazole | 40 mg AM | 14 | 58 |
| 12. Fass (2000) | Omeprazole | 40 mg AM and 20 mg PM | 14 | 14 |
| 13. Juul-Hansen (2001) | Lansoprazole | 60 mg AM | 5 | 56 |
| 14. Schenk (1997) | Omeprazole | 40 mg AM | 14 | 41 |
| 15. Juul-Hansen (2003) | Lansoprazole | 60 mg AM | 7 | 52 |
| 16. Fass (1999) | Omeprazole | 40 mg AM and 20 mg PM | 7 | 42 |

- Non-cardiac chest pain patients are one of the best candidates, if their pain is related to acid reflux.
- *The suggested therapeutic trial is 2 weeks for a double dose of PPI, and the response should be >50% healing of symptoms. It still must be determined which symptoms should be considered: heartburn, regurgitation or both?*

## Upper Gastrointestinal Endoscopy

Upper gastrointestinal endoscopy (UGIE) is the most commonly used diagnostic technique. It is an important tool to determine whether the phenotype of the disease is NERD or erosive oesophagitis. UGIE detects oesophagitis, strictures and Barrett's oesophagus. It also allows to take biopsy, particularly for the diagnosis of eosinophilic oesophagitis, and it is useful for differential diagnoses, particularly in PPI refractory patients. However, in patients with non-peptic symptoms, the yield is low.

LA Grades C, D and possibly B oesophagitis are sufficient for the diagnosis [10]. However, note that oesophagitis A can be observed in a minority of asymptomatic patients. Oesophageal histology has limited value except for Barrett's oesophagus and eosinophilic oesophagitis. Narrow band imaging, confocal laser endomicroscopy and similar new endoscopic techniques do not add more information to the diagnosis [11]. Dilated intercellular spaces and microscopic oesophagitis are observed more in NERD and ERD; however, routine biopsy of the oesophagus and histopathology are not recommended.

### Indications for First Upper Gastrointestinal Endoscopy
- Upper gastrointestinal tract cancer or Barrett's oesophagus in first-degree relatives.
- Alarm symptoms; dysphagia, odynophagia, unexplained weight loss, anaemia, vomiting.
- If peptic symptoms start in patients older than 50 years of age.
- A symptom duration >5 years.
- A <50% response rate after 8 weeks of PPI therapy.

### Indications for Follow-Up Upper Gastrointestinal Endoscopy
- The presence of Barrett's oesophagus.
- In patients with severe erosive oesophagitis: after high-dose PPI therapy for 4–8 weeks to evaluate for possible Barrett's oesophagus.

## 24-h Ambulatory pH or pH-Impedance Monitoring

Traditionally, 24-h pH monitoring has been accepted as the gold standard diagnostic method for GORD. Although this technique is important, "the gold standard" concept is questionable. A 24-h conventional pH testing failed to diagnose abnormal acid exposure in up to 40% of patients with erosive oesophagitis when the percentage total time for pH < 4 was used as the only criterion. This technology has many limitations. It measures only acid reflux episodes; however, weak and possibly non-acid reflux episodes might be responsible for some symptoms, particularly in patients with extraoesophageal symptoms or PPI refractories. Indeed, it has been suggested that acidic reflux is not the major precipitant of airway disease. Patients cannot maintain their regular daily activities and having meals with a catheter in their noses and throats. The day-to-day variation is high, and only reflux at the fifth centimeter within the oesophagus is measured. Lack of a diagnostic gold standard for gastroesophageal reflux disease is also a problem when measuring the exact sensitivity and specificity of the technique. Therefore, there is a strong need for better technologies [7].

Recently, a new technology was added for pH-monitoring, and now we have 24-h impedance-pH monitoring. This technology allows the detection of acidic, weakly acidic, and non-acid reflux, as well as liquid and gaseous refluxates [10]. There is still a strong need for more healthy control studies with equipment from different companies to detect normative thresholds. Many new metrics have been proposed over the years; however, baseline impedance is a good reflection of mucosal integrity and can be used. However, low baseline impedance makes it difficult to interpret pH-impedance studies. Automated analysis may be sufficient; however, in the case of a significant number of weak and/or non-acid reflux events, it is advisable to perform a manual analysis. Addition to these major metrics, it is important to evaluate the symptom-reflux association [12].

*Symptom-reflux association* is an interesting approach to diagnose some GORD phenotypes, such as oesophageal hypersensitivity and functional heartburn. Currently two metrics are used: symptom index and symptom association probability.

$$Symptom\,index = number\,of\,reflux - related\,symptom\,episodes\,/\,(total\,number\,of\,symptom\,episodes) \times 100$$

Symptom association probability is calculated by dividing the 24-h data into 2-min segments. Then, for each 2-min segment, it is possible to determine whether the reflux occurred and a symptom was reported. At least three events per symptom episode must be reported to calculate these tests.

These tests should be used together, and if two metrics are positive, then the diagnosis is oesophageal hypersensitivity; if the metrics are negative, then the diagnosis is functional heartburn.

## Indications for 24-h Impedance-pH Monitoring
- Patients with non-erosive reflux disease and who are refractory to PPI therapy (the procedure should be performed off-PPI in patients with no response at all. However, an on-PPI test is suggested for patients who demonstrate a partial response).
- Extraoesophageal symptoms, particularly cough, to identify the reflux-cough relationship (pharyngeal pH measurements are possibly not useful).
- Belching and rumination.

- Select patients undergoing anti-reflux surgery and with post-fundoplication symptoms.
- Evaluation of anti-reflux treatment failure.
- Non-cardiac chest pain.

**Wireless pH Monitoring**

In this capsule-based study, the placement of the wireless pH capsule was performed in the outpatient endoscopy unit, following an upper GI endoscopy.

The distance from the incisors to the oesophagogastric junction was measured during the upper GI endoscopy, then the endoscope was removed, and the capsule was transorally advanced with an applicator deployed 6 cm proximal to the junction. It measured the pH level until the capsule fell, which generally took 2–9 days. This procedure is preferable in patients who are intolerant of a catheter-based measurement. When the symptom-reflux relationship occurs is important; however, symptoms (such as NCCP) rarely occur. Therefore, it is preferable to measure them for as long as possible. In our department, we prefer to analyse the data on a daily basis, and when sufficient evidence is obtained for a GORD diagnosis, the PPI therapy is immediately initiated to observe the PPI response. The major drawbacks of the procedure are the cost and need for an upper GI endoscopy [13, 14].

**Oesophageal Manometry**

Oesophageal manometry does not have any direct diagnostic value for GORD; however, it has different utilizations to support the diagnosis. Patients who are refractory to PPIs should be evaluated to eliminate other diseases, such as achalasia and other motor disorders of the oesophagus. Other indications are preoperative evaluation of the patient and localization of LES for the placement of pH catheters.

New technologies, such as high-resolution manometry, have a higher diagnostic value than conventional manometry and should be preferred. Indeed, some patients with 'idiopathic' airway symptoms have been diagnosed with oesophageal dysmotility. This technology can be used to assess the size of the hiatal hernia, as well as the peristaltic reserve [15].

**Other Tests**

A barium swallow and scintigraphy cannot be recommended to diagnose GORD. Endoluminal functional lumen imaging probe (Endo FLIP) is a new diagnostic tool that can be used to measure the distensibility of LES. Achalasia dilatation and anti-reflux fundoplication are possible indications for the technique; however, its value is not established yet for the diagnose of the disease. The measurement of pepsin in the saliva is a promising tool and will be discussed in the following chapters.

## Medical, Endoscopic and Surgical Therapy

The major aim of current GORD therapy is symptom relief. The possibility of curing symptoms is low, which increases the importance of GORD-related quality of life as a major therapeutic target.

## Lifestyle Modifications

Despite their common use, lifestyle modifications have limited effects but should be advised according to a patient's history and experience [16, 17]. If a patient defines some foods or drinks responsible for symptoms, a particular dietetic modification can be arranged. According to the meta-analysis, only some modifications are significant;

- Obesity is one of the most important factors, and losing weight is crucial. The association between obesity and GORD was evaluated in a systematic review, which found a positive association between a BMI > 25 kg and GORD symptoms (odds ratio 1.43, 95% CI 1.16–1.77). A similar increase was also shown for oesophagitis and obesity (1.76, 1.16–2.68) [18].
- Chocolate, fatty food, sodas should be avoided. Salt and white-wheat bread might be related to symptoms. Personal differences are encountered with different foods.
- Low volume, protein-rich and high-fibre food should be preferred. Controlled data, however, are greatly lacking and inconclusive [19].
- Heavy exercise might increase the risk.
- Smoking, in terms of the consumption rate, is a risk factor that has been reported in basic science and epidemiologic studies. Alcohol consumption is noxious on the oesophageal epithelium in basic science studies; however, the risk is unclear in epidemiologic studies. The cessation of both is advisable [20].
- Left lateral position and head elevation are important to protect against night-time reflux but difficult to adapt and disruptive to the quality of sleep [21]. Their long-term effects are not clear.

Interestingly and contrary to dogma, the speed of eating does not impact reflux episodes in normal weight [22] and obese populations [23].

## Medical Therapy

GORD medications can be classified as follows:

I Acid neutralization or inhibition:
  1. Antacids neutralize secreted acids and are primarily used for mild peptic symptoms. The onset of action is rapid; however, the effects are short lived. Despite the widespread use of antacids, even the studies compared to placebo

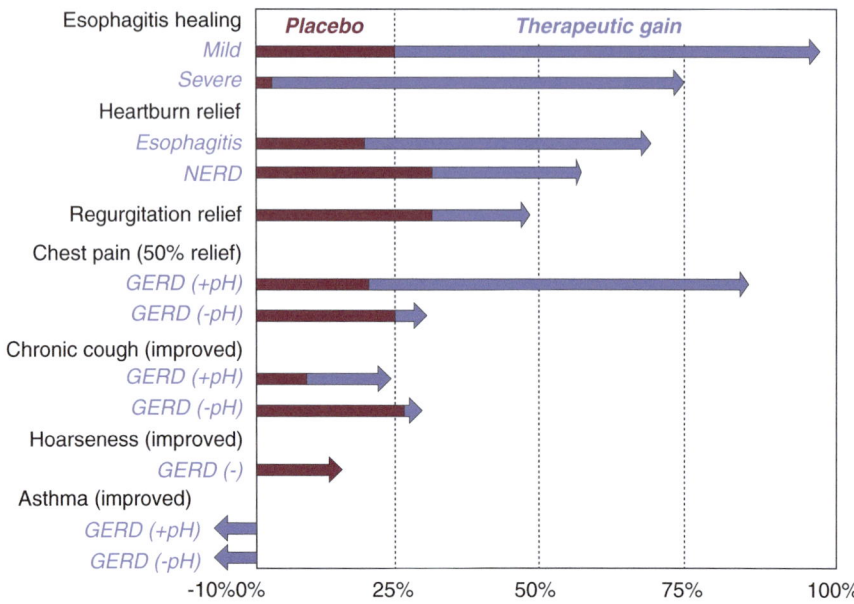

**Fig. 2.2** PPI efficacy for potential manifestations of GERD [28]

provided conflicting results. Their therapeutic benefit in the treatment of GORD is limited by the lack of well-designed, large, placebo-controlled trials. Thus, it is unlikely that these drugs will have a major effect on the disease [24]. Because they act locally, antacids are considered to be a first line therapy with alginates for GORD in pregnancy [25]. However, magnesium-containing agents should be avoided, and calcium content should be taken into consideration especially for the overdose.

2. H2 receptor antagonists inhibit acid production in the parietal cell on H2 receptors. Cimetidine, ranitidine, famotidine, and nizatidine are still widely use worldwide, particularly for night-time reflux, because of their inhibitory effect on basal acid stimulation [17]. All H2RAs have a similar efficacy in symptom relief and the healing of oesophagitis. This drug group has a good safety record, with few side effects. However, some limitations exist, such as a relatively short duration of action, incomplete inhibition of meal-induced acid secretion, and the development of tolerance (as common as 50% within 2 weeks, possibly related to the down-regulation of H2-receptors) [26].

3. Proton pump inhibitors irreversibly inhibit acid secretion through H+/K+ adenosine triphosphatase (ATPase), the proton pump of the parietal cell responsible for acid production. They have superior efficacy compared to histamine H2 receptor antagonists and are currently the most effective therapeutic option [27]. The healing rates for oesophagitis are summarized in Fig. 2.2 [28]. According to

**Table 2.5** The possible reasons for the ineffectuality of PPIs

- Diagnostic problems such as functional dyspepsia, IBS, cancers, achalasia, eosinophilic esophagitis
- Compliance problems such as postprandial consumption of medications
- Inadequate dosing
- Acid regurgitation
- Fast metabolizers
- Concomitant medications
- Malabsorptions,
- Hypersensive oesophagus, functional heartburn
- Weak/nonacid reflux
- Pscyhiatric comordidities, fear of cancer
- PPI resistance in time
- Delayed gastric emptying, gastric outflow obstructions
- Gastric acid hypersecretion
- Extraesophageal symptoms
- Nocturnal acid breakthrough

    the standard dose treatment, compared to placebo, the highest response rate can be achieved with mild oesophagitis. In terms of heartburn relief, patients with oesophagitis have a higher success rate compared to non-erosive reflux patients [17]. However, it should be noted that the PPI unresponsiveness rate reaches 30–40% in erosive or NERD groups [29]. Regurgitation, which is the most common symptom in non-Western countries, has an even lower response rate (<50%) [30]. The lowest response rates are seen for extraoesophageal symptoms, such as hoarseness, asthma and chronic cough. The possible reasons for the ineffectuality of these drugs are summarized in Table 2.5. The complications of long-term PPI consumption are always worrying [31]. Of the many possible side effects, only a minority has been found to be significant: bone fractures (osteoporosis), clostridium difficile infection, bacterial overgrowth, and spontaneous bacterial peritonitis. The latter has the highest risk. This is a hot topic now, and many new studies are being published. Patients who need these drugs for long-term or continue therapy should be monitored carefully. However, there is no consensus on the concept of "long-term" therapy in terms of time and dosage.

II Barrier forming agents, such as alginate-based formulations, appear to act through a unique mechanism, a mechanical barrier. In the presence of gastric acid, alginates precipitate, forming a gel. In the presence of gastric acid, bicarbonate is converted to carbon dioxide, which becomes entrapped within the gel precipitate and converts into foam, floating on the surface of the gastric contents, much like a raft on water [32]. The alginate-based raft remains in the upper part of the stomach, suppressing the acid pocket [33]. It also binds or filters pepsin and bile, removing them from the refluxate. These drugs primarily reduce acid and then non-acid reflux events (and on the height of proximal extent of reflux events along the oesophagus in some studies). However, the gaseous component of reflux is not controlled [34].

III Prokinetic agents increase lower oesophageal sphincter pressure, accelerate gastric emptying, and increase the amplitude of oesophageal contractions. Their effects vary from one agent to another. The adverse-event profile of these agents must be weighed against any clinical benefit and most classical agents, such as bethanechol, metoclopramide, domperidone, and cisapride, either out of market or under supervision (by reason of cardiac side effects, particularly fatal arrhythmia). However, safety studies, particularly those with domperidone, are questionable and clearly metoclopramide is much riskier [35]. Care should be taken in patients older than 65 years of age; long QT syndromes or medications prolong the QT, with arrhythmia, >30 mg/day.

IV Mucosal protectives. Sucralfate, is a mucosal-protective agent that binds to inflamed tissue, producing a protective barrier, inhibiting the noxious effects of pepsin and bile. GORD studies are limited, with small numbers of participants, primarily compared to placebo [36]. Because of the high confidence interval, the effect is not superior to placebo. Currently, its use is limited to GORD in pregnancy, pill oesophagitis, caustic ingestion, etc.

V Other options. Tricyclic antidepressants and selective serotonin reuptake inhibitors can be used in some subgroups, such as oesophageal hypersensitivity and functional heartburn [17]. This is a new and exciting era for these GORD phenotypes.

## Endoluminal Therapies

Different endoluminal therapies have been developed in recent years, and many have disappeared because of either inefficiency or complications. Endoluminal therapies have been categorized in four different types: (1) fixation, (2) ablation, (3) injection, and (4) mucosal excision and suturing. Currently, only two techniques are widely available. Stretta is an anti-reflux device that consists of a four-channel radiofrequency-generating catheter delivering thermal energy, without reaching the ablation values into the muscularis propria within the oesophagus at four levels and cardia at two levels. A recent meta-analysis has shown that 49% of patients are off PPI following the procedure [37]. A long-term study has also revealed that the 5-year follow up results are consistent with the 10-year follow up results. The procedure certainly improves health-related quality of life and the pooled heartburn standardized score, reduces oesophageal acid exposure, and increases lower oesophageal sphincter basal pressure, although the last two features were not normalized. EsophyX (transoral incisionless fundoplication; TIF) is used to restore the angle of His by delivering multiple full thickness, nonabsorbable fasteners, and it creates a valve at the oesophagogastric junction [17].

## Anti-reflux Surgery

Laparoscopic anti-reflux surgery is an effective long-term therapy option. It restores the mechanical barrier and improves LES pressure, decreases reflux episodes, and improves symptoms and quality of life [38]. It can be safely performed with minimal perioperative morbidity and mortality. Shorter follow-up studies (<3 years) have observed better outcomes (90%) [39].

It is advisable that all NERD patients should be evaluated with oesophageal (high-resolution) manometry and 24 h pH (-impedance) or capsule pH monitoring study before surgery [10]. The best candidates are patients with good responses to PPIs and fewer functional gastrointestinal symptoms, such as bloating, belching or psychological co-morbidity. Patients with inadequate symptom control represent another group with difficulties, and they should be carefully evaluated before surgery for possible explanations for their failure to respond to medications. Typical symptoms respond better than atypical symptoms, and only patients with atypical symptoms should be carefully evaluated before the surgery and avoided if possible. Severe regurgitation (generally accompanied by hiatal hernia) and medication side-effects. Barrett's oesophagus and peptic structure can be treated surgically; however, there is no absolute indication in these groups.

Nissen was the most common choice between surgeons; however, partial fundoplication has attracted more attention in recent years because of the fewer postoperative complications, particularly dysphagia and bloating [38]. An interesting approach is to perform partial fundoplication in patients with preoperative major depression, as it may lead to better outcomes. Morbid obesity is a concern for higher surgery failures. For morbidly obese patients (BMI > 35 kg/m$^2$), gastric bypass should be the procedure of choice when treating GORD.

## Summary of the Therapeutic Approach

Lifestyle changes, particularly weight loss, smoking cessation and possibly alcohol cessation, should be the first line approach in all cases. Strict dietary restrictions should be avoided because of the negative impact on quality of life. Many algorithms and approaches have been published. As shown in Fig. 2.3, as suggested by the Turkish consensus group, and the therapeutic approach was divided into three different categories: primary health care (first level), internists (second level) and gastroenterologists (third level) [40]. In the presence of the mild symptoms (less than three times a week, minimal impact on quality of life, short duration), on-demand therapy with any effective medication, such as antacids, alginate or antacid/alginate combination, H2 RA, and low dose of PPI, can be initiated. Moderate symptoms need a single dose of PPI; however, in cases of severe symptoms, a double dose of PPI with the combination of prokinetics or alginate is advisable. If upper gastrointestinal endoscopy is performed, the severity of findings should direct the dose, meaning that in cases of erosive oesophagitis A or B require a single dose, and C or D cases require a double dose of PPI. In patients who are unresponsive to the therapy, further diagnostic modalities, such as oesophageal manometry (high resolution if possible) and 24 h pH (impedance) monitoring, are advised [41]. While they are undergoing ambulatory pH-impedance recordings, patients should be carefully advised to describe their symptoms because some

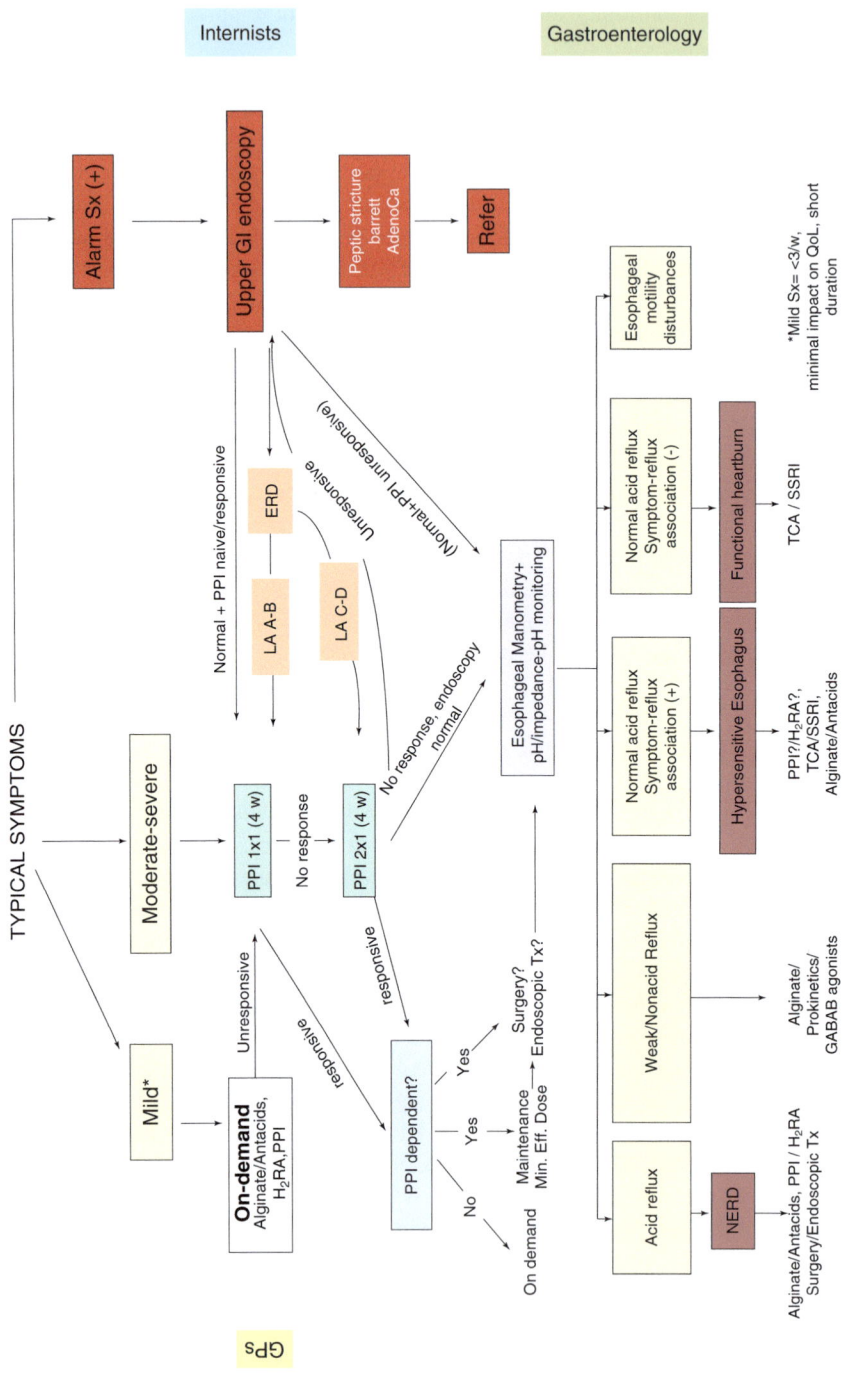

**Fig. 2.3** Therapeutic algorithm inpatients with typical GERD symptoms [40]

GORD phenotypes, such as oesophageal hypersensitivity, are diagnosed based only on their reports. Those modalities are difficult to treat and generally do not response to classical GORD medications, especially anti-reflux surgery. They define more psychiatric co-morbidities compared to NERD and erosive patients. These subgroups and patients with functional heartburn need extensive evaluations of their psychiatric conditions, and tricyclics or SSRIs are commonly prescribed, as well as prokinetics.

The discontinuation of PPIs is possible, according to different studies, ranging from 14% to 64%, without deteriorating symptom control for a one-year period. Tapering may be a better approach than abrupt discontinuation [42].

## Status of Newer Medications

Different new medications are currently under investigation. Here, some new achievements are summarized;

## Improved Acid Suppression

In terms of better inhibition of gastric acid secretion, novel long-lasting PPIs and potassium-competitive acid blockers (P-CABs) are being developed.

*Tenatoprazole and S-Tenatoprazole are* imidazopyridine-based PPIs with a prolonged plasma half-life. It has been under development for years [43]. A Phase 2 study has been conducted in S Korea, and Phase 1 was conducted in the European Union and India.

*Rabeprazole extended release 50 mg:* Phase 3 has been completed and discontinued in some countries. It is registered in Turkey, and Phase 3 study is running.

Omeprazole+succinic acid (an acid pump activator VB 101; Vecam): A Phase 2 study was completed in 2011. Vecam, a combination of a PPI and succinic acid (an acid pump activator, VB101), is a drug that has meal-independent anti-secretory effect [44].

*Ilaprazole* (P-CAB) has been studied in phase III clinical trials, in which it failed to show superiority over esomeprazole in erosive oesophagitis and NERD [45]. It is registered in S. Korea, and at the Phase 2 level in China.

Vonoprazan is a new, potent and long-lasting acid inhibitory drug that exerts a direct and targeted effect on the parietal cell. It produces rapid, reversible, and long-lasting inhibition of the gastric $H+, K+$-ATPase. It has a reversible inhibitory effect on gastric acid secretion by competing with $K+$ on the luminal surface of the proton pump. The inhibitory effect acid secretion is independent of the secretory state of the $H+, K+$-ATPase. The efficacy of vonoprazan in patients with erosive oesophagitis was evaluated in a multicentre, randomized, double-blind, parallel-group, dose-ranging study. Vonoprazan at 5, 10, 20, and 40 mg doses was compared to PPI lansoprazole 30 mg for healing of EE at 4 and 8 weeks. The percent of EE healing at 4 weeks for vonoprazan was between 92.3% and 97.0%

and was dose-dependent, compared with 93.2% for lansoprazole [46]. It may play a potent role in patients' refractory to PPIs; however, it merits more and extensive research [47].

## *Helicobacter pylori* and GORD

This issue is controversial, and deserves a special mention. The relationship between *Helicobacter pylori* and GORD is not clear. This topic is particularly important in countries with a high prevalence of HP. The Turkish GORD consensus group evaluated the literature, and the following statements were suggested [48];

- There is no clear association between HP and GORD [49, 50].
- The eradication of HP does not have any impact on either the appearance or exacerbation of GORD symptoms.
- Long-term PPI consumption does not have any impact on gastric atrophy in HP-positive cases [51, 52].
- The presence of HP might be protective for the development of Barrett oesophagus and oesophageal adeno cancer, particularly in cagA positive patients [53, 54].
- The screening and eradication of HP should be decided independently of the presence of GORD.

## References

1. Bor S. World gastroenterology organization. Heartburn handbook. Worldwide epidemiology of gastroesophageal disease; 2015. p. 12–4. http://www.worldgastroenterology.org/UserFiles/file/WDHD-2015-handbook-final.pdf
2. Akyuz F, Mutluay Soyer O. How is gastroesophageal reflux disease classified? Turk J Gastroenterol. 2017;28(Suppl 1):S10–1.
3. Klauser AG, Schindlbeck NE, Muller-Lissner A. Symptoms in gastro-oesophageal reflux disease. Lancet. 1990;335:205–8.
4. Bor S, Sarıtaş Yüksel E. How is the gastroesophageal reflux disease prevalence, incidence, and frequency of complications (stricture/esophagitis/Barrett's esophagus/carcinoma) in Turkey compared to other geographical regions globally? Turk J Gastroenterol. 2017;28(Suppl 1):S4–9.
5. Bor S, Kitapcioglu G, Kasap E. Prevalence of gastroesophageal reflux disease in a country with a high occurrence of *Helicobacter pylori*. World J Gastroenterol. 2017;23(3):525–53.
6. Bor S, Lazebnik LB, Kitapcioglu G, Manannikof I, Vasiliev Y. Prevalence of gastroesophageal reflux disease in Moscow. Dis Esophagus. 2016;29(2):159–65.
7. Hirano I, Richter JE, Practice Parameters Committee of the American College of Gastroenterology. ACG practice guidelines: esophageal reflux testing. Am J Gastroenterol. 2007;102(3):668–85.
8. Fass R, Ofman JJ, Sampliner RE, Camargo L, Wendel C, Fennerty MB. The omeprazole test is as sensitive as 24-h oesophageal pH monitoring in diagnosing gastro-oesophageal reflux disease in symptomatic patients with erosive oesophagitis. Aliment Pharmacol Ther. 2000;14(4):389–96.

9. Vardar R, Keskin M. What is the place of empirical proton pump inhibitor testing in the diagnosis of gastroesophageal reflux disease? (description, duration, and dosage). Turk J Gastroenterol. 2017;28(Suppl 1):S12–5.
10. Roman S, Gyawali CP, Savarino E, Yadlapati R, Zerbib F, Wu J, Vela M, Tutuian R, Tatum R, Sifrim D, Keller J, Fox M, Pandolfino JE, Bredenoord AJ, GERD consensus group. Ambulatory reflux monitoring for diagnosis of gastro-esophageal reflux disease: update of the Porto consensus and recommendations from an international consensus group. Neurogastroenterol Motil. 2017;29(10):1–15.
11. Reddymasu SC, Sharma P. Advances in endoscopic imaging of the esophagus. Gastroenterol Clin N Am. 2008;37(4):763–74.
12. Abdul-Hussein M, Zhang C, Castell D. Symptom index or symptom association probability? A closer look at symptom association in suspected GERD patients. J Clin Gastroenterol. 2018;52(1):e7–e10.
13. Vardar R, Keskin M. Indications of 24-h esophageal pH monitoring, capsule pH monitoring, combined pH monitoring with multichannel impedance, esophageal manometry, radiology and scintigraphy in gastroesophageal reflux disease? Turk J Gastroenterol. 2017;28(Suppl 1):S16–21.
14. Kessels SJM, Newton SS, Morona JK, Merlin TL. Safety and efficacy of wireless pH monitoring in patients suspected of gastroesophageal reflux disease: a systematic review. J Clin Gastroenterol. 2017;51(9):777–88.
15. Gyawali CP, Roman S, Bredenoord AJ, Fox M, Keller J, Pandolfino JE, Sifrim D, Tatum R, Yadlapati R, Savarino E, International GERD Consensus Working Group. Classification of esophageal motor findings in gastro-esophageal reflux disease: conclusions from an international consensus group. Neurogastroenterol Motil. 2017;29(12). https://doi.org/10.1111/nmo.13104.
16. Holtmann G, Adam B, Liebregts T. Review article: the patient with gastro-oesophageal reflux disease-lifestyle advice and medication. Aliment Pharmacol Ther. 2004;20(Suppl 8):24–7.
17. Sandhu DS, Fass R. Current trends in the management of gastroesophageal reflux disease. Gut Liver. 2018;12(1):7–16.
18. Hampel H, Abraham NS, El-Serag HB. Meta-analysis: obesity and the risk for gastroesophageal reflux disease and its complications. Ann Intern Med. 2005;143:199–211.
19. Nilsson M, Johnsen R, Ye W, Hveem K, Lagergren J. Lifestyle related risk factors in the aetiology of gastro-oesophageal reflux. Gut. 2004;53:1730–5.
20. Zheng Z, Nordenstedt H, Pedersen NL, Lagergren J, Ye W. Lifestyle factors and risk for symptomatic gastroesophageal reflux in monozygotic twins. Gastroenterology. 2007;132:87–95.
21. Khan BA, Sodhi JS, Zargar SA, et al. Effect of bed head elevation during sleep in symptomatic patients of nocturnal gastroesophageal reflux. J Gastroenterol Hepatol. 2012;27:1078–82.
22. Bor S, Bayrakci B, Erdogan A, Yildirim E, Vardar R. The influence of the speed of food intake on multichannel impedance in patients with gastro-oesophageal reflux disease. United European Gastroenterol J. 2013;1:346–50.
23. Bor S, Bayrakci B, Erdogan A, Yildirim E, Vardar R. The impact of the speed of food intake on intraesophageal reflux events in obese female patients. Dis Esophagus. 2017;30(1):1–6.
24. Koop H. Medical therapy of gastroesophageal reflux disease. In: Granderath FA, Kamolz T, Pointner R, editors. Gastroesophageal reflux disease; principles of disease, diagnosis, and treatment. Wien: Springer; 2006. p. 103–11.
25. Katz PO, Castell DO. Gastroesophageal reflux disease during pregnancy. Gastroenterol Clin N Am. 1998;27:153–67.
26. Tougas G, Armstrong D. Efficacy of H2-receptor antagonists in the treatment of gastroesophageal reflux disease and its symptoms. Can J Gastroenterol. 1997;11(suppl B):51–4.
27. Donnellan C, Sharma N, Preston C, Moayyedi P. Medical treatments for the maintenance therapy of reflux oesophagitis and endoscopic negative reflux disease. Cochrane Database Syst Rev. 2004;4:CD003245.
28. Boeckxstaens G, El-Serag HB, Smout AJ, Kahrilas PJ. Symptomatic reflux disease: the present, the past and the future. Gut. 2014;63(7):1185–93.

29. Fass R, Sifrim D. Management of heartburn not responding to proton pump inhibitors. Gut. 2009;58(2):295–309.
30. Kahrilas PJ, Jonsson A, Denison H, Wernersson B, Hughes N, Howden CW. Impact of regurgitation on health-related quality of life in gastro-oesophageal reflux disease before and after short-term potent acid suppression therapy. Gut. 2014;63(5):720–6.
31. Vaezi MF, Yang YX, Howden CW. Complications of proton pump inhibitor therapy. Gastroenterology. 2017;153:35–48.
32. Vardar R, Keskin M, Valitova E, Bayrakçı B, Belen E, Bor S. Effect of alginate in patients with GERD; hiatal hernia matters. Dis Esophagus. 2017;30(10):1–7.
33. Kwiatek MA, Roman S, Fareeduddin A, Pandolfino JE, Kahrilas PJ. An alginate-antacid formulation (Gaviscon Double Action Liquid) can eliminate or displace the postprandial 'acid pocket' in symptomatic GERD patients. Aliment Pharmacol Ther. 2011;34:59–66.
34. Leiman DA, Riff BP, Morgan S, Metz DC, Falk GW, French B, Umscheid CA, Lewis JD. Alginate therapy is effective treatment for gastroesophageal reflux disease symptoms: a systematic review and meta-analysis. Dis Esophagus. 2017;30(2):1–8.
35. Arana A, Johannes CB, McQuay LJ, Varas-Lorenzo C, Fife D, Rothman JK. Risk of out-of-hospital sudden cardiac death in users of Domperidone, proton pump inhibitors, or metoclopramide: a population-based nested case-control study. Drug Saf. 2015;38:1187–99.
36. Elsborg L, Beck B, Stubgaard M. Effect of sucralfate on gastroesophageal reflux in esophagitis. Hepato-Gastroenterology. 1985;32:181–4.
37. Fass R, Cahn F, Scotti DJ, Gregory DA. Systematic review and meta-analysis of controlled and prospective cohort efficacy studies of endoscopic radiofrequency for treatment of gastroesophageal reflux disease. Surg Endosc. 2017;31(12):4865–82.
38. Schijven MP, Gisbertz SS, van Berge Henegouwen MI. Laparoscopic surgery for gastroesophageal acid reflux disease. Best Pract Res Clin Gastroenterol. 2014;28(1):97–109.
39. Peters JH. Laparoscopic treatment of gastroesophageal reflux. In: Talamini MA, editor. Advanced therapy in minimally invasive surgery. Oxford: B.C. Decker; 2006. p. 111–20.
40. Celebi A, Yilmaz H. What is proton pump inhibitors unresponsiveness in gastroesophageal reflux disease? How should these cases be managed? Turk J Gastroenterol. 2017;28(Suppl 1):S71–2.
41. Ates F, Francis DO, Vaezi MF. Refractory gastroesophageal reflux disease: advances and treatment. Expert Rev Gastroenterol Hepatol. 2014;8(6):657–67.
42. Haastrup P, Paulsen MS, Begtrup LM, Hansen JM, Jarbøl DE. Strategies for discontinuation of proton pump inhibitors: a systematic review. Fam Pract. 2014;31(6):625–30.
43. Hunt RH, Armstrong D, Yaghoobi M, James C. The pharmacodynamics and pharmacokinetics of S-tenatoprazole-Na 30 mg, 60 mg and 90 mg vs. esomeprazole 40 mg in healthy male subjects. Aliment Pharmacol Ther. 2010;31(6):648–57.
44. Chowers Y, Atarot T, Pratha VS, Fass R. The effect of once daily omeprazole and succinic acid (VECAM) vs once daily omeprazole on 24-h intragastric pH. Neurogastroenterol Motil. 2012;24:426–31.
45. Xue Y, Qin X, Zhou L, Lin S, Wang L, Hu H, Xia J. A randomized, double-blind, active-controlled, multi-center study of Ilaprazole in the treatment of reflux esophagitis. Clin Drug Investig. 2016;36(12):985–92.
46. Ashida K, Sakurai Y, Nishimura A, et al. Randomised clinical trial: a dose-ranging study of vonoprazan, a novel potassium competitive acid blocker, vs. lansoprazole for the treatment of erosive oesophagitis. Aliment Pharmacol Ther. 2015;42:685–95.
47. Scott DR, Marcus EA, Sachs G. Vonoprazan: MarKed competition for PPIs? Dig Dis Sci. 2016;61(7):1783–4.
48. Mungan Z, Pınarbaşı Şimşek B. Gastroesophageal reflux disease and the relationship with *Helicobacter pylori*. Turk J Gastroenterol. 2017;28(Suppl 1):S61–7.
49. Cremonini F, Di Caro S, Delgado-Aros S, et al. Meta-analysis: the relationship between *Helicobacter pylori* infection and gastrooesophageal reflux disease. Aliment Pharmacol Ther. 2003;18:279–89.

50. Yaghoobi M, Farrokhyar F, Yuan Y, Hunt RH. Is there an increased risk of GERD after *Helicobacter pylori* eradication? A meta-analysis. Am J Gastroenterol. 2010;105:1007–13.
51. Kuipers EJ, Nelis GF, Klinkenberg-Knol EC, et al. Cure of *Helicobacter pylori* infection in patients with reflux oesophagitis treated with long term omeprazole reverses gastritis without exacerbation of reflux disease: results of a randomised controlled trial. Gut. 2004;53:12–20.
52. Yang HB, Sheu BS, Wang ST, Cheng HC, Chang WL, Chen WY. *H. pylori* eradication prevents the progression of gastric intestinal metaplasia in reflux esophagitis patients using long-term esomeprazole. Am J Gastroenterol. 2009;104:1642–9.
53. Islami F, Kamangar F. Helicobacter pylori and esophageal cancer risk: a meta-analysis. Cancer Prev Res (Phila). 2008;1:329–38.
54. Xie FJ, Zhang YP, Zheng QQ, et al. Helicobacter pylori infection and esophageal cancer risk: an updated meta-analysis. World J Gastroenterol. 2013;19:6098–107.

# Chemical Composition of Refluxate

**3**

Iain A. Brownlee

**Abstract**

The reflux of gastric contents into the aerodigestive tract has been linked to a variety of oesophageal, oral, airways and respiratory diseases. The composition of refluxate is not merely secreted gastric juice and instead represents a complex mixture of gastrointestinal secretions and exogenous factors. Within the stomach, gastric juice mixes with proximal (saliva) and distal (pancreatic juice, bile) gastrointestinal secretions. New microbes enter the stomach via ingested food, saliva and other aerodigestive secretions and join the gastric microbial community. Ingestion of food may itself drive a number of physiological actions that are linked to the occurrence of reflux.

Digestive enzymes, acid and bile may cause direct damage to the unprotected mucosal tissues of the aerodigestive tract. Further from this, the processes of digestion within the stomach may release new antigen that have the potential to cause an immunological response. The gastric microbiome is largely similar to that of the aerodigestive tract, so its role in damage as a result of reflux is unclear. The complex interplay between all of the above factors is not currently well understood, although is likely to play a role both in the damaging potential of refluxate as well as the frequency and volume of reflux events.

## Introduction

The secretions of the stomach have vital physiological roles in the enzymatic and chemical processes of digestion and also act as a barrier that limits the number of microbes entering the distal gut [1]. During the gastric phase of digestion, the

I. A. Brownlee
Newcastle Research and Innovation Institute, Newcastle University, Singapore, Singapore
e-mail: iain.brownlee@csiro.au

circular, longitudinal and oblique smooth muscle layers surrounding the stomach act to homogenise ingested food into a creamy paste known as chyme. This action allows for easier passage of digesta through into the narrower duodenum but also better mixes enzymes with the target substrates. The release of chyme into the duodenum through the pyloric sphincter is phased. Previous evidence would suggest that pyloric sphincter opening is affected by the chemical composition of the material within the gastric lumen, which is sensed by endocrine cells within the gastric mucosa. These cells release neurohumoral factors with act within the stomach, other parts of the gut and systemically to orchestrate the processes of digestion [2, 3].

The stomach is well protected against its own digestive secretions by the presence of a continuous mucus barrier that covers the gastric luminal surface [4]. There is increasing evidence to suggest that the inappropriate movement of gastric content to proximal parts of the gastrointestinal tract of into the respiratory tree (where it would be considered refluxate) can damage these less well protected tissues, potentially resulting in damage, obstruction, inflammation or immune responses, dependent on the chemical composition of refluxed material.

As the exposure of tissues to refluxate is believed to be the key mediating factor in the onset a number of diseases of the oesophagus, mouth and upper and respiratory tract (discussed in other chapters within this edition), there are at least three postulates for why some individuals suffer from these conditions while other do not: (1) Exposure is more frequent or over longer periods of time in the diseased state, (2) Individuals are pre-disposed to the diseased state as a result of limited protection from refluxate exposure or (3) The chemical composition of refluxate is different within the diseased state. Within all of these postulates, it appears that the composition of refluxed material is a key determinant of the damaging potential of reflux events. This chapter therefore aims to describe the major components that can occur within refluxate, highlight factors that affect the composition of refluxate and examine how factors within refluxate could be potentially damaging to the aerodigestive tract.

## Overview of Gastric Secretions

Gastric glands are organised units of the epithelium that produce a range of exocrine secretions from different epithelial cell types. Alongside cells that produce various exocrine secretions, the gastric epithelium also contains a range of cell types that produce endocrine secretions to mediate local and systemic control of the processes of digestion. These endocrine cells are discussed in further detail in the section "Control of Gastric Secretion below". In order to ensure that the epithelium is integral and that proper epithelial function is maintained, stem cells must be present within the gastric pits. Stem cells are pluripotent cells that differentiate into the variety of different cells types necessary to maintain the endocrine and exocrine functions of the gastric epithelium effectively. It appears as though stem cells occur in a niche within the epithelial surface at the top of each gastric gland just below the opening of the pit [5, 6]. This organisation is different from intestinal crypt units, where stem cells are found nearer the base of the crypt in both the small and large intestine [7]. Therefore, within the gastric glands, differentiated cells must migrate either towards the gland base or towards the luminal opening.

Hydrogen ions are secreted into the gastric lumen by the parietal cells that occur at the base of the gastric pit. This occurs as a result of the action of the ATP-driven basolateral Na/K antiporter and the luminal H/K antiporter, resulting in an approximate million-fold concentration of hydrogen ions across the epithelium. The presence of high acidity within the gastric milieu activates digestive enzymes [8] and represents an innate defence mechanism against swallowed microbes [9, 10]. Stomach acid also acts to denature dietary proteins, which allows better homogenisation of gastric contents and also improves access to sites of cleavage on peptide chains by proteolytic enzymes.

Stomach acid has historically been perceived as a major causative factor of reflux diseases. In the same way that the low pH of gastric juice causes the denaturation of dietary proteins, acid would be expected to initially cause damage to membrane-bound proteins on the luminal membrane the oesophageal epithelium before potentially infiltrating the mucosa and causing further structural damage. A number of therapies for peptic ulcer and reflux disease have focused on limiting the secretion of hydrogen ions by parietal cells by competitively inhibiting histamine-induced secretion or by acting to inhibit the apical potassium-hydrogen ATPase that greatly increases luminal $H^+$ concentration. Such therapies appear to be have been successful in improving symptomology in peptic reflux oesophagitis patients [11]. However, these studies highlight a high frequency of placebo effects (>30%) in the control group, symptoms still persist in those in whom they are abated and long-term PPI usage has been associated with increased infection rates (possibly due to the removal of the gastric acid barrier) and increased risk of fracture, possibly due to inhibiting the molecular processes involved in bone remodelling [12]. The pH of the gastric juice also controls the activity of the enzymes there within. While a low pH is ideal for gastric enzymes to work at, higher pH will tend to increase the activity of enzymes initially secreted into the intestine and mouth that may subsequently end up in the stomach.

A series of aspartate proteases, referred to as "pepsins", are secreted in their inactive form (pepsinogen) by the chief cells situated towards the base of the gastric pits. At low pH (below 5) a conformational change occurs in the pepsinogen chain that results in the peptide chain covering the active site swivelling into the catalytic cleft and being cleaved off. Active pepsin is important in the initial stage of protein digestion, producing shorter chains from polypeptides in a relatively non-specific manner [8].

The exposure of the *in vitro* porcine or *in vivo* canine larynx to pepsin plus acid or even pepsin alone at higher pH leads to increased damage than acidic solutions [13, 14]. Recent work has also highlighted that human pepsins remains active over a relatively wide pH range (up to pH 7.0 in the case of pepsin 3B) and pepsin that has been inactivated at lower pH (down to pH 8.0) can be reactivated again in the presence of an acidic milieu [15]. Previous *in vitro* studies also suggest that pepsin proteins may have cancer-promoting effects on laryngeal cells and tissues under conditions that would not be expected to cause damage to the epithelial surface [16, 17].

Mucin is secreted by gastric mucus cells (situated in higher number towards the top of the gastric gland) and rapidly swells in the aqueous environment to form mucus [18]. Gastric mucus is believed to exist in a functional bilayer, with the outermost layer being loosely adherent and easily removed by shear stress, while the inner layer is firmer and more resistant to removal [19]. The outer layer therefore acts as a functional lubricant to reduce mechanical damage to the underlying mucosa. Mucins degraded by shear stress or other processes will end up within the luminal bulk content. Higher rates of gastric mucolysis have been historically hypothesised to be a factor in the aetiology of peptic ulcer disease [20]. While it is unlikely that mucin monomers in refluxate would have any damaging potential, further degradation of the mucins by endogenous or bacterial enzymes could result in the release of peptide fragments that might represent novel antigen challenges to tissues that refluxate contacts.

While the chemical composition of gastric content changes greatly before and during meals, previous observations suggest the presence of considerable interindividual variation in the fasted state. In healthy adults, fasting gastric volume appears to vary from almost zero to as much as 40 ml while the pH of this content varied from over pH 6 to less than pH 1.5 [21]. Higher fasting volumes (with some measured as higher than 100 ml) were noted in a previous study, along with an estimated mean of pepsin concentration 0.5 (±SD 0.31) mg/ml [22].

Until recently, it was generally accepted that the contents of the stomach tended to become homogenous during gastric mixing. However, it appears as though there is a degree of compartmentalisation within the stomach itself. The gradual flow of contents out of the pyloric region and patterns of contractility has previously been evidenced to cause a phenomenon termed "gastric sieving". More fully homogenised and digested content is able to pass the funnel-like structure of the pylorus, whereas larger material is retained within the body of the stomach for further digestion [23]. Recent advances in intragastric imaging have also revealed that during gastric digestion, a distinct region of acidic fluid can occur in the near the gastro-oesophageal junction, termed the acid pocket [24]. This low pH fluid does not appear to become mixed into the partially homogenised material occurring distally.

## Control of Gastric Secretion

All exocrine secretions of the stomach tend to be stimulated by the release of acetylcholine from vagal efferent fibres. Alongside this, positive or negative feedback can be provided from neurohumoral agents released by endocrine cells with the gastric or intestinal epithelium. Neurohumoral release within the gastric and intestinal phases of digestion tends to be driven by the chemical composition of the digesta within the gut lumen and the mechanical stress this digesta imparts on the underlying tissue [25].

Acid secretion occurs as a result of cholinergic stimulation of parietal cells by vagal efferents during both the cephalic and gastric phases of digestion but is also stimulated as a result of release of both histamine and gastrin by enteroendocrine cells within the gastric mucosa [26]. Somatostatin-producing D cells provide negative feedback to acid production as a result of low pH being sensed within the gastric lumen. The action of somatostatin appears to inhibit further stimulation of parietal secretion [27]. Previous research has suggested that increasing luminal concentrations of a number of dietary factors could be important in driving gastric acid secretion include luminal calcium, high concentration of digested proteins (particularly free amino acids) mixed dietary fat, glucose, caffeine and capsaicin [2, 28–30].

Pepsinogen secretion is stimulated by vagal cholinergic activity and a range of other neurohumoral mediators, particularly immediately after the ingestion of food [31]. Mucus secretion is also governed by cholinergic stimulation but is also modulated by the release of gastrin or secretin and can be rapidly increased within gastric tissues in the presence of noxious agents, such as alcohol [4].

## The Gastric Microbiome

A large body of recent literature has highlighted the importance of the large intestinal microflora to colonic and systemic health. A more limited range of research has been carried out on the importance of the gastric microbiome and its roles in health and pathophysiology. The total number of microbial cells that exist within the stomach is relatively low. Recent estimates suggest that the human stomach contains approximately 1000 colony forming units/ml of fluid [32]. As in other parts of the gut, the gastric microbiome can interact with luminal contents and the mucosal lining in ways that are potentially positive or negative to health.

Previous studies have highlighted similar microbes appear to occur within the buccal cavity, respiratory tract and gastric niches [33]. This suggests that the resident microflora across the aerodigestive tract could be shared. While reflux events could act to bring microbes resident in the gastric contents into the other areas of the aerodigestive tract, the action of mucociliary clearance would also lead to inhaled microbes being swallowed and potentially surviving within the stomach. The most abundant species of bacteria found in the stomach appear to be *Streptococcus* and *Prevotella* [34]. *Helicobacter pylori* is frequently associated with gastric pathologies and been evidenced to exist in other aerodigestive niches [35]. However, there is no causal evidence to suggest that *H. pylori* has arrived into other areas of the aerodigestive tract as a result of initial gastric infection and subsequent retrograde flow of refluxate.

Within a previous study that observed the 16s ribosomal RNA sequences present in gastric samples collected from six healthy individuals, it was noted that the three individuals who were *Helicobacter pylori* negative had more diverse bacterial communities, with H. pylori accounting for the high proportion (c. 95%) of the total bacteria. In both cases, the percentage of unclassifiable bacteria was low (<1%). It must be noted that such techniques only allow characterisation of bacteria present and not fungi or viruses [36]. While *Candida albicans* and other fungi might be involved in secondary infection of damage to gastric mucosa [37], there is no evidence linking these other micro-organisms to the occurrence or pathogenicity of reflux.

## Refluxate and Other Non-gastric Secretions

The material that is refluxed into the upper aerodigestive tract from the stomach will also contain digestive secretions proximal secretions that have moved into the stomach (e.g. saliva and mucus from the upper respiratory tract and pulmonary system) which could drive translocation of microbes [36]. Saliva secretion around meal times is likely to be high in volume and bicarbonate concentration which might directly neutralise gastric acidity. Saliva eases the passage of boluses of food down the oesophagus and may act both as a clearance mechanism as well as a neutralising agent that could reduce the damaging potential of refluxate.

Swallowed saliva is also likely to contain low concentrations of two microbial metabolites of the oral bacteria that could also impact on reflux. The first is nitrite, which is produced by the reduction of salivary nitrate by oral microbes [38]. When nitrite reaches the acidic conditions in the stomach, nitrite is further reduced to produce nitric oxide, the majority of which is absorbed in the small intestine. Nitric oxide is a major mediator of relaxation of the lower oesophageal sphincter which could increase the occurrence of reflux events [39]. However, recent evidence suggests that amounts of nitrite that reach the stomach in saliva do not appear to affect the occurrence of reflux [40].

Short-chain fatty acids, produced as a by-product of metabolism of energy sources within the buccal cavity may also impact on the occurrence of reflux events. Previous evidence suggests that short-chain fatty acids produced in (or hypothetically reaching the colon) could also cause increased occurrence of transient lower oesophageal relaxations, resulting in increased frequency of reflux events [41]. However, there is currently no evidence to support the idea that this happens as a result of oral production of short chain fatty acids.

Duodenogastric reflux describes the movement of duodenal contents proximally into the stomach. This event appears to occur physiologically in healthy individuals [42]. The resultant movement of bile and pancreatic enzymes into the lumen of the stomach and aerodigestive tract has the potential to expand the range of injurious factors that occur within refluxate. While the movement of duodenal contents into the stomach might be expected to result in a reduction in pH of the gastric milieu, there is still strong evidence associating the occurrence of duodenogastric reflux can result in faster disease progression. For example, the presence of bile acids in the post-transplant lung has been linked to impairment of the innate pulmonary immune system [43]. Bile acids are believed to act as damaging agents in refluxate, as they may act to disrupt cell membranes of mucosal cells lining the aerodigestive tract. Trypsin and other pancreatic enzymes also have the potential to digest mucosal surfaces they come into contact with in the digestive tract. However, unlike pepsin, their optimal activity occurs at pHs close to neutral, so these enzymes could be more active under the conditions that would be expected to occur in the aerodigestive tract.

## Dietary Intake and Reflux

While information given to patients around the world would highlight the potential for foods consumed to trigger reflux, the evidence suggesting this is frequently rarely above the level of anecdotal. Specific phytochemicals like capsaicin or caffeine have been suggested to be associated with worse symptomology in reflux oesophagitis and such factors are simple to test within challenge meals in an appropriately blinded fashion. However, whole foods are rather more difficult to hide from the participant or researcher, so experimental design becomes more difficult. High fat and high protein intake are also suggested as being linked to reflux occurrence. A previous study looking at a holistic dietary approach to reduce intake of "acidic" foods has been evidenced to benefit symptoms in laryngopharyngeal reflux patients who showed no symptom improvement on pharmacological therapy [44]. It is likely that an overarching approach to diets and lifestyle management will be of more benefit to reduction of the frequency and length of reflux events in those affected by symptoms. The clearest evidence currently exists for central adiposity being linked to reflux (likely as a result of increased intra-abdominal pressure). Weight-loss interventions have been evidenced to be successful in reducing the occurrence of reflux events and improving symptoms in patient groups [45, 46]. A previous systematic review highlighted that recommendations for reduction of intake of citrus fruits, tomatoes/tomato products, chocolates, caffeinated beverages and fatty foods to improve reflux symptomology was not well founded [47]. A further observational study noted that adherence to guidelines to avoid putatively "refluxogenic" foods in gastro-oesophageal reflux disease patients was low [48].

Causal evidence of individual dietary components impacting reflux is limited. One previous study noted that reducing dietary fat consumption and increasing fruit and vegetable intake over a 3-year period did not improve histological findings in Barrett's oesophagus [49]. Some previous evidence highlights suggests that thickened infant formulae reduce the oesophageal acid exposure but do not necessarily reduce the total number of reflux events [50, 51]. Allergy to cow's milk has long been associated with the occurrence of reflux/regurgitation in infants. A recent open, crossover trial evaluating reflux occurrence in children with clinically-substantiated cow's milk allergy noted that the total number of reflux events was 60% higher during feeding with cow's milk formula than an amino acid-based control, with a large proportion of weekly-acidic reflux events seemingly the cause for the increase in total number of reflux events. A recent study in patients with functional dyspepsia who did not have endoscopically-assessed symptoms of gastro-oesophageal reflux, reduced meal size was associated with faster gastric emptying and lower gastric volume [52]. These effects could be assumed to reduce the incidence of reflux events in frequent refluxers.

While weight management strategies appear to be effective in improving reflux symptoms, there appears to be a need to further elucidate dietary factors that may or may not be refluxogenic to improve the quality of evidence supporting dietary management of reflux. Further mechanistic studies assessing whether these dietary factors directly trigger symptoms, result in a change in gastric juice composition resulting in a higher damaging potential, or are affecting gastric motility, gastric emptying, lower oesophageal sphincter tone or other physiological events that may drive the occurrence of reflux. Such studies may be more feasible when non-invasive measures of reflux occurrence are employed (e.g. Peptest™) but should be carefully controlled (by meal composition and content) to avoid false-positive findings from the intake of specific dietary factors.

## Summary

From the above, it is clear that the content of the gastric lumen does simply originate from the gastric glands. Due to the mixing action of the stomach, the gastric and other gastrointestinal secretions, microbiota and dietary factors will come into contact with each other in the stomach and may interact in a number of ways. Figure 3.1 below shows a number of hypothetical ways that these compositional components could interact to affect the occurrence of reflux events or the damaging potential of refluxate.

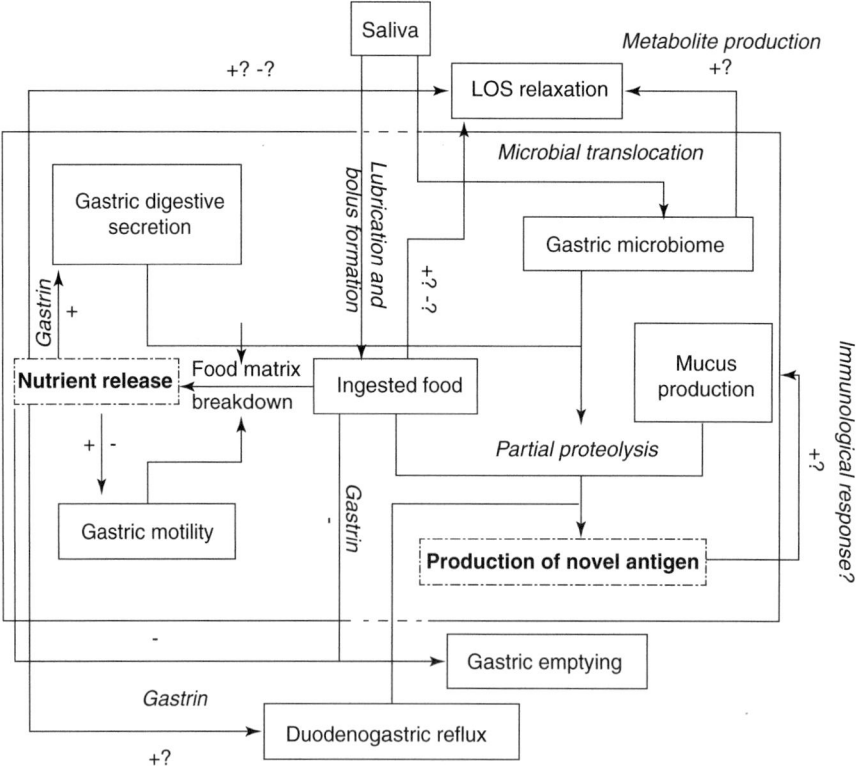

**Fig. 3.1** Hypothetical model of the interactions between compositional components of gastric contents and some physiological factors governing the chemical composition of refluxate. "+" and "−" represent an increase or decrease in the event the arrow points to, while a question mark is used to highlight where an outcome is unknown or not well-evidenced

# References

1. Shafik A, El Sibai O, Shafik AA, Shafik IA. Mechanism of gastric emptying through the pyloric sphincter: a human study. Med Sci Monit. 2007;13(1):CR24–CR9.
2. Kidd M, Hauso Ø, Drozdov I, Gustafsson BI, Modlin IM. Delineation of the chemomechanosensory regulation of gastrin secretion using pure rodent G cells. Gastroenterology. 2009;137(1):231–41.e10.
3. Lee CS, Perreault N, Brestelli JE, Kaestner KH. Neurogenin 3 is essential for the proper specification of gastric enteroendocrine cells and the maintenance of gastric epithelial cell identity. Genes Dev. 2002;16(12):1488–97. https://doi.org/10.1101/gad.985002.
4. Allen A, Flemström G. Gastroduodenal mucus bicarbonate barrier: protection against acid and pepsin. Am J Physiol Cell Physiol. 2005;288(1):C1–C19.
5. Barker N, Huch M, Kujala P, van de Wetering M, Snippert HJ, van Es JH, et al. Lgr5+ve stem cells drive self-renewal in the stomach and build long-lived gastric units in vitro. Cell Stem Cell. 2010;6(1):25–36. https://doi.org/10.1016/j.stem.2009.11.013.
6. Mills JC, Shivdasani RA. Gastric epithelial stem cells. Gastroenterology. 2011;140(2):412–24. https://doi.org/10.1053/j.gastro.2010.12.001.
7. Barker N, Van Oudenaarden A, Clevers H. Identifying the stem cell of the intestinal crypt: strategies and pitfalls. Cell Stem Cell. 2012;11(4):452–60. https://doi.org/10.1016/j.stem.2012.09.009.
8. Pearson JP, Parikh S, Robertson AGN, Stovold R, Brownlee IA. Pepsins. In: Johnston N, Toohill RJ, editors. Effects, diagnosis and management of extra-esophageal reflux. New York: Nova Science Publishers; 2012. p. 29–41.
9. Howell MD, Novack V, Grgurich P, Soulliard D, Novack L, Pencina M, et al. Iatrogenic gastric acid suppression and the risk of nosocomial Clostridium difficile infection. Arch Intern Med. 2010;170(9):784–90.
10. Lombardo L, Foti M, Ruggia O, Chiecchio A. Increased incidence of small intestinal bacterial overgrowth during proton pump inhibitor therapy. Clin Gastroenterol Hepatol. 2010;8(6):504–8.
11. Van Pinxteren B, Numans ME, Lau J, De Wit NJ, Hungin APS, Bonis PAL. Short-term treatment of gastroesophageal reflux disease: a systematic review and meta-analysis of the effect of acid-suppressant drugs in empirical treatment and in endoscopy-negative patients. J Gen Intern Med. 2003;18(9):755–63. https://doi.org/10.1046/j.1525-1497.2003.20833.x.
12. Ali T, Roberts DN, Tierney WM. Long-term safety concerns with proton pump inhibitors. Am J Med. 2009;122(10):896–903. https://doi.org/10.1016/j.amjmed.2009.04.014.
13. Koufman JA. The otolaryngologic manifestations of gastroesophageal reflux disease (Gerd): a clinical investigation of 225 patients using ambulatory 24-hour pH monitoring and an experimental investigation of the role of acid and pepsin in the development of laryngeal injury. Laryngoscope. 1991;101(4):1–78.
14. Bulmer DM, Ali MS, Brownlee IA, Dettmar PW, Pearson JP. Laryngeal mucosa: its susceptibility to damage by acid and pepsin. Laryngoscope. 2010;120(4):777–82. https://doi.org/10.1002/lary.20665.
15. Johnston N, Dettmar PW, Bishwokarma B, Lively MO, Koufman JA. Activity/stability of human pepsin: implications for reflux attributed laryngeal disease. Laryngoscope. 2007;117(6):1036–9. https://doi.org/10.1097/MLG.0b013e31804154c3.
16. Johnston N, Yan JC, Hoekzema CR, Samuels TL, Stoner GD, Blumin JH, et al. Pepsin promotes proliferation of laryngeal and pharyngeal epithelial cells. Laryngoscope. 2012;122(6):1317–25.
17. Kelly EA, Samuels TL, Johnston N. Chronic pepsin exposure promotes anchorage-independent growth and migration of a hypopharyngeal squamous cell line. Otolaryngol Head Neck Surg. 2014;150(4):618–24. https://doi.org/10.1177/0194599813517862.
18. Harada S, Tanaka S, Takahashi Y, Matsumura H, Shimamoto C, Nakano T, et al. Inhibition of Ca2+-regulated exocytosis by levetiracetam, a ligand for SV2A, in antral mucous cells of guinea pigs. Eur J Pharmacol. 2013;721(1–3):185–92.

19. Phillipson M, Johansson MEV, Henriksnäs J, Petersson J, Gendler SJ, Sandler S, et al. The gastric mucus layers: constituents and regulation of accumulation. Am J Physiol Gastrointest Liver Physiol. 2008;295(4):G806–G12.
20. Younan F, Pearson J, Allen A, Venables C. Changes in the structure of the mucous gel on the mucosal surface of the stomach in association with peptic ulcer disease. Gastroenterology. 1982;82(5 Pt 1):827–31.
21. Goudra BG, Singh PM, Carlin A, Manjunath AK, Reihmer J, Gouda GB, et al. Effect of gum chewing on the volume and pH of gastric contents: a prospective randomized study. Dig Dis Sci. 2015;60(4):979–83. https://doi.org/10.1007/s10620-014-3404-z.
22. Hirschowitz BI. Gastric acid and pepsin secretion in patients with Barrett's esophagus and appropriate controls. Dig Dis Sci. 1996;41(7):1384–91. https://doi.org/10.1007/BF02088563.
23. Janssen P, Vanden Berghe P, Verschueren S, Lehmann A, Depoortere I, Tack J. Review article: the role of gastric motility in the control of food intake. Aliment Pharmacol Ther. 2011;33(8):880–94.
24. Beaumont H, Bennink RJ, De Jong J, Boeckxstaens GE. The position of the acid pocket as a major risk factor for acidic reflux in healthy subjects and patients with GORD. Gut. 2010;59(4):441–51. https://doi.org/10.1136/gut.2009.178061.
25. Brownlee IA. The impact of dietary fibre intake on the physiology and health of the stomach and upper gastrointestinal tract. Bioact Carbohydr Diet Fibre. 2014;4(2):155–69. https://doi.org/10.1016/j.bcdf.2014.09.005.
26. Schubert ML, Peura DA. Control of gastric acid secretion in health and disease. Gastroenterology. 2008;134(7):1842–60.
27. Isackson H, Ashley CC. Secretory functions of the gastrointestinal tract. Surgery (United Kingdom). 2014;32(8):396–403.
28. Brownlee IA. The physiological roles of dietary fibre. Food Hydrocoll. 2011;25(2):238–50.
29. Saqui-Salces M, Dowdle WE, Reiter JF, Merchant JL. A high-fat diet regulates gastrin and acid secretion through primary cilia. FASEB J. 2012;26(8):3127–39.
30. Torii K, Uneyama H, Nakamura E. Physiological roles of dietary glutamate signaling via gut-brain axis due to efficient digestion and absorption. J Gastroenterol. 2013;48(4):442–51.
31. Fiorucci S, Distrutti E, Federici B, Palazzetti B, Baldoni M, Morelli A, et al. PAR-2 modulates pepsinogen secretion from gastric-isolated chief cells. Am J Physiol Gastrointest Liver Physiol. 2003;285(3):G611–G20.
32. Lopetuso LR, Scaldaferri F, Franceschi F, Gasbarrini A. The gastrointestinal microbiome - functional interference between stomach and intestine. Best Pract Res Clin Gastroenterol. 2014;28(6):995–1002. https://doi.org/10.1016/j.bpg.2014.10.004.
33. Bassis CM, Erb-Downward JR, Dickson RP, Freeman CM, Schmidt TM, Young VB, et al. Analysis of the upper respiratory tract microbiotas as the source of the lung and gastric microbiotas in healthy individuals. mBio. 2015;6(2):e00037-15. https://doi.org/10.1128/mBio.00037-15.
34. Wang ZK, Yang YS. Upper gastrointestinal microbiota and digestive diseases. World J Gastroenterol. 2013;19(10):1541–50. https://doi.org/10.3748/wjg.v19.i10.1541.
35. Deng B, Li Y, Zhang Y, Bai L, Yang P. *Helicobacter pylori* infection and lung cancer: a review of an emerging hypothesis. Carcinogenesis. 2013;34(6):1189–95. https://doi.org/10.1093/carcin/bgt114.
36. Scarpellini E, Ianiro G, Attili F, Bassanelli C, De Santis A, Gasbarrini A. The human gut microbiota and virome: potential therapeutic implications. Dig Liver Dis. 2015;47(12):1007–12. https://doi.org/10.1016/j.dld.2015.07.008.
37. Gong YB, Zheng JL, Jin B, Zhuo DX, Huang ZQ, Qi H, et al. Particular *Candida albicans* strains in the digestive tract of dyspeptic patients, identified by multilocus sequence typing. PLoS One. 2012;7(4):e35311. https://doi.org/10.1371/journal.pone.0035311.
38. Lundberg JO, Weitzberg E, Gladwin MT. The nitrate-nitrite-nitric oxide pathway in physiology and therapeutics. Nat Rev Drug Discov. 2008;7(2):156–67. https://doi.org/10.1038/nrd2466.

39. Kessing BF, Conchillo JM, Bredenoord AJ, Smout AJPM, Masclee AAM. Review article: the clinical relevance of transient lower oesophageal sphincter relaxations in gastro-oesophageal reflux disease. Aliment Pharmacol Ther. 2011;33(6):650–61. https://doi.org/10.1111/j.1365-2036.2010.04565.x.
40. Seenan JP, Wirz AA, Robertson EV, Clarke AT, Manning JJ, Kelman AW, et al. Effect of nitrite delivered in saliva on postprandial gastro-esophageal function. Scand J Gastroenterol. 2012;47(4):387–96. https://doi.org/10.3109/00365521.2012.658854.
41. Piche T, Zerbib F, Bruley Des Varannes S, Cherbut C, Anini Y, Roze C, et al. Modulation by colonic fermentation of LES function in humans. Am J Physiol Gastrointest Liver Physiol. 2000;278(4):G578–G84.
42. Fuchs KH, Maroske J, Fein M, Tigges H, Ritter MP, Heimbucher J, et al. Variability in the composition of physiologic duodenogastric reflux. J Gastrointest Surg. 1999;3(4):389–96.
43. D'Ovidio F, Mura M, Ridsdale R, Takahashi H, Waddell TK, Hutcheon M, et al. The effect of reflux and bile acid aspiration on the lung allograft and its surfactant and innate immunity molecules SP-A and SP-D. Am J Transplant. 2006;6(8):1930–8. https://doi.org/10.1111/j.1600-6143.2006.01357.x.
44. Koufman JA. Low-acid diet for recalcitrant laryngopharyngeal reflux: therapeutic benefits and their implications. Ann Otol Rhinol Laryngol. 2011;120(5):281–7.
45. Singh M, Lee J, Gupta N, Gaddam S, Smith BK, Wani SB, et al. Weight loss can lead to resolution of gastroesophageal reflux disease symptoms: a prospective intervention trial. Obesity. 2013;21(2):284–90. https://doi.org/10.1038/oby.2012.180.
46. Smith JE, Morjaria JB, Morice AH. Dietary intervention in the treatment of patients with cough and symptoms suggestive of airways reflux as determined by hull airways reflux questionnaire. Cough. 2013;9(1):27. https://doi.org/10.1186/1745-9974-9-27.
47. Kaltenbach T, Crockett S, Gerson LB. Are lifestyle measures effective in patients with gastroesophageal reflux disease? An evidence-based approach. Arch Intern Med. 2006;166(9):965–71.
48. Kubo A, Block G, Quesenberry CP, Buffler P, Corley DA. Dietary guideline adherence for gastroesophageal reflux disease. BMC Gastroenterol. 2014;14(1):144. https://doi.org/10.1186/1471-230X-14-144.
49. Kristal AR, Blount PL, Schenk JM, Sanchez CA, Rabinovitch PS, Odze RD, et al. Low-fat, high fruit and vegetable diets and weight loss do not affect biomarkers of cellular proliferation in Barrett esophagus. Cancer Epidemiol Biomarkers Prev. 2005;14(10):2377–83. https://doi.org/10.1158/1055-9965.EPI-05-0158.
50. Corvaglia L, Aceti A, Mariani E, Legnani E, Ferlini M, Raffaeli G, et al. Lack of efficacy of a starch-thickened preterm formula on gastro-oesophageal reflux in preterm infants: a pilot study. J Matern Fetal Neonatal Med. 2012;25(12):2735–8. https://doi.org/10.3109/14767058.2012.704440.
51. Xinias I, Mouane N, Le Luyer B, Spiroglou K, Demertzidou V, Hauser B, et al. Cornstarch thickened formula reduces oesophageal acid exposure time in infants. Dig Liver Dis. 2005;37(1):23–7. https://doi.org/10.1016/j.dld.2004.07.015.
52. Delgado-Aros S, Camilleri M, Cremonini F, Ferber I, Stephens D, Burton DD. Contributions of gastric volumes and gastric emptying to meal size and postmeal symptoms in functional dyspepsia. Gastroenterology. 2004;127(6):1685–94. https://doi.org/10.1053/j.gastro.2004.09.006.

# Pathological Processes

Jeffrey P. Pearson, Adil Aldhahrani, Peter I. Chater, and Matthew D. Wilcox

A key factor in many lung diseases and in lung allograft deterioration is an inflammatory response leading to fibroproliferation. What is the evidence for gastroduodenal reflux and aspiration being a driver of these processes? The potential damaging agents in aspirated refluxate are food particles, and microbes (particularly when patients are treated with proton pump inhibitors (PPI) and microbial overgrowth of the stomach occurs). In addition gastric juice contains enzymes e.g. pepsin and lipase and gastric acid which all have the potential to damage airway mucosa [1]. If duodenal reflux into the stomach has occurred then the gastric juice will contain conjugated bile acids, bilirubin, phospholipids and digestive enzymes in particular trypsin, chymotrypsin and lipases. These pancreatic enzymes could survive in the stomach retaining activity if the pH has been elevated by the alkaline refluxate coming from the duodenum, or in patients on PPI treatment. For example trypsin retains functionality when exposed to pepsin at pH 4.0 for 6 h but was denatured by incubation with pepsin at pH 2.2 for 4 h [2].

## Putative Mechanisms for Reflux/Aspiration Leading to Inflammation

### Animal Models

Rat gastroduodenal reflux models have been used to demonstrate the link between repetitive aspiration and respiratory diseases. Que et al. [3] used a surgical technique to separate the bottom of the oesophagus from the stomach at the cardiac sphincter leaving the pylorus connected to the duodenum. The bottom of the

J. P. Pearson (✉) · A. Aldhahrani · P. I. Chater · M. D. Wilcox
Institute of Cell and Molecular Biosciences, Newcastle University,
The Medical School, Newcastle upon Tyne, UK
e-mail: Jeffrey.Pearson@newcastle.ac.uk

© Springer International Publishing AG, part of Springer Nature 2018
A. H. Morice, P. W. Dettmar (eds.), *Reflux Aspiration and Lung Disease*,
https://doi.org/10.1007/978-3-319-90525-9_4

oesophagus was then joined to the jejunum. This leads to gastroduodenal contents flowing back into the oesophagus producing reflux and aspiration. This model can only assess the effect of gastroduodenal reflux and not gastric reflux alone. In addition the gastric secretions will be modified as no food enters the stomach directly.

Be that as it may the effects of aspiration were assessed at 10 and 20 weeks after surgery. Haematoxylin and eosin staining of lung tissue showed areas of inflammation with cell infiltrates and there were examples of partial or complete lung collapse. The severity of these effects increased at 20 compared to 10 weeks. Higher magnification showed that the lung alveolar spaces and small airways contained neutrophilic infiltrates, macrophages and multinucleated giant cells. There was also an increase in PAS/Alcian blue staining indicating goblet cell hyperplasia again greater at 20 weeks. There was also evidence of an increase in smooth muscle layer thickness confirmed by evidence of myofibroblast formation with increases in alpha-smooth muscle actin ($\alpha$-SMA) levels. In addition bronchial obliterans (BO) like lesions showing narrowing of the lumen of the bronchioles by filling with granulation tissue containing fibrous connective tissue and CD68 positive macrophages. Bile acids in the aspirate in this animal model may in part explain the pulmonary damage as they can cause cytotoxicity by disrupting plasma membranes and transporter activity. This study has demonstrated how gastroduodenal reflux followed by aspiration could result in the pathology involved in several respiratory diseases. Asthma where there is a characteristic increase in the goblet cell population and a concomitant increase in mucus secretion and where airway inflammation involving lymphocytic infiltration is involved in exacerbations [4, 5]. Chronic obstructive pulmonary disease (COPD) where exacerbations are often caused by infection of the lungs and gastro-oesophageal reflux (GOR) followed by aspiration may be a significant route for microbial entry. The evidence of BO like lesions in the rats may provide a link between reflux/aspiration and deterioration of allografts post transplantation.

Animal models have been developed by Duke University to investigate the effects of aspiration of gastric fluid on pulmonary allografts to determine the link between chronic aspiration and obliterative bronchiolitis (OB) leading to graft failure. Tang et al. [6] addressed the question as to the role of pH in lung damage using this rat lung transplantation model [7, 8]. They exposed the transplant to eight weekly lavages with pooled rat gastric juice either at the pH collected 2.5 or with juice neutralized with NaOH to pH 7.4, normal saline was used as a control. Based on histological examination both pH 2.5 and pH 7.4 gastric juice treated lungs showed damage characteristic of OB with parenchymal and peribronchiolar fibrosis and complete or partial small airway occlusion. The saline treated lungs showed no such damage. An important message from this study is that there are damaging agents in gastric juice other than acid. Therefore reduction of gastric acid secretion via the use of PPIs will not prevent the potential damage that could be caused by reflux and aspiration of gastric juice at a pH at or close to neutral.

## Cell Models

Cell models have been used to try and understand the cellular mechanisms driving the pathological changes in lung disease. These models have used whole gastric juice or the components of gastric juice. Cheng et al. [9] used a murine macrophage cell line (RAW264.7) to investigate the mechanism pertaining to chronic inflammatory lung disease, a part of which would involve macrophage activation. Gastric juice was collected from BALB/cJ mice. This could not be directly applied to the cells as it was cytotoxic, consequently they used 1% or lower levels of gastric juice diluted with culture medium. This diluted gastric juice applied to the macrophages activated the nuclear factor kappa light chain enhancer of activated B cells (NF-κB) signal transduction pathway as demonstrated by upregulation of the nuclear proteins p50 and p65. This pathway can also explain the observed increase in macrophage migration as its activation will lead to the production of monocyte chemoattractant protein MCP-1 [10]. The diluted juice also produced an increase in TNFα production in a toll like receptor (TLR-4) dependant manner, indicating that bacterial components e.g. Lipopolysaccharide (LPS) in gastric juice could be involved in macrophage activation. However at high concentrations of gastric juice tumor necrosis factor alpha (TNFα) production was increased in a non TLR-4 dependant manner. In addition the matrix metalloproteinases MMP2 and MMP9 were elevated although not as much as with direct stimuli with LPS. Finally macrophages express large amounts of protease-activated receptor 1 (PAR-1) activated by proteolysis and these receptors are linked to increased migration [11]. It is unlikely that any pepsin activity would be present in the gastric juice at neutral pH but the presence of any duodenal juice in the stomach could mean that trypsin/chymotrypsin shown to survive gastric conditions [2] could have an important role in PAR activation. These data again show the potential damaging effect of gastric juice at neutral pH. The group of Cheng et al. [12] have also investigated the effect of gastric juice on airway smooth muscle cells in an attempt to define the role of reflux/aspiration in airway remodelling a key process in airway disease e.g. asthma [13]. They applied rat gastric juice onto rat tracheal smooth muscle cells in primary culture. Again as in their previous work the gastric juice was used at a 1% dilution with culture media. Forty eight hour incubation in diluted gastric juice induced the secretion of cytokines IL-4 and IL-6 which are T helper type 2 cytokines [14]. Gastric juice also increased secretion of cytokines between 1.9 and 399 fold. These included LIX/CXCL 5 (lipopolysaccharide-induced CXC chemokine), fractalkine (CX3CL1), Cytokine induced neutrophil chemoattractant 2 (CINC-2), CINC-3 and CNTF (ciliary neurotrophic factor). The upregulation of fractalkine may have a role in attracting T cells and monocytes to the airways and promoting adhesion of leucocytes to activated endothelial cells [15]. Fractalkine could be involved in the crosstalk between smooth muscle cells (SMC) and macrophages both activated by exposure to gastric juice. SMC migration is one key process in airway remodelling [16] and migration is associated with focal adhesion kinase (FAK) activation [17]. The results of Chiu et al. [12] demonstrate activation of FAK and SMC migration is promoted by exposure to gastric juice. These in vitro experiments clearly implicate aspiration of gastric juice in promoting airway smooth muscle inflammation and remodelling and that is linked to macrophage activation by gastric juice (Fig. 4.1). Other researchers have attempted to investigate specific components of refluxate/aspirate and their role in airway inflammation. Bathoorn et al. [18] studied the effect

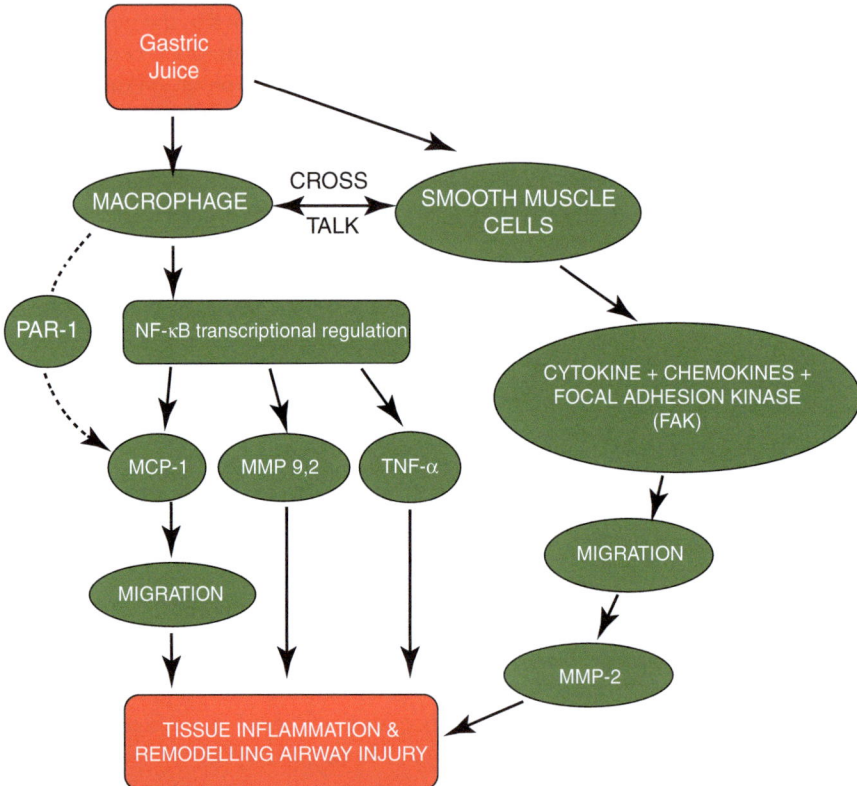

**Fig. 4.1** Macrophages and smooth muscle cells activation by gastric juice and their role in airway inflammation and remodelling. Gastric juice applied to macrophages will induce the NF-κB signal transduction pathway leading to the production of monocyte chemoattractant protein (MCP1), Tumour necrosis factor α (TNFα) and matrix metalloproteinases (MMP) 2 and 9. PAR1 (protease-activated receptor) are activated by proteolysis from the gastric juice and increase macrophage migration. This cascade of events leads to tissue inflammation and remodelling. There is crosstalk between the macrophages and smooth muscle cells activated by gastric juice leading to cytokine, chemokine and MMP2 production and smooth muscle cell migration adding to the inflammation and remodelling

of pepsin and acid on SV-40 transformed human bronchial epithelial cells (16HBE). Five minutes exposure to low pH with or without pepsin followed by incubation in normal cell culture conditions demonstrated pepsin plus acid had greater cytotoxic and inflammatory effects than acid alone. Cytotoxicity being assessed by lactate dehydrogenase release and methylene blue staining and inflammation by release of Il-6 and 8. These studies give some insight into the potential effects on the lungs of aspirated gastric juice, however these studies were carried out at pH 1.5, 2.0 and 2.5. These pHs are unlikely to be achieved in vivo with the refluxate more likely to reach the lung at pH 3.0 and above, due to mixing with oesophageal and laryngeal secretions. It would therefore be important to carry out studies at higher pHs at which pepsin will still be active [19] and this could allow longer exposure times than 5 min. Also assays for metabolic activity such as celltiter-blue or MTT could be used to assess cell viability.

Bile acids have been implicated with a role in inflammation and remodelling. Studies with human primary alveolar cells by Su et al. [20] investigated changes in epithelial permeability which is a signature of acute lung injury [21, 22]. Chenodeoxycholic acid (CDCA) (a primary bile acid) at a concentration of 200 µmol/l caused a significant decrease in transepithelial resistance (TER) which persisted up to 6 h. This was associated with a 40% reduction in cell viability. Lower levels of bile acids (100–150 µmol/l) caused a non-significant fall in TER but had no effect on cell viability. Suggesting that the effect of the highest concentration of bile acids on TER was caused by the presence of dead cells in the monolayer. CDCA levels of between 100–150 µmol/l in the non-cytotoxic range also produced a significant increase in prostaglandin $E_2$ ($PGE_2$) production by the cells. The authors then showed that $PGE_2$ alone applied to the cells (100 ng/ml) caused a transient significant decrease in TER, suggesting a link between CDCA mediated $PGE_2$ production and the fall in TER. This link was further investigated in terms of intracellular signalling molecules and proteins involved in tight junction formation. 150 µmol/l of CDCA caused a large increase in p38 and JNK phosphorylation (mitogen activated protein kinases). In addition mRNA levels for cytosolic phospholipase $A_2$ and cyclooxogenase-2 are increased by CDCA. The final piece of the jigsaw is that CDCA treatment at 150 µmol/l down regulated zonula occludens-1 (ZO-1) and E cadherin. These effects can be linked to show how CDCA opens tight junctions and could increase epithelial cell permeability in lung disease (Fig. 4.2). Although these effects are interesting some caution must be exercised as the concentrations of CDCA used were very high, considering the same group reported levels for total bile acids in the sputum of asthma patients with gastroesophageal reflux of ~5 µmol/l [23]. Also we have shown that CDCA is potentially cytotoxic to lung epithelial cell lines BEAS-2B, NCI-H292 and Calu-3 at 100 µmol/l (Fig. 4.3) and is cytotoxic at lower levels to primary human lung epithelial cells. Another mechanism by which bile acids could be linked to airway inflammation is via hypoxia-inducible factor 1. HIF-1 is made up of two subunits α and β, for activity

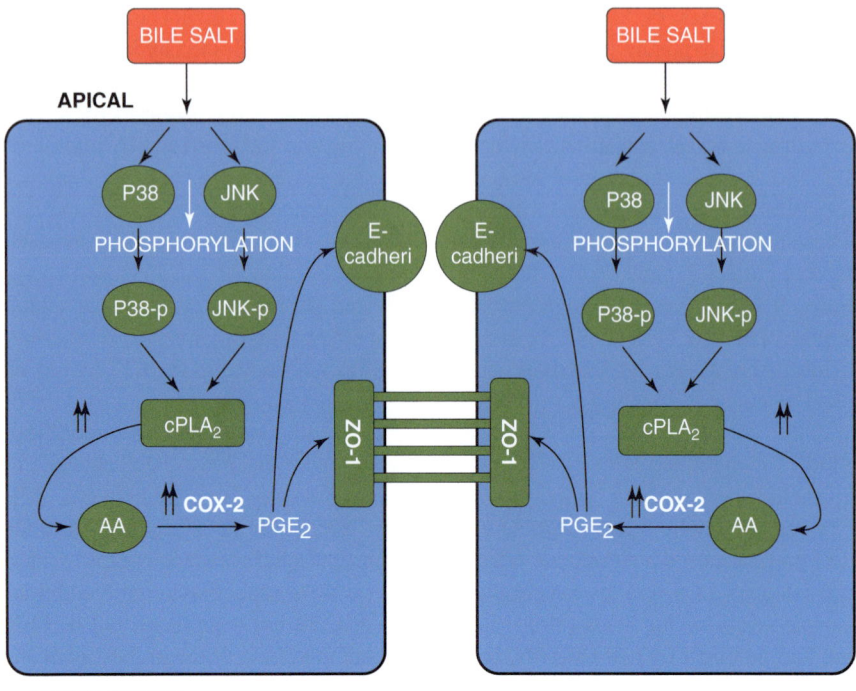

**Fig. 4.2** Effect of bile acids on human alveolar epithelial cells. 150 μmol/l chenodeoxycholic acid applied to the apical surface caused an increase in the levels of mitogen activated kinases P38 and JNK, which become phosphorylated leading to an increase in cytosolic phospholipase $A_2$ (cPLA$_2$) releasing arachidonic acid which is converted to PGE$_2$ via the increased levels of cyclooxygenase-2 (COX-2). The PGE$_2$ increase effects the levels of E-cadherin and Zonula occludens (ZO-1) leading to a relaxation of the tight junctions

HIF-1α must be stabilized. HIF-1β is constitutively expressed but the levels of HIF-1α are regulated by the action of prolyl hydroxylase domain proteins (PHD) which hydroxylate HIF-1α, which leads to its degradation. Hypoxia inhibits PHD hydroxylase activity thus stabilizing HIF-1α. In addition chronic inflammation and bacterial infection e.g. *Pseudomonas aeruginosa* can inhibit PHD activity increasing the levels of HIF-1α. HIF-1 at increased levels will stimulate the release of cytokines, NO and antimicrobial peptides from immune and epithelial cells [24]. HIF-1α is a main regulator in the response to infection and inflammation [25–27]. Legendre et al. [28] demonstrated that chenodeoxycholate and deoxycholate but not cholate caused a dose dependent down regulation of HIF-1α levels. This leads to a different expression of cytokines with down regulation of Il-8 and upregulation of Il-6 shifting from an acute to a chronic inflammatory response (Fig. 4.4).

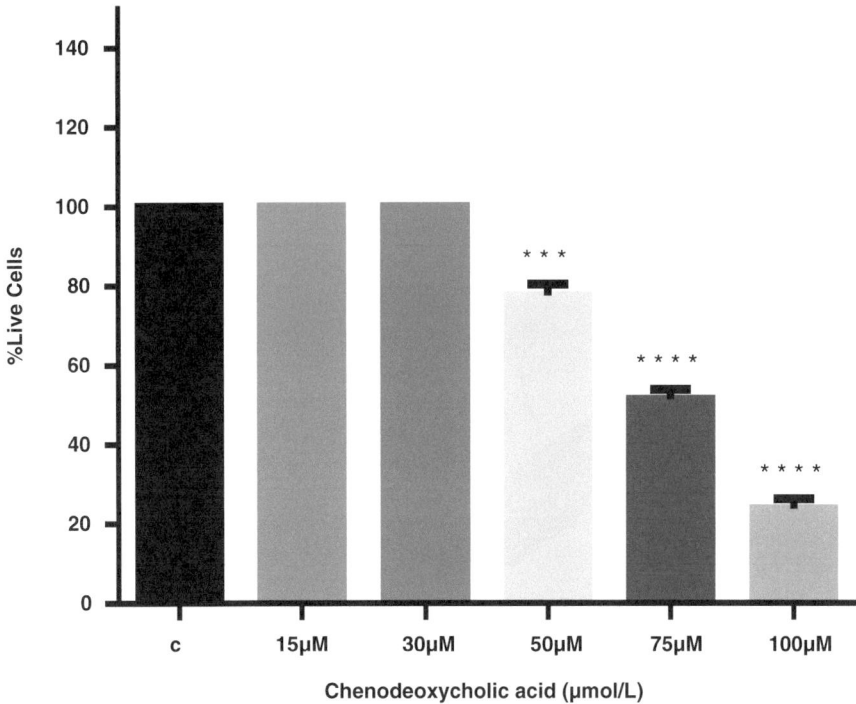

**Fig. 4.3** Cytotoxicity of chenodeoxycholic acid with BEAS-2B cells. Significant cell death is shown at 50, 75 and 100 µmol/l as measured using the Celltiter-blue assay after 48 h incubation. BEAS-2B is a human lung epithelial cell line. The data is displayed as a percentage of the normal control. Negative controls were methanol fixed cells. Significance was set at $p \leq 0.05$, n = 12. Similar results were found for 16HBE14-o cells (a human bronchial epithelial cell line) and Calu-3 a lung cancer cell line with epithelial morphology

Interestingly conjugated bile acids did not elicit this response. Therefore in vivo they would require bacterial de-conjugation to effect the levels of HIF-1α. De-conjugation of bile acids would normally occur in the ileum and colon but could occur in the stomach of patients on PPI treatment were bacterial overgrowth can occur. Consequently patients with lung disease and gastroesophageal reflux on PPIs could be aspirating unconjugated bile acids into the lungs with the implied effects on HIF-1.

As well as bile acids producing host cell responses it has been demonstrated that whole bile can alter the growth characteristics of respiratory pathogens [29]. The authors showed that bile at high concentrations could push *Pseudomonas aeruginosa* into a biofilm mode as opposed to planktonic growth. As evidenced by increased pellicle formation and increased expression of quorum sensing molecules key to switching growth characteristics. This effect was also induced in

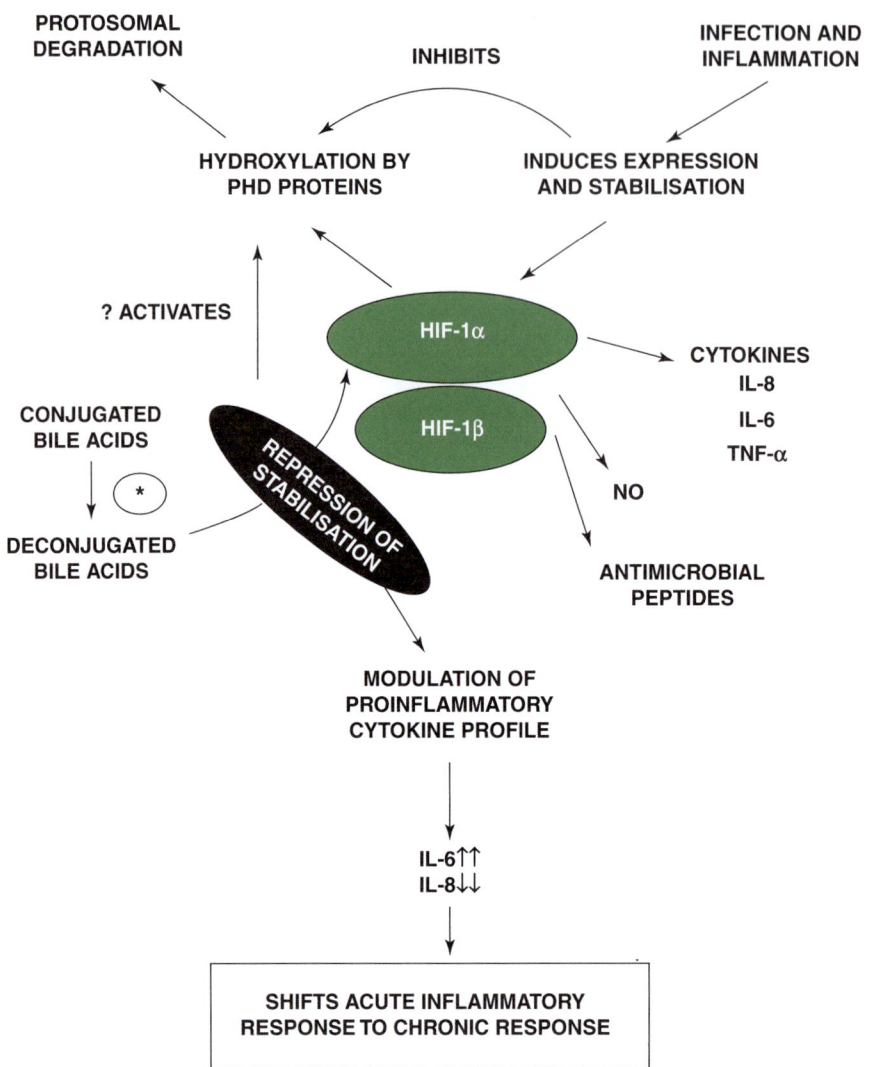

**Fig. 4.4** Effect of bile acids on hypoxia inducible factor-1 (HIF-1) in airway epithelial cells. The levels of HIF-1 are controlled by stabilization or degradation. Infection and inflammation stabilizes HIF-1 and inhibits its breakdown by PHD (prolpyl hydroxylase domain proteins) hydroxylase activity and that will lead to an acute inflammatory response. (*) Deconjugated but not conjugated bile acids promote degradation of HIF-1, changing the cytokine profile to a chronic inflammatory response

*Burkholderia cepacia* and *Staphylococcus aureus*. This growth modification has serious implications in cystic fibrosis where reflux/aspiration is prevalent [30] and patients are often infected with *Pseudomonas aeruginosa* [31]. Bacteria in biofilm form are much more difficult to eradicate with antibiotics a situation seen in cystic fibrosis.

## Human Studies

Human studies have been carried out to examine the role of reflux/aspiration in disease progression and how anti-reflux therapy could slow or stop that progression. Idiopathic pulmonary fibrosis (IPF) is a condition where gastro-oesophageal reflux is highly prevalent. With oesophageal pH monitoring suggesting a prevalence of distal reflux between 67 and 88% and proximal reflux between 30 and 71%. This high level of proximal reflux being the most important as once the refluxate is at the top of the oesophagus it is a small step to envisage the reflux leaving the oesophagus and being aspirated into the lungs [32–34]. A study involving 204 IPF patients [35], demonstrated that there was an association between gastroesophageal reflux and lung fibrosis score. In that PPI or $H_2$ antagonist therapy was associated with a lower fibrosis score. In addition anti-reflux therapy was an independent predictor of longer survival time.

Another study [36] has attempted to link a biomarker of reflux related lung disease (pepsin) to pathological gastroesophageal reflux in children with chronic cough or asthma. Fifty patients were included in the study and the presence of pepsin determined in lung lavage samples collected at bronchoscopy. The subjects were then divided into 22 positive for pepsin and 28 negative for pepsin. The presence of pathologic reflux was determined using oesophagogastroduodenoscopy and multichannel intraluminal impedance. Non-acid reflux had a positive correlation with pepsin positivity and it is important to note that pepsin retains activity above pH 4.0, above which a refluxate is often defined as non-acidic [2, 19, 37]. The authors concluded "Lung pepsin cannot predict pathologic reflux in the oesophagus but its correlation with lung inflammation suggests pepsin may be an important biomarker for reflux-related lung disease" [36]. This conclusion could be revised if one considers any reflux between pH 1 and 7 as potentially pathologic to the oesophagus based on pepsins ability to remain active over that pH range. Also if the refluxate is non-acidic it may be a result of gastroduodenal reflux containing bile salts which can be linked to oesophageal damage. However, 'airway reflux' may result in epithelial damage through other mechanisms. Attempts have been made to link reflux with pulmonary disease/function by comparing patients with and without gastroesophageal reflux disease. The classical sequence of events is reflux followed by microaspiration which can cause inflammation and pulmonary fibrosis leading to decreased gas exchange caused by damage to the alveolocapillary membrane. In addition neuronally mediated bronchoconstriction occurs [38–40]. However the paper by Bonacin et al. [41] suggested another pathway to loss of respiratory function. That is reflux/microaspiration can increase the pulmonary dead space. The refluxate in the lung can cause damage to surfactant. This could result from the action of bile salts which have been demonstrated in the lung lavage of transplant patients [42, 43]. The damage to surfactant then results in alveolar collapse (microatelectasis) leading to an increase in $Q_S/Q_T$ indicating an increase in intrapulmonary venous shunt.

The remaining human studies described in this chapter deal with lung transplantation but the pathology of damage can shed some light on all reflux related lung damage. Because of the poor long term survival of lung allografts most studies have concentrated on mediators of bronchiolitis obliterans syndrome (BOS). One such mediator is type V collagen sensitization. Collagen V is found as heterotypic fibrils with collagen I and collagen V is not exposed on the surface of the fibril [44]. When the fibril is exposed to pepsin and or acid the outer collagen I is degraded and the collagen V exposed. An auto-immune type reaction is initiated with monocytes and T-helper 17 cells directed against the α I chain of collagen V [45, 46]. This leads to fibroproliferation and the development of BOS (Fig. 4.5). This pathway was investigated by Bobadilla et al. [47] who showed that transplant recipients with GORD had significantly higher sensitivity to Collagen V as assessed by the trans vivo delayed type hypersensitivity reaction and had a significant reduction in BOS free survival time. Several further studies have investigated GORD after lung transplantation with reference to pathophysiology and implications for treatment. In a study of 35 patients Davis et al. [48] demonstrated that the prevalence of GORD was 51% and significantly more of the GORD positive patients had defects in oesophageal motility compared to transplant patients without GORD. Also 36% of the GORD positive patients had delayed gastric emptying and 12% Barrett's oesophagus.

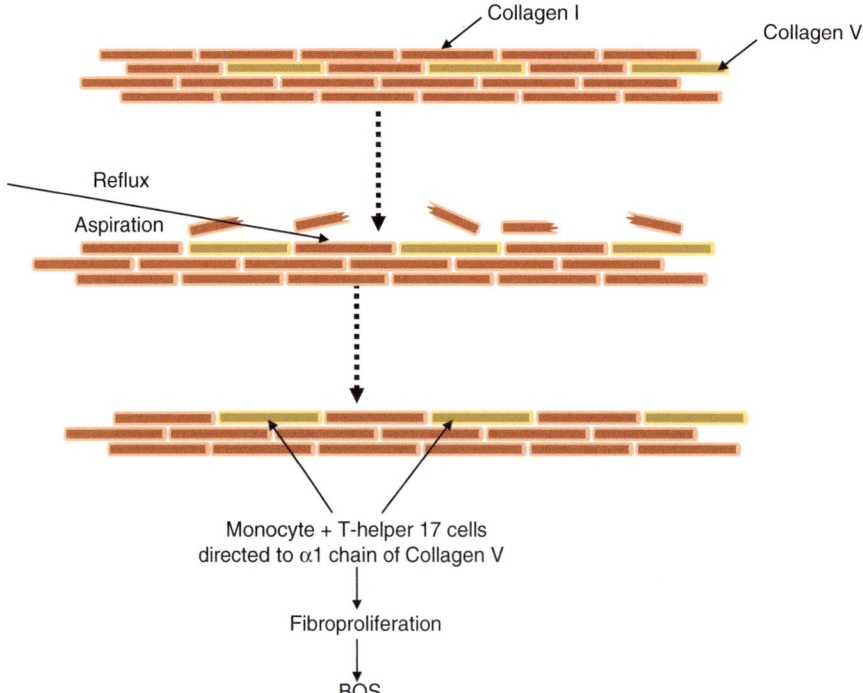

**Fig. 4.5** Collagen V as a cryptic self-antigen in the lung. Collagen V is positioned in the middle of a collagen I/V heterotypic fibril. Reflux/aspiration containing pepsin and or acid degrades the surface collagen I exposing collagen V. Collagen V is recognised by immune cells leading to damage and fibroproliferation and bronchiolitis obliterans syndrome

Based on proximal pH sensor data the GORD group had significantly higher proximal reflux. These data demonstrate the potential for a substantial risk from reflux/aspiration damage to the lungs in lung transplant patients with GORD and early anti-reflux surgery should be considered to protect the allograft [49–51].

A small study of eight lung transplant patients with GORD and a pathological white cell population demonstrated that laparoscopic anti-reflux surgery could correct the immune changes seen pre-surgery to a more physiological state. Measurement of the white cell population and several cytokines were made 4 weeks before anti-reflux surgery, 4 weeks after and 12 months after anti-reflux surgery. Four weeks after surgery the neutrophil levels fell significantly from 6.6% to 2.8%. The lymphocytes fell from 10.4% to 2.4% and the macrophages increased from 74.8% to 94.6%. In addition Interleukin 1β levels fell and interferon γ rose [52]. It has also been shown that the levels of CD8 cytotoxic cells are significantly reduced in lung transplant patients after fundoplication [53].

## Summary

This chapter discusses three approaches to study the pathological processes involved in lung disease. Firstly animal models where gastroduodenal reflux is generated by surgically connecting the jejunum to the oesophagus in rats. This model can demonstrate how reflux followed by aspiration can produce the pathology seen in asthma, COPD and BOS seen post lung transplantation. Lung allograft models have been developed to study the role of acid and pepsin in the development of BO.

Secondly cell models have allowed us to try and tease out the intracellular mechanisms leading to lung pathology. Such as; an increase in epithelial permeability a signature of acute lung injury, Macrophage and smooth muscle cell migration and tissue remodelling, and the role of HIF-1 in controlling the epithelial response to aspirate.

Thirdly human studies that have demonstrated the links between reflux/aspiration and fibrosis and tissue remodelling. Furthermore the effect of anti-reflux surgery on halting/reversing the pathological processes is considered.

## References

1. Brownlee IA, et al. From gastric aspiration to airway inflammation. Monaldi Arch Chest Dis. 2010;73:54–63.
2. Pearson JP, Parikh S. Nature and properties of gastro-oesophageal and extra- oesophagel refluxate. Aliment Pharmacol Ther. 2011;33(suppl 1):1–7.
3. Que K, et al. Histological examination of the relationship between respiratory disorders and repetitive microaspiration using a rat gastro-duodenal contents reflux model. Exp Anim. 2011;60(2):141–50.
4. Harding SM. Gastroesophageal reflux: a potential asthma trigger. Immunol Allergy Clin North Am. 2005;25:131–48.
5. Aikawa T, et al. Marked goblet cell hyperplasia with mucus accumulation in the airways of patients who died of severe acute asthma attack. Chest. 1992;101:916–21.

6. Tang T, et al. Aspiration of gastric fluid in pulmonary allografts: effects of pH. J Surg Res. 2013;181:E31–8.
7. Li B, et al. Chronic aspiration of gastric fluid induces the development of obliterative bronchiolitis in rat lung transplants. Am J Transplant. 2008;8:1614–21.
8. Hartwig MG, et al. Chronic aspiration of gastric fluid accelerates pulmonary dysfunction in a rat model of lung transplantation. J Thorac Cardiovasc Surg. 2006;131:209–17.
9. Cheng CM, et al. Macrophage activation by gastric fluid suggests MMP involvement in aspiration-induced lung disease. Immunobiology. 2010;215:173–81.
10. Cho NH, et al. Induction of the gene encoding macrophage chemoattractant protein 1 by orientia tsutsugamushi in human endothelial cells involves activation of transcription factor activator protein 1. Infect Immun. 2002;70:4841–50.
11. Chen D, et al. Protease activated receptor 1 activation is necessary for monocyte chemoattractant protein 1 dependent leucocyte recruitment in vivo. J Exp Med. 2008;205:1739–46.
12. Chiu HY, et al. Study of gastric fluid induced cytokine and chemokine expression in airway smooth muscle cells and airway remodelling. Cytokine. 2011;56:726–31.
13. Doherty T, Broide D. Cytokines and growth factors in airway remodelling in asthma. Curr Opin Immunol. 2007;19:676–80.
14. Barbas AS, et al. Chronic aspiration shifts the immune response from Th1 to Th2 in a murine model of asthma. Eur J Clin Invest. 2008;38:596–602.
15. Imai T, et al. Identification and molecular characterisation of fractalkine receptor CX3CR1 which mediates both leucocyte migration and adhesion. Cell. 1997;91:521–30.
16. Murphy DM, O'Byrne PM. Recent advances in the pathophysiology of asthma. Chest. 2010;137:1417–26.
17. Lan H, et al. The PTEN tumor suppressor inhibits human airway smooth muscle cell migration. Int J Mol Med. 2010;26:893–9.
18. Bathoorn E, et al. Cytotoxicity and induction of inflammation by pepsin and acid in bronchial epithelial cells. Int J Inflamm. 2011;2011:569416. https://doi.org/10.4061/2011/569416.
19. Bulmer DM, et al. Laryngeal mucosa: its susceptibility to damage by acid and pepsin. Laryngoscope. 2010;120:777–82.
20. Su KC, et al. Bile acids increase alveolar epithelial permeability via mitogen-activated protein kinase, cytosolic phospholipase $A_2$, cyclooxygenase-2, prostaglandin $E_2$ and junctional proteins. Respirology. 2013;18:848–56.
21. Ware LB, Matthay MA. The acute respiratory distress syndrome. N Engl J Med. 2000;342:1334–49.
22. Matthay MA, et al. Lung epithelium fluid transport and the resolution of pulmonary edema. Physiol Rev. 2002;82:569–600.
23. Perng DW, et al. Exposure of airway epithelium to bile acids associated with gastroesophageal reflux symptoms. Chest. 2007;132:1548–56.
24. Peyssonnaux C, et al. HIF-1alpha expression regulates the bactericidal capacity of phagocytes. J Clin Invest. 2005;115:1806–15.
25. Eltzschig HK, Carmeliet P. Hypoxia and inflammation. N Engl J Med. 2011;364:656–65.
26. Cramer T, et al. HIF-1alpha is essential for myeloid cell-mediated inflammation. Cell. 2003;112:645–57.
27. Nizet V, Johnson RS. Interdependence of hypoxic and innate immune responses. Nat Rev Immunol. 2009;9:609–17.
28. Legendre C, et al. Bile acids repress hypoxia-inducible factor 1 and modulate the airway immune response. Infect Immun. 2014;82:3531–41.
29. Reen FJ, et al. Respiratory pathogens adopt a chronic lifestyle in response to bile. PLoS One. 2012;7:e45978.
30. Brodlie M, et al. Bile acid aspiration in people with cystic fibrosis before and after lung transplantation. Eur Respir J. 2015;46(6):1820–3.

31. Goss CH, Burns JJ. Exacerbations in cystic fibrosis. 1: Epidemiology and pathogenesis. Thorax. 2007;62:360–7.
32. Raghu G, et al. High prevalence of abnormal acid gastro-oesophageal reflux in idiopathic pulmonary fibrosis. Eur Respir J. 2006;27:136–42.
33. Salvioli B, et al. Gastro-oesophageal reflux and interstitial lung disease. Dig Liver Dis. 2006;38:879–84.
34. Sweet MP, et al. Gastro-oesophageal reflux in patients with idiopathic pulmonary fibrosis referred for lung transplantation. J Thorac Cardiovasc Surg. 2007;133:1078–84.
35. Lee JS, et al. Gastroesophageal reflux therapy is associated with longer survival in patients with idiopathic pulmonary fibrosis. Am J Crit Care Med. 2011;184:1390–4.
36. Rosen R, et al. The presence of pepsin in the lung and its relationship to pathologic gastroesophageal reflux. Neurogastroenterol Motil. 2012;24:129–e85.
37. Ali MS, et al. Bile acids in Laryngopharyngeal refluxate: will they enhance or attenuate the action of pepsin? Laryngoscope. 2012;123:434–9.
38. Parsons JP, Mastronarde JG. Gastroesophageal reflux disease and asthma. Curr Opin Pulm Med. 2010;16:60–3.
39. Ravelli AM, Panarotto MB, Verdoni L, et al. Pulmonary aspiration shown by scintigraphy in gastroesophageal reflux-related respiratory disease. Chest. 2006;130:1520–6.
40. Araujo AC, Aprile LR, Dantas RO, et al. Bronchial responsiveness during esophageal acid infusion. Lung. 2008;186:123–8.
41. Bonacin D, Fabijanic D, Rasic M, et al. Gastroesophageal reflux disease and pulmonary function: a potential role of dead space extension. Med Sci Monit. 2012;18:CR271–5.
42. D'Ovidio F, Mura M, Ridsdale R, et al. The effect of reflux and bile acid aspiration on the lung allograft and its surfactant and innate immunity molecules SP-A and SP-D. Am J Transpl. 2006;6:1930–8.
43. Blondeau K, Mertens V, Vanaudenaerde BA, et al. Gastro-oesophageal reflux and gastric aspiration in lung transplant patients with or without chronic rejection. Eur Respir J. 2008;31:707–13.
44. Birk DE. Type V collagen: heterotypic type I/V collagen interactions in regulation of fibril assembly. Micron. 2001;32:223–37.
45. Burlingham WJ, Love RB, Jankowska-Gan E, et al. Il-17-depenent cellular immunity to obliterative bronchiolitis in human lung transplants. J Clin Invest. 2007;117:3498–506.
46. Yoshida S, haque A, Mizobuchi T, et al. Anti-type V collagen lymphocytes that express Il-17 and IL-23 induce rejection pathology in fresh and well healed lung transplants. Am J Transplant. 2006;6:724–35.
47. Bobadilla JL, Jankowska-Gan E, Quingyong X, et al. Reflux-induced collagen type V sensitization. Chest. 2010;138:363–70.
48. Davis SD, Shankaran V, Kovacs EJ, et al. Gastroesophageal disease after transplantation: Pathophysiology and implications for treatment. Surgery. 2010;148:737–45.
49. Cantu E, Appel JZ, Hartwig MG, et al. Early fundoplication prevents chronic allograft dysfunction in patients with gastroesophageal reflux disease. Ann Thorac Surg. 2004;78:1142–51.
50. Robertson AGN, Shenfine J, Ward C, et al. A call for standardization of anti-reflux surgery in the lung transplant population. Transplantation. 2009;87:1112–4.
51. Robertson AGN, Ward C, Pearson JP, et al. Lung transplantation, gastroesophageal reflux, and fundoplication. Ann Thorac Surg. 2010;89:653–60.
52. Fisichella PM, Davis CS, Lowery E, et al. Pulmonary immune changes early after laparoscopic antireflux surgery in lung transplant patients with gastroesophageal reflux disease. J Surg Res. 2012;177:E65–73.
53. Neujahr DC, Mohammed A, Ulukpo O, et al. Surgical correction of gastroesophageal reflux in lung transplant patients is associated with decreased effector CD8 cells in lung lavages: a case series. Chest. 2010;138:937–43.

# Pathophysiology in the Lung

Chris Ward, Rhys Jones, Mellissa Friel, Eoin Hunt, and Des Murphy

## Gastro Oesophageal Reflux and Aspiration Occurs Normally in Humans

This chapter discusses selected aspects of reflux, aspiration and pathophysiology in the lung. It is complimented by reviews that exist in this broad area dealing with adult [1–3] and paediatric patients [4–6].

Gastro Oesophageal reflux (GOR) describes the retrograde flow of stomach content into the oesophagus. Aspiration is a potentially dangerous scenario, where refluxed material enters the airway and lung.

The amount of material that enters the airway and lung, frequency of the challenge and the activity of clearance mechanisms are important determinants of the response to injury in individuals. The terms aspiration and micro aspiration are used, the latter denoting smaller quantities of aspiration, which may be chronic and deleterious, over time.

Individuals are predisposed to aspiration by decreased consciousness, compromised airway clearance and dysregulated swallowing. Gastroesophageal reflux or re-occurent vomiting are also risks. Aspiration into the airways and lung can therefore cause a wide range of pulmonary problems. These range from aspiration pneumonia, through to asthma and the bronchiolitis obliterans syndrome in lung allograft recipients. Micro aspiration has increasingly been implicated as a contributing

C. Ward (✉)
Institute of Cellular Medicine, Newcastle University, Newcastle upon Tyne, UK
e-mail: chris.ward@newcastle.ac.uk

R. Jones
Northern Oesophago-Gastric Unit, Royal Victoria Infirmary, Newcastle upon Tyne, UK

M. Friel
Department of Respiratory Medicine, Galway University Hospitals, Galway, Ireland

E. Hunt · D. Murphy
Department of Respiratory Medicine, Cork University Hospitals, Cork, Ireland

factor to airways disease [7]. It is of interest that a number of studies indicate that such aspiration is often clinically occult, and there is potential that this is an under recognised and under diagnosed injury in respiratory medicine [7, 8].

Broadly there are two mechanisms by which GOR is thought to produce lung pathophysiology. In the first, direct mechanism gastric contents leaves the stomach and refluxes above the upper oesophagus. Movement of stomach content into the upper airway is variously described as laryngopharyngeal reflux (LPR), silent reflux or airway reflux. This can lead to extra-oesophageal reflux symptoms and upper airway injury and if aspirated into the tracheobronchial tree can produce airway and lung disease. In addition to direct mechanisms of reflux associated damage, reflex neural mechanisms are also thought to occur during reflux events. This indicates that reflux can have effects in the distal airway and lung, which do not involve 'direct' contact with refluxate. This is covered in more depth in other Chapters of this book.

It is important to recognise that GOR occurs in people without lung disease and a degree of reflux is recognised as 'normal'. In pH studies an oesophageal acid exposure of <4.5% is considered in the normal range [9]. In a 'normal' population of 72 healthy French and Belgian volunteers, mean age 35, with no known gastrointestinal disease or thoracic/abdominal history, a study showed an average of 40 reflux events in 24 h [10].

It has also long been recognised that as well as refluxing, healthy adults may aspirate oropharyngeal secretions, especially during reclined sleep. An indium111 chloride study from 1978 showed that 45% of normal subjects aspirated during deep sleep. In patients with "depressed consciousness", aspiration was detectable in 70% of patients [11].

This study noted the potential for bacterial pneumonia as a result of failed clearance of aspirated bacteria. More recently pepsin, a putative marker of gastric aspiration, has been shown to be detectable in control populations, both by our group and independently by a number of international centres, using a range of assay systems [12, 13].

Some level of reflux and aspiration may therefore be regarded as normal or physiological. A valuable quantitative study by Gleeson et al. employed infusion of 2 mL/h radioactive 99mTc tracer into the nasopharynx to estimate the quantity of occult aspiration of nasopharyngeal secretions during sleep in normal humans. This showed that aspiration was common, occurring in 50% of healthy young men during sleep, and was variable within subjects studied on more than one occasion. The aspiration measured was 0.01–0.2 mL. This quantitation was noted as being consistent with a potentially significant bacterial inoculum [14]. Normally cough and ciliary transport protect the airways and this indicates the vital role of normal airway homeostasis and clearance. A fuller understanding of lung pathophysiology associated with reflux and aspiration therefore requires integrating an understanding of GOR, aspiration and the homeostasis of an integrated aerodigestive compartment. This is a challenge, since traditionally the GI and Respiratory systems have separate literatures, healthcare teams and research groupings. A multi-disciplinary approach is therefore required.

Both GOR and aspiration are recognised potential sources of acute lung injury and frank airway damage. It is of interest that the quantitative study of aspiration in normals cited above was performed to contextualise the known association between aspiration and pneumonia both outside and inside hospital/healthcare facilities. Early concepts involved Herb Reynolds [15], an influential and notable North American respiratory clinical academic who also pioneered early bronchoscopic studies. The established literature linking aspiration and pneumonia is a consideration relevant to the potential role for GOR and aspiration in other, chronic lung disease. Cross reference may therefore be useful.

With age and functional decline, reflux may increase and defence mechanisms become impaired: Fragile elders are recognised as being more vulnerable to developing aspiration, and pneumonia is notably more common in the elderly. Cognitive impairment, stroke, or other conditions that cause incompetent swallowing are risk factors for aspirating foreign material. Again these are more common in the elderly and frail, who may also have abnormal levels of GOR and chronic lung disease. The Iatrogenic potential of oral and inhaled corticosteroid treatment, use of antibiotics and treatments that alter normal gastric physiology including proton pump inhibitors [16, 17] are factors that may also be important in complex real world patients. A number of factors can lead to overall lung injury and pathophysiology and this complexity may be underestimated and requires further research. On the other hand the pleiotropic effect of PPI therapy has recently been shown to lead to suppression of lung inflammation and fibrosis in a rat model of bleomycin-induced lung injury [18]. Given the common use of PPIs and 'over the counter' availability in many countries, there is a need for further work in this area, interpreted in the whole patient setting.

## Lung Diseases Associated with GOR and Aspiration

### Parenchymal Disease (See Also Chap. 16)

Interstitial lung diseases have consistently been associated with GOR and aspiration. Idiopathic Pulmonary Fibrosis (IPF) may be regarded as an exemplar of this. IPF is a chronic, progressive lung disease, with median survival figures of 2.5–5 years from diagnosis. This manifests in patients over 60 years old with, has a male preponderance and comorbidities are common [19]. There are few effective treatments except lung transplantation, for which few patients are eligible and this is an internationally recognised area in need of further research. It is currently postulated that identification and treatment of comorbidities, including GOR, may have a clinically significant impact and an overall outcome that's is meaningful for IPF patients where treatment options are limited [19].

An association between IPF and Gastro Oesophageal Reflux (GOR) was demonstrated in an early study by Mays et al., which noted that hiatus hernia is common in IPF patients. Hiatus Hernia is a consistently implicated risk factor in reflux [20]. Reflux in IPF has been highlighted by international consensus as a priority for research. The limited available data have demonstrated, through pH monitoring, that GOR is significantly increased in patients with IPF as compared to normal subjects, but may be clinically occult of peptic symptoms [21]. Recently this has been confirmed by Raghu et al., demonstrating GOR on 24-h pH monitoring in 87% of their subjects [22]. The literature is variable however with a recent systematic review indicating that the prevalence of abnormal GOR in 23 studies ranged from 0 to 94%. Methodological considerations are clearly important. The prevalence of no abnormal GOR was among 20 IPF patients participating in a study into mechanisms of sleep-disordered breathing, with no history of GER recorded. The figure of 94% came from a single North American group who studied consecutive, patients with IPF who were newly diagnosed.

Until recently GOR assessment, including the few IPF studies performed to date, focused on using conventional pH monitoring, limited to detecting acid refluxing from the stomach. Newer technology based on measurement of electrical conductivity in oesophageal catheters may advance understanding. Such impedance measurements allow quantification of both acid and non-acid reflux and normal ranges have been established. However, impedance has several methodological problems. Work evaluating pepsin and bile salts as markers of aspiration in healthy individuals and patients with lung disease has also been performed [8, 13, 23, 24].

An influential retrospective study showed that GOR therapy including surgery was associated with longer survival in IPF and a lower radiologic fibrosis score, emphasising the need for further careful study [25]. Patients with IPF can experience acute exacerbations in their respiratory status leading to loss of lung function, morbidity and mortality. Occult aspiration of gastric contents has been proposed as a possible mechanism. A study from the University of California [26] showed that levels of lavage pepsin were correlated with clinical features and disease course. Pepsin levels were an indicator of acute exacerbation status and on average, pepsin appeared higher in patients with acute exacerbations compared with stable controls although pepsin level was not an independent predictor of survival time. These results suggested that occult aspiration may play a role in some cases of acute exacerbation of idiopathic pulmonary fibrosis. Reflux and aspiration have also been implicated in IPF with the finding that some patients with IPF have marked asymmetry of their lung disease on high-resolution CT (HRCT), potentially suggestive of aspiration from the gastrointestinal (GI) tract [27]. These patients showed an increased prevalence of acute exacerbations, with increased reflux symptoms.

The potential for combining physiological evaluation of reflux by pH impedance, manometry and bronchoscopic investigation of BAL markers of aspiration were also evaluated in a study by Savarino et al. [28]. IPF patients were found to have higher levels of proximal reflux events than non-IPF patients and healthy volunteers, in association with higher levels of BAL bile acids and pepsin. This was often 'asymptomatic' of typical symptoms of GOR; i.e. heartburn/regurgitation. The authors' discussion included wide ranging interpretation. The findings were reported to be consistent with a previous report suggesting that IPF patients who underwent Nissen fundoplication "had an additional benefit in terms of life survival" [25]. Savarino et al. called for "outcome studies with intense anti-reflux therapy" [28].

This an area that would benefit from timely and open research and discussion. It is of potential concern that the current literature includes increasing numbers of statements supporting surgical treatment for IPF. This is despite the lack of evidence from trials. For example Allaix et al. concluded that "because there is no effective therapy for IPF, it makes sense to treat the abnormal reflux by a well proven therapy for GERD, a laparoscopic fundoplication" [29]. A conclusion that would seem extrapolated from the experience of fundoplication in a non IPF population [30]. This is potentially made more complex by the suggestion that the label of IPF may mean different things in different centres, due to diagnostic and methodological variation [19].

IPF is a disease that is more common in the elderly and patients can be frail with significant co-morbidities [19]. It is understandable that there is enthusiasm for treatments that may benefit the overall pathophysiology of IPF. This should also take into consideration the potential iatrogenic consequences of treatment however, especially when 'elective'. In a series of four patients from Johns Hopkins Hospital with acute exacerbations in IPF, two of three patients who underwent video-assisted thoracoscopic surgery (VATS) lung biopsy had a fatal outcome. A fourth patient survived an acute exacerbation after a total knee replacement but had a fatal outcome after a subsequent coronary artery bypass graft surgery. This illustrates that both lung and nonlung surgical procedures have a high degree of risk in patients with IPF, indicating the need for very careful patient selection [31]. VATS lung biopsies are rarely carried out in our regional centre. It is therefore valuable that there is a current trial of surgical fundoplication that is estimated to finish in Dec 2016 ClinicalTrials.gov Identifier: NCT01982968.

Chronic cough is a persisting and dominant clinical feature of IPF, which has not been sufficiently studied. Interviews with IPF patients have revealed that cough has an extremely significant impact on patients' quality of life (QoL). IPF cough is dry, non-productive and hacking, with significant physical and social impacts. It has been suggested that cough affects 73–86% of cases [32]. A recent study from the Manchester group (see Chap. 25) objectively quantified cough in IPF. They confirmed that cough is a major, distressing and disabling symptom. There was a strong correlation between objective cough counts and cough-related QoL measures [32].

Reflux and microaspiration have been postulated as a possible cause of cough in IPF. The fact that cough receptors are expressed proximally, whereas the pathological changes in IPF involve the parenchyma, lends physiological potential for a link between GOR and cough in IPF.

Despite the narrative outlined above, prospective studies of antireflux treatment in IPF are lacking. Our group has initiated a pilot randomised placebo controlled trial of Omeprazole in IPF. ClinicalTrials.gov Identifier: NCT02085018. The primary outcome is the change in frequency of objectively measured cough from beginning of the study to the end of treatment.

Consideration of the potential role of reflux in IPF illustrates a potentially important conundrum relevant to IPF and other parenchymal pathophysiologies:

the question of *how* GOR and aspiration may result in anatomical changes in the periphery and interstitium of the lung. Direct contact injury mediated by microsaspirate may not be consistent with the recognised alveolar/lung pathophysiology of IPF. A possibility is that microsaspirate may in some way be converted into a liquid aerosol, since it is recognised that particulate aerosols are able to reach the alveolar spaces of the lung. This is exploited for therapeutic purposes in nebulised medication but the biophysical principle is also relevant to human lung injury. In animal models gastric juice is found to have rapid distribution in the lungs and is detected in the subpleural zones within 20s following instillation in the main bronchus of dogs [33].

Reflex neural mechanisms are also thought to occur during reflux events, indicating that reflux could have effects in the distal airway and lung which do not involve 'direct'; contact with refluxate.

In contrast to the potential puzzle linking aspiration and peripheral lung diseases such as IPF, it is conceptually more straightforward to understand how aspiration may be linked with airway disease. Indeed, in our work evaluating a potential role for GOR and aspiration in respiratory disease, we have noted that some patients undergoing bronchoscopy have direct evidence of movement of liquid into the airway, consistent with a potential injury, which can be visualised in real time at bronchoscopy. Contact of aspirate with airway may represent an important injury. GOR and aspiration have therefore been linked to a number of airway pathophysiologies.

## Airways Disease

### COPD

Reflux is a recognised co morbidity in COPD [34, 35]. Reviews of oesophageal pH testing confirmed that reflux is present in 49–62% of COPD clinic patients [36, 37].

Potential mechanisms that predispose patients with COPD may include smoking, obesity as well as exaggerated intrathoracic pressure shifts, increased coughing and diaphragmatic flattening. The use of $\beta 2$-agonists may also have an effect on sphincter tone, [38] and predispose to people with airways disease who routinely need to use inhalers to reflux.

Because lung function is not regained, exacerbations are recognised pivotal events in the progression of many chronic lung disease including COPD. In an influential study the frequency and associations of exacerbation in 2138 patients enrolled in the Evaluation of COPD Longitudinally to Identify Predictive Surrogate Endpoints (ECLIPSE) study were evaluated in a multivariate model [39]. This included an exacerbation during the previous year with an odds ratio (95% CI) of 5.72 (4.47–7.31), supporting the hypothesised "frequent exacerbation phenotype". Of interest, the second best independent predictor in the model was peptic symptoms of reflux or heartburn, with an OR of 2.07 (1.58–2.72).

It seems reasonable to speculate that the type of patient history in the ECLIPSE study favoured the reporting of "acid reflux". Arguably this may therefore systematically underestimate the role of overall reflux in COPD. This is because nonacid components of refluxate, such as bile are damaging, potentially aspirated, but are not necessarily denoted by symptoms associated with acid reflux [40].

A potential related concern from such work, not derived from the authors own conclusions, was that the reported association might be used to over emphasise the role of an antiacid therapy. This might be predicted to relieve symptoms associated with acid reflux but possibly be less effective on overall reflux. The need for further research in COPD was marked by interest and correspondence [41] and further research has been stimulated.

In a South Korean study of 118 patients, symptoms of laryngopharyngeal reflux (LPR) in patients with COPD were significant predictors for severe acute exacerbation of COPD, associated with diffuse oedema, erythema, and hyperaemia on laryngeal examination. The potential interest of this finding is that LPR symptoms are thought to relate to extra-oesophageal reflux, and a potential precursor to aspiration [42].

## Asthma

The equivalent of 1 in every 12 adults and 1 in every 11 children have asthma in the UK and in Ireland asthma prevalence is the fourth highest in the world. In 2012, 1242 people died from asthma in the UK, one of the highest asthma death rates in Europe. The economic and social impact of asthma is therefore huge.

A relationship between GOR and airways disorders such as asthma has been long postulated. Several risk factors have been identified as occurring in association with a more severe asthma phenotype including female sex, obesity, tobacco exposure and GOR [43]. Hence, asthma and GOR share potential risk factors. Whether any association between aspiration and asthma severity is the result of confounding or is due to a direct independent effect remains unknown.

In keeping with this, previous studies suggest that GOR, often asymptomatic, is common in asthma. Preliminary prospective data from our group suggest that 8/16 severe asthmatics attending a dedicated clinic had evidence of GOR on Barium swallow, a further patient had undergone a fundoplication while 69% reported GOR symptoms, with 14/16 patients on proton pump inhibitors. Extensive trials examining the potential of proton pump inhibitors to improve airways disease in asthma have had mixed findings [44, 45]. Current evidence does not support the routine use of these agents to improve outcomes in asthma. If non-acid reflux is an important component of airway injury then proton pump inhibitors might be expected to be of limited clinical efficacy or indeed increase the risk of aspiration. Studies which evaluate the potential response to injury of different reflux components may therefore have a role in guiding individual treatment strategies in respiratory patients with reflux and aspiration.

## Cystic Fibrosis (CF)

Gastro-oesophageal reflux is known to occur frequently in children and adults with CF and estimates of prevalence range from 55 to 90% [46]. The presence of reflux-induced cough and reported gastro-oesophageal reflux have both been associated with reduced lung function [46]. High levels of pepsin, a gastric protease, have been described in bronchoalveolar lavage (BAL) samples from children with CF [12]. People with CF are predisposed to reflux as a result of both primary and secondary mechanisms and abnormal gastrointestinal motility. Reflux of duodenal contents back in to the stomach is also common. Consistent with these observations high concentrations of bile acids have been described in saliva and sputum of both adults and children with CF [46, 47].

Reflux is also a common finding in lung transplant recipients, who may receive the operation as a result of end stage CF lung disease [24]. Microaspiration of refluxate has been implicated in the pathogenesis of bronchiolitis obliterans syndrome (BOS) [48]. Blondeau et al. found bile acids in 60% of BAL samples from people with CF post-lung transplantation in addition to a series of other studies from the Leuven group indicating a potential role for bile acid aspiration in the pathophysiology of BOS [46].

We have previously shown that extraction followed by tandem mass spectrometry was necessary to document the low levels of bile acids produced by dilution effects in human BAL [49]. In pilot work we detected bile acids in the lower airways of nine people homozygous for Phe508del with advanced CF lung disease at the time of lung transplantation [23]. We subsequently hypothesised that bile acids were present in the lower airways of people with CF before and after lung transplantation. To investigate we used mass spectrometry to detect and identify bile acids in lower airway samples and oesophageal pH-impedance studies to provide physiological measurements of reflux. Combined 24-h ambulatory pH impedance was performed to investigate reflux [50].

We found that bile acids were detected in samples from the explanted lungs of all 19 participants with CF and in all BAL samples from the same individuals post-lung transplantation. Of this group 9/19 had oesophageal pH-impedance studies performed post-transplant. These studies identified abnormal overall reflux in seven (78%) patients [50].

Our data therefore confirm that bile acids are present in the lower airways of people with advanced CF lung disease, consistent with our previous observations restricted to Phe508del homozygotes [23]. Longitudinal follow up showed that bile acids continue to be detectable in the lower airways post-lung transplantation. Furthermore, we found abnormal levels of reflux in most people with CF tested post-transplant. At a physiological level this rare longitudinal information indicates that reflux and aspiration is not simply a function of factors associated with chronic lung disease, such as abnormal cardiothoracic pressure gradients caused by chronic disease; our data demonstrate persistence post-transplantation, where cough is attenuated and thoracic mechanical changes, caused by advanced lung disease, are corrected.

CF is a multi-system disorder that involves both the respiratory and gastrointestinal tract. Our work and that of others indicate that duodeno-gastro-oesophageal reflux and subsequent microaspiration may be an under recognised contributor to airway injury in CF lung disease. Treatments for reflux exist and a very limited literature has advocated fundoplication in CF. In a recent small open study of adult CF patients there was a fall in cough and exacerbation events reduced by 50% post-fundoplication [51]. Fundoplication in children with CF has also been undertaken but results have been varied [52].

Post-transplantation people with CF have comparable levels of BOS with patients transplanted for other indications. However, the CF population post-transplantation is heterogeneous and some individuals develop BOS with an aggressive onset and this is now recognised as a complex, alloimmune and non-alloimmune response to injury. Colonisation of CF allografts with Pseudomonas aeruginosa has been associated with bile aspiration and neutrophilic airway inflammation by the Leuven group [53]. In turn, infection and inflammation, associated with bile aspiration, has been linked to BOS and death in 260 lung transplant recipients in a recent University of California series [54]. Further studies are therefore required in greater numbers of patients. There is potential that outcomes of lung transplantation in CF, already comparable with other indications on average, could be further improved. This 'aerodigestive' approach may have therapeutic implications in a disease where available treatments are limited.

### Non-cystic Fibrosis Bronchiectasis (NCFB)

Non-cystic fibrosis bronchiectasis (NCFB) is defined by structural remodelling and dilatation of the airways, visible on high resolution computed tomography (HRCT). Patients suffer from repeated episodes of bronchitis and chest infections and NCFB has numerous causes. Around 50% of patients have no causative factor identified however [55].

GORD may be a potential risk factor for NCFB. Studies utilising questionnaire pH monitoring, show symptomatic and clinically silent reflux in 26–75% of patients. Symptomatic GORD is also associated with reduced lung function, exacerbation frequency and reduced quality of life in NCFB [56, 57].

The association between hiatal hernias (HH) and GORD has previously been evaluated and increased prevalence has been reported in lung disease and GORD [20, 58]. A HH follows disruption of the anti-reflux barrier at the gastro-oesophageal junction such that part of the stomach protrudes into the thoracic cavity through the oesophageal hiatus of the diaphragm. These anatomical changes lead to the development of reflux [59].

With no studies of prevalence rate in NFCB patients we estimated the prevalence of HH on HRCT among well-defined patients [60]. We compared clinical indices in hiatal hernia-positive (HH+) and hiatal hernia-negative (HH−) patients in a retrospective observational cross-sectional cohort study of 100 consecutive bronchiectasis patients. Imaging was assessed in a blinded fashion by an independent specialist thoracic radiologist to determine the presence of HH and the extent of bronchiectatic disease.

Eighty-one patients had adequate imaging and 36% were confirmed to have HH on CT. HH-positive patients tended to have high BMI and had significantly increased frequency of cystic bronchiectasis. An increased number of bronchiectatic lobes were affected. This cohort therefore showed that HH a known risk for GORD correlated with increased extent and severity of radiological disease [60].

In preliminary, supporting cell work we showed that bile acids may cause inflammation and injure airway epithelium in challenge experiments of human bronchial epithelial cells. Challenge with bile acids led to both IL-6, IL-8 and TGF-B release [61]. This was attenuated by incubation of the cells with azithromycin and provided potential mechanistic insights linking GORD and potential aspiration to the clinical characteristics of NCFB [62].

### BOS Post Lung Transplantation

This is a subject of Chap. 14 and we have contributed studies in this area. The role of reflux and aspiration early post lung transplantation is of potential importance but research in this setting is rare and challenging. Non-alloimmune injuries have been increasingly recognised as risk factors for the Bronchiolitis Obliterans Syndrome (BOS), consistently a major barrier to long term allograft success and function [63]. It is therefore hypothesised that early post transplant non-alloimmune injuries may play a key role in predisposing the allograft to BOS, Chronic aspiration, secondary to extra-oesophageal reflux, may be a significant non alloimmune injury to lung allografts [8, 13, 53, 63]. Up to 75% of patients have demonstrable gastro-oesophageal reflux disease (GERD) following lung transplantation.

The practical importance of a more detailed understanding of reflux and aspiration injury in lung allografts is that treatments are possible. Anti-reflux surgery may be associated with an increased survival and improved lung function [64]. This is currently used in our centre in carefully selected patients. In particular, it has been suggested that fundoplication within 3 months of transplant may significantly reduce the incidence of BOS [12].

Since no previous studies had assessed lung transplant recipients for reflux/aspiration in the immediate post-transplant period, we evaluated whether assessment was feasible in the immediate post-transplant setting in the first prospective study immediately post-transplantation to date [24]. Eighteen lung transplant recipients, were recruited. Eight had abnormal oesophageal peristalsis and five had abnormal levels of extra oesophageal reflux, despite the use of PPIs. Pepsin was detected in 11 of 15 BAL samples, signifying aspiration. Bile salts were undetectable, using spectrophotometry and only detectable in two patients using a more sensitive tandem mass spectrometry approach [24].

This study therefore indicated that lung transplant recipients can be assessed for reflux/aspiration within the first month post-transplant. Reflux/aspiration was present early post-operatively in some patients. These investigations are used in our centre to contribute to clinical decisions regarding fundoplication of selected patients post transplant. This has led to an integrated 'aerodigestive' mixed disciplinary team (MDT) clinical initiative in Newcastle [65].

## The Role of a Mixed Disciplinary Aerodigestive Team Approach

In Newcastle patients with chronic lung disease where GOR is thought be a significant comorbidity have been reviewed by a newly established, formal, "aerodigestive" mixed disciplinary team (MDT) [65]. We now have 2 years of experience with this approach. The MDT includes gastroesophageal surgical representation, respiratory physicians and anaesthetists. Day to day organisation is by a clinical fellow (RJ) working closely with hospital secretarial staff for the respective consultants. Prior to MDT discussion, each patient has oesophageal manometry, pH-impedance testing, spirometry, high resolution thoracic CT, BAL results and notes collated. Meetings are held in venues allowing group assessment of high quality imaging. Action points for reflux treatment and further investigations are discussed, decided and implemented by the MDT. This is documented by letter (MDT chair), with notification of actions to the patient referral source.

In this setting we have investigated reflux and aspiration in over a hundred patients. This has included an unselected IPF cohort of 35 patients. Oesophageal manometry suggested normal oesophageal function in only 46%. pH-impedance demonstrated supranormal GOR in 24 patients (69%). In nine the combination of clinical history and structured questionnaire revealed no evidence of GORD. BAL pepsin concentrations were significantly higher than those measured in four healthy volunteer controls. Our preliminary experience therefore suggests that acid reflux and weakly acid reflux was common and frequently asymptomatic in IPF patients, [65] but not found to the same extents as the higher levels reported in the IPF literature [19].

This supports the need for carefully integrated assessments to inform potential treatment of reflux in IPF, which may be facilitated by the MDT review. In addition to patients with IPF our ongoing aerodigestive MDT has considered adult and paediatric patients. Patients with IPF, CF, Bronchiectasis and from the transplant clinic have been studied to date with this integrated approach.

## Questions Raised by This Chapter

The potential relationships between reflux, aspiration and lung disease and issues discussed in this chapter suggest a number of questions for further research. The potential from better understanding is that patient treatment may be personalised and improved.

## What Is Normal?

Established normal ranges for levels of reflux and markers of aspiration and standardisation of methodology are required. Reflux data from an older age range would be particularly helpful in diseases of the elderly such as IPF. This would help inform the question of what is the clinical relevance of events-both severity and frequency of events. Near patient testing of markers of aspiration may be useful in this setting.

## The Importance of the Microbiome

With the increasing recognition of the importance of the human microbiome in health and disease the understanding of the potential for reflux and aspiration to affect the lung/GI microbiome is required. The relevance of this is suggested by work from our centre indicating that biofilm forming Pseudomonas aeruginosa can be common in the lungs and gastric juice of patients with CF [66]. The effects of common therapies such as proton pump inhibitors on the microbiome require further investigation.

## Understanding Therapy

The effects of therapies on reflux, aspiration and overall lung pathophysiology require further work and open minded appraisal. Examples are the potential effects of antibiotics, PPIs and commonly used inhaled medications on aerodigestive (patho)physiology. Potential iatrogenic effects may be under recognised e.g. the effects of PPI, inhalers and antibiotic therapy on aerodigestive microbiome homeostasis. For example is the change in organisms responsible for pneumonia in the infirm (hospital acquired, nursing home etc.) due to colonisation or aspiration? This may be very relevant in terms of antibiotic choice and patient care.

## Interrelationships Between Lung and Gastrointestinal Pathophysiology: The Chicken and Egg of Reflux and Aspiration

A potential theory that may account for the high prevalence of GORD in advanced lung disease is related to the exaggerated pressure fluctuations between the thorax and abdomen seen in pulmonary disease; this may challenge the normal gastro-oesophageal barrier and predispose to the movement of stomach contents up the oesophagus. Further research into whether reflux and aspiration leads to lung disease or is a consequence of lung disease could benefit understanding.

## The Role of Surgical Fundoplication

Surgical fundoplication requires careful consideration in all patients and especially the frail and groups with comorbidities. For example surgery in patients with IPF is known to associate with death and acute exacerbations of lung disease.

## References

1. Harding SM, Allen JE, Blumin JH, Warner EA, Pellegrini CA, Chan WW. Respiratory manifestations of gastroesophageal reflux disease. Ann N Y Acad Sci. 2013;1300:43–52.
2. Morehead RS. Gastro-oesophageal reflux disease and non-asthma lung disease. Eur Respir Rev. 2009;18(114):233–43.
3. Sweet MP, Patti MG, Hoopes C, Hays SR, Golden JA. Gastro-oesophageal reflux and aspiration in patients with advanced lung disease. Thorax. 2009;64(2):167–73.
4. Trinick R, Johnston N, Dalzell AM, McNamara PS. Reflux aspiration in children with neurodisability – a significant problem, but can we measure it? J Pediatr Surg. 2012;47(2):291–8.

5. Blake K, Teague WG. Gastroesophageal reflux disease and childhood asthma. Curr Opin Pulm Med. 2013;19(1):24–9.
6. Mousa HM, Woodley FW. Gastroesophageal reflux in cystic fibrosis: current understandings of mechanisms and management. Curr Gastroenterol Rep. 2012;14(3):226–35.
7. Hu X, Lee JS, Pianosi PT, Ryu JH. Aspiration-related pulmonary syndromes. Chest. 2015;147(3):815–23.
8. Ward C, Forrest IA, Brownlee IA, Johnson GE, Murphy DM, Pearson JP, et al. Pepsin like activity in bronchoalveolar lavage fluid is suggestive of gastric aspiration in lung allografts. Thorax. 2005;60(10):872–4.
9. DeMeester TR, Wang CI, Wernly JA, Pellegrini CA, Little AG, Klementschitsch P, et al. Technique, indications, and clinical use of 24 hour esophageal pH monitoring. J Thorac Cardiovasc Surg. 1980;79(5):656–70.
10. Zerbib F, des Varannes SB, Roman S, Pouderoux P, Artigue F, Chaput U, et al. Normal values and day-to-day variability of 24-h ambulatory oesophageal impedance-pH monitoring in a Belgian-French cohort of healthy subjects. Alimentary Pharmacol Ther. 2005;22(10):1011–21.
11. Huxley EJ, Viroslav J, Gray WR, Pierce AK. Pharyngeal aspiration in normal adults and patients with depressed consciousness. Am J Med. 1978;64(4):564–8.
12. McNally P, Ervine E, Shields MD, Dimitrov B, El Nazir B, Taggart CC, et al. High concentrations of pepsin in bronchoalveolar lavage fluid from children with cystic fibrosis are associated with high interleukin-8 concentrations. Thorax. 2011;66(2):140–3.
13. Stovold R, Forrest IA, Corris PA, Murphy DM, Smith JA, Decalmer S, et al. Pepsin, a biomarker of gastric aspiration in lung allografts: a putative association with rejection. Am J Respir Crit Care Med. 2007;175(12):1298–303.
14. Gleeson K, Eggli DF, Maxwell SL. Quantitative aspiration during sleep in normal subjects. Chest. 1997;111(5):1266–72.
15. Gleeson K, Reynolds HY. Pneumonia in the intensive care unit setting. J Intensive Care Med. 1992;7(1):24–35.
16. Shah NH, LePendu P, Bauer-Mehren A, Ghebremariam YT, Iyer SV, Marcus J, et al. Proton pump inhibitor usage and the risk of myocardial infarction in the general population. PLoS One. 2015;10(6):e0124653.
17. Abraham NS. Proton pump inhibitors: potential adverse effects. Curr Opin Gastroenterol. 2012;28(6):615–20.
18. Ghebremariam YT, Cooke JP, Gerhart W, Griego C, Brower JB, Doyle-Eisele M, et al. Pleiotropic effect of the proton pump inhibitor esomeprazole leading to suppression of lung inflammation and fibrosis. J Transl Med. 2015;13:249.
19. Raghu G, Amatto VC, Behr J, Stowasser S. Comorbidities in idiopathic pulmonary fibrosis patients: a systematic literature review. Eur Respir J. 2015;46(4):1113–30.
20. Mays EE, Dubois JJ, Hamilton GB. Pulmonary fibrosis associated with tracheobronchial aspiration. A study of the frequency of hiatal hernia and gastroesophageal reflux in interstitial pulmonary fibrosis of obscure etiology. Chest. 1976;69(4):512–5.
21. Tobin RW, Pope CE 2nd, Pellegrini CA, Emond MJ, Sillery J, Raghu G. Increased prevalence of gastroesophageal reflux in patients with idiopathic pulmonary fibrosis. Am J Respir Crit Care Med. 1998;158(6):1804–8.
22. Raghu G, Freudenberger TD, Yang S, Curtis JR, Spada C, Hayes J, et al. High prevalence of abnormal acid gastro-oesophageal reflux in idiopathic pulmonary fibrosis. Eur Respir J. 2006;27(1):136–42.
23. Aseeri A, Brodlie M, Lordan J, Corris P, Pearson J, Ward C, et al. Bile acids are present in the lower airways of people with cystic fibrosis. Am J Respir Crit Care Med. 2012;185(4):463.
24. Griffin SM, Robertson AG, Bredenoord AJ, Brownlee IA, Stovold R, Brodlie M, et al. Aspiration and allograft injury secondary to gastroesophageal reflux occur in the immediate post-lung transplantation period (prospective clinical trial). Ann Surg. 2013;258(5):705–11. Discussion 11-2.
25. Lee JS, Ryu JH, Elicker BM, Lydell CP, Jones KD, Wolters PJ, et al. Gastroesophageal reflux therapy is associated with longer survival in patients with idiopathic pulmonary fibrosis. Am J Respir Crit Care Med. 2011;184(12):1390–4.

26. Lee JS, Song JW, Wolters PJ, Elicker BM, King TE Jr, Kim DS, et al. Bronchoalveolar lavage pepsin in acute exacerbation of idiopathic pulmonary fibrosis. Eur Respir J. 2012;39(2):352–8.
27. Tcherakian C, Cottin V, Brillet PY, Freynet O, Naggara N, Carton Z, et al. Progression of idiopathic pulmonary fibrosis: lessons from asymmetrical disease. Thorax. 2011;66(3):226–31.
28. Savarino E, Carbone R, Marabotto E, Furnari M, Sconfienza L, Ghio M, et al. Gastro-oesophageal reflux and gastric aspiration in idiopathic pulmonary fibrosis patients. Eur Respir J. 2013;42(5):1322–31.
29. Allaix ME, Fisichella PM, Noth I, Herbella FA, Borraez Segura B, Patti MG. Idiopathic pulmonary fibrosis and gastroesophageal reflux. Implications for treatment. J Gastrointest Surg. 2014;18(1):100–4. Discussion 4-5.
30. Allaix ME, Fisichella PM, Noth I, Mendez BM, Patti MG. The pulmonary side of reflux disease: from heartburn to lung fibrosis. J Gastrointest Surg. 2013;17(8):1526–35.
31. Ghatol A, Ruhl AP, Danoff SK. Exacerbations in idiopathic pulmonary fibrosis triggered by pulmonary and nonpulmonary surgery: a case series and comprehensive review of the literature. Lung. 2012;190(4):373–80.
32. Key AL, Holt K, Hamilton A, Smith JA, Earis JE. Objective cough frequency in idiopathic pulmonary fibrosis. Cough. 2010;6:4.
33. Lee JS, Collard HR, Raghu G, Sweet MP, Hays SR, Campos GM, et al. Does chronic microaspiration cause idiopathic pulmonary fibrosis? Am J Med. 2010;123(4):304–11.
34. Eryuksel E, Dogan M, Olgun S, Kocak I, Celikel T. Incidence and treatment results of laryngopharyngeal reflux in chronic obstructive pulmonary disease. Eur Arch Otorhinolaryngol. 2009;266(8):1267–71.
35. Pacheco-Galvan A, Hart SP, Morice AH. Relationship between gastro-oesophageal reflux and airway diseases: the airway reflux paradigm. Arch Bronconeumol. 2011;47(4):195–203.
36. Andersen LI, Jensen G. Prevalence of benign oesophageal disease in the Danish population with special reference to pulmonary disease. J Intern Med. 1989;225(6):393–402.
37. Casanova C, Baudet JS, del Valle Velasco M, Martin JM, Aguirre-Jaime A, de Torres JP, et al. Increased gastro-oesophageal reflux disease in patients with severe COPD. Eur Respir J. 2004;23(6):841–5.
38. Tottrup A, Forman A, Madsen G, Andersson KE. The actions of some beta-receptor agonists and xanthines on isolated muscle strips from the human oesophago-gastric junction. Pharmacol Toxicol. 1990;67(4):340–3.
39. Hurst JR, Vestbo J, Anzueto A, Locantore N, Mullerova H, Tal-Singer R, et al. Susceptibility to exacerbation in chronic obstructive pulmonary disease. N Engl J Med. 2010;363(12):1128–38.
40. Perng DW, Chang KT, Su KC, Wu YC, Wu MT, Hsu WH, et al. Exposure of airway epithelium to bile acids associated with gastroesophageal reflux symptoms: a relation to transforming growth factor-beta1 production and fibroblast proliferation. Chest. 2007;132(5):1548–56.
41. Ward C, Ryan V, Pearson J. Susceptibility to exacerbation in COPD. N Engl J Med. 2010;363(27):2671. Author reply.
42. Jung YH, Lee DY, Kim DW, Park SS, Heo EY, Chung HS, et al. Clinical significance of laryngopharyngeal reflux in patients with chronic obstructive pulmonary disease. Int J Chron Obstruct Pulm Dis. 2015;10:1343–51.
43. Jarjour NN, Erzurum SC, Bleecker ER, Calhoun WJ, Castro M, Comhair SA, et al. Severe asthma: lessons learned from the National Heart, Lung, and Blood Institute Severe Asthma Research Program. Am J Respir Crit Care Med. 2012;185(4):356–62.
44. American Lung Association Asthma Clinical Research C, Mastronarde JG, Anthonisen NR, Castro M, Holbrook JT, Leone FT, et al. Efficacy of esomeprazole for treatment of poorly controlled asthma. N Engl J Med. 2009;360(15):1487–99.
45. Kiljander TO, Junghard O, Beckman O, Lind T. Effect of esomeprazole 40 mg once or twice daily on asthma: a randomized, placebo-controlled study. Am J Respir Crit Care Med. 2010;181(10):1042–8.
46. Blondeau K, Dupont LJ, Mertens V, Verleden G, Malfroot A, Vandenplas Y, et al. Gastro-oesophageal reflux and aspiration of gastric contents in adult patients with cystic fibrosis. Gut. 2008;57(8):1049–55.

47. Hallberg K, Fandriks L, Strandvik B. Duodenogastric bile reflux is common in cystic fibrosis. J Pediatr Gastroenterol Nutr. 2004;38(3):312–6.
48. Mertens V, Blondeau K, Van Oudenhove L, Vanaudenaerde B, Vos R, Farre R, et al. Bile acids aspiration reduces survival in lung transplant recipients with BOS despite azithromycin. Am J Transpl. 2011;11(2):329–35.
49. Parikh S, Brownlee IA, Robertson AG, Manning NT, Johnson GE, Brodlie M, et al. Are the enzymatic methods currently being used to measure bronchoalveolar lavage bile salt levels fit for purpose? J Heart Lung Transpl. 2013;32(4):418–23.
50. Brodlie M, Aseeri A, Lordan JL, Robertson AG, McKean MC, Corris PA, Griffin SM, Manning NJ, Pearson JP, Ward C. Bile acid aspiration in people with cystic fibrosis before and after lung transplantation. Eur Respir J. 2015;46(6):1820–3.
51. Fathi H, Moon T, Donaldson J, Jackson W, Sedman P, Morice AH. Cough in adult cystic fibrosis: diagnosis and response to fundoplication. Cough. 2009;5:1.
52. Boesch RP, Acton JD. Outcomes of fundoplication in children with cystic fibrosis. J Pediatr Surg. 2007;42(8):1341–4.
53. Vos R, Blondeau K, Vanaudenaerde BM, Mertens V, Van Raemdonck DE, Sifrim D, et al. Airway colonization and gastric aspiration after lung transplantation: do birds of a feather flock together? J Heart Lung Transpl. 2008;27(8):843–9.
54. Gregson AL, Wang X, Weigt SS, Palchevskiy V, Lynch JP 3rd, Ross DJ, et al. Interaction between Pseudomonas and CXC chemokines increases risk of bronchiolitis obliterans syndrome and death in lung transplantation. Am J Respir Crit Care Med. 2013;187(5):518–26.
55. McShane PJ, Naureckas ET, Tino G, Strek ME. Non-cystic fibrosis bronchiectasis. Am J Respir Crit Care Med. 2013;188(6):647–56.
56. Mandal P, Morice AH, Chalmers JD, Hill AT. Symptoms of airway reflux predict exacerbations and quality of life in bronchiectasis. Respir Med. 2013;107(7):1008–13.
57. Tsang KW, Lam WK, Kwok E, Chan KN, Hu WH, Ooi GC, et al. Helicobacter pylori and upper gastrointestinal symptoms in bronchiectasis. Eur Respir J. 1999;14(6):1345–50.
58. Noth I, Zangan SM, Soares RV, Forsythe A, Demchuk C, Takahashi SM, et al. Prevalence of hiatal hernia by blinded multidetector CT in patients with idiopathic pulmonary fibrosis. Eur Respir J. 2012;39(2):344–51.
59. Bredenoord AJ, Pandolfino JE, Smout AJ. Gastro-oesophageal reflux disease. Lancet. 2013;381(9881):1933–42.
60. McDonnell MJ, Ahmed M, Das J, Ward C, Mokoka M, Breen DP, et al. Hiatal hernias are correlated with increased severity of non-cystic fibrosis bronchiectasis. Respirology. 2015;20(5):749–57.
61. McDonnell MJ, O'Toole D, Rutherford R, De Soyza A, Lordan J, Pearson J, Ward C, Laffey JG. Bile acids cause direct inflammation and injury and worsen acid induced injury in the pulmonary epithelium. Am J Respir Crit Care Med. 2015;191:A1292.
62. McDonnell MJ, Ward C, Rutherford RM, Verdon B, Pearson JP, Aldharani A, Lordan J, De Soyza A, Laffey JG, O Toole D. Azithromycin attenuates release of bile acid-mediated neutrophilic and remodeling factors in bronchiectasis airway epithelial cells. Am J Respir Crit Care Med. 2018;197:A2841.
63. Robertson AG, Griffin SM, Murphy DM, Pearson JP, Forrest IA, Dark JH, et al. Targeting allograft injury and inflammation in the management of post-lung transplant bronchiolitis obliterans syndrome. Am J Transpl. 2009;9(6):1272–8.
64. Hartwig MG, Anderson DJ, Onaitis MW, Reddy S, Snyder LD, Lin SS, et al. Fundoplication after lung transplantation prevents the allograft dysfunction associated with reflux. Ann Thorac Surg. 2011;92(2):462–8. Discussion 8-9.
65. Jones RT, Krishnan A, Zeybel GL, Pearson JP, Simpson AJ, Griffin SM, et al. P276 characterisation of reflux and aspiration in idiopathic pulmonary fibrosis; an integrated approach. Thorax. 2014;69(Suppl 2):A194.
66. Krishnan A, Perry A, Robertson A, Brodlie M, Perry J, Corris P, et al. Identical biofilm forming strains of pseudomonas aeruginosa occur in lung allograft BAL and gastric juice from CF patients with gastro oesophageal reflux. J Heart Lung Transpl. 2013;32(4):S28.

# Effect of Reflux on Cough Sensitivity and Bronchial Responsiveness

Peter V. Dicpinigaitis

## Abstract

Gastroesophageal reflux is an extremely common condition often associated with chronic cough, dyspnea, laryngeal discomfort, and other extraesophageal symptoms. A considerable body of evidence has established an association of reflux with the presence of cough reflex hypersensitivity and/or bronchial hyperresponsiveness. However, the demonstration of such airway hyperreactivity does not uniformly predict the presence of underlying pathology nor the occurrence of symptoms. Furthermore, treatment aimed at suppressing cough reflex sensitivity or bronchial responsiveness, even when successful, often fails to ameliorate associated symptoms. Given that reflux, cough, and asthma are all very common conditions, the association of reflux with cough reflex hypersensitivity and bronchial hyperresponsiveness is likely causal in some individuals and coincidental in others. Adequately performed clinical trials evaluating the presence of pathological reflux, its effect on cough reflex sensitivity, airway responsiveness and pulmonary symptoms, as well as objective and symptomatic response to therapeutic interventions, will be most useful in elucidating the pathophysiologic manifestations of reflux on the respiratory system.

## Introduction

Gastroesophageal reflux (GERD) is a ubiquitous clinical problem that is associated not only with the classic symptoms of heartburn and dyspepsia, but also with extraesophageal manifestations such as cough, laryngeal discomfort, and dyspnea. Despite the documentation of enhanced cough reflex sensitivity and bronchial hyperresponsiveness (BHR) in association with GERD, studies of pharmacological

P. V. Dicpinigaitis
Albert Einstein College of Medicine and Montefiore Medical Center, Bronx, NY, USA

treatment of reflux have failed to demonstrate a clinically relevant, therapeutic benefit in chronic cough [1, 2] and asthma [3–5].

This chapter will focus on basic and clinical studies examining the effect of reflux on cough reflex sensitivity and on bronchial responsiveness. The association of reflux and asthma is reviewed elsewhere in this book.

## Reflux and Cough Reflex Sensitivity

Preclinical studies have suggested a variety of mechanisms through which acid and non-acid refluxate may affect esophageal function and thereby enhance cough reflex sensitivity. In a model of hydrochloric acid (HCl) and pepsin-induced acute esophagitis in ferrets, investigators observed increased sensitivity of capsaicin-activated inhibitory pathways affecting lower esophageal sphincter function, apparently mediated by neurokinin (NK)-1 receptors [6]. In a model of ovalbumin-sensitized guinea pigs undergoing esophageal mast cell activation by in vivo ovalbumin inhalation, intraluminal acid infusion activated esophageal nociceptive C-fibers, suggesting that mast cell activation renders esophageal epithelium more permeable to acid, thereby increasing esophageal vagal nociceptive C-fiber activation [7]. In a recent study employing an ex vivo guinea pig esophageal-vagal preparation with intact nerve endings in the esophagus, acid perfusion activated jugular, but not nodose C fibers and inhibited both responses to esophageal distention. This inhibitory effect was thought mediated mainly through transient receptor potential vanilloid-1 (TRPV-1) receptors, and may be relevant to esophageal sensory and motor dysfunction in clinical acid reflux disease [8].

Numerous clinical trials have documented the association of reflux with enhanced cough reflex sensitivity. Most have employed capsaicin, the pungent extract of the red hot chili pepper, as the provocative tussive agent. Indeed, capsaicin remains the most widely used tussive agent in clinical cough research, given its established record of safe, dose-dependent, and reproducible induction of cough [9]. In an elegant study of the effect of esophageal HCl infusion on capsaicin cough sensitivity, investigators compared two groups of patients with GERD: those with and without chronic cough. Only in patients with associated chronic cough did acid infusion enhance cough reflex sensitivity; those with GERD but without chronic cough, as well as a group of healthy volunteers, were not affected [10]. An earlier study of distal esophageal acid infusion compared with saline infusion in patients with asthma provided similar findings of enhanced cough reflex sensitivity to capsaicin, though no changes were observed in pulmonary function parameters [11]. Interestingly, one of the earliest studies in this field demonstrated that patients with GERD, but without cough or other respiratory symptoms, did indeed have enhanced cough reflex sensitivity to inhaled capsaicin compared with non-GERD subjects, thus suggesting that reflux is necessary but not sufficient for the induction of cough in this patient population, and that other associated factor(s) are necessary [12]. Two recent studies have compared cough reflex sensitivity between patients with acid- and non-acid reflux, demonstrating no difference in capsaicin cough sensitivity between the two types of GERD [13, 14], but enhanced sensitivity compared with healthy volunteers [13]. One pediatric study demonstrated similar findings to adults; children with a confirmed diagnosis of GERD, by 24-h esophageal pH monitoring, had significantly enhanced capsaicin cough sensitivity compared with healthy children [15]. Furthermore, cough reflex hypersensitivity was noted only in the subjects with significant distal, not proximal, acid exposure [15].

Several studies have evaluated the effect of reflux treatment on the associated enhanced cough reflex sensitivity, with discordant results. In a group of 29 asthmatics with reflux confirmed by 24-h pH monitoring, a short course of therapy with omeprazole (20 mg twice daily for 12 days) decreased cough and cough reflex sensitivity to capsaicin, with the decrease being positively correlated with proximal acid exposure. Bronchial responsiveness to methacholine was not affected, though asthma symptoms were improved in subjects with proximal reflux [16]. In a study of 21 patients with reflux esophagitis and digestive symptoms, a 60-day course of omeprazole resulted in decreased capsaicin cough threshold, digestive symptoms, as well as cough and laryngeal symptoms in the subgroup of patients with those complaints [17]. In a study of patients presenting for evaluation of chronic cough, cough severity as measured by visual analogue scale (VAS) as well as cough sensitivity to capsaicin were noted to be diminished in a subgroup of patients who responded to specific treatment of underlying GERD [18]. On the other hand, two studies failed to show inhibition of cough reflex sensitivity with treatment. In a group of 13 patients with chronic cough associated with GERD, a course of therapy with omeprazole (40 mg daily for 14 days) led to significant symptomatic improvement based on the Leicester Cough Questionnaire, yet pH levels in exhaled breath condensate (EBC) and capsaicin cough response were not affected [19]. In a study of 101 patients with chronic cough, 35 patients with associated GERD did not demonstrate suppression of cough reflex hypersensitivity to capsaicin after a 3-month course of therapy [20].

As noted above, capsaicin inhalation cough challenge is commonly used to assess cough reflex sensitivity [9]. Often, measurements are made to compare different subject populations, or, to measure the effect of a pharmacological or other intervention on the cough reflex in a single subject. Several studies have evaluated the effect of presentation of capsaicin to the gastrointestinal tract in terms of induction of symptoms of reflux. Two trials have demonstrated that the intraesophageal administration of capsaicin induces esophageal and gastric symptoms of reflux in patients with GERD as well as in healthy volunteers [21, 22]. Postprandial heartburn symptoms were also induced in 11 GERD patients when capsaicin was administered orally in the form of a 5 mg gelatin capsule [23]. Another study employing intraesophageal administration of capsaicin in 12 subjects with GERD and ineffective esophageal motility demonstrated that capsaicin induced significant improvement in esophageal body contractility, suggesting a potential therapeutic role for capsaicin as a prokinetic agent in this patient population [24].

Citric acid is a long established provocative agent for cough challenge testing, but in recent decades has been used much less frequently than capsaicin [9]. Nevertheless, cough reflex sensitivity to citric acid has also been shown to be enhanced in subjects with reflux relative to healthy volunteers [25, 26]. Studies evaluating the effect of a therapeutic intervention on citric acid cough threshold in patients with GERD have yielded discordant results. In a group of elderly, institutionalized subjects with GERD, 1 month of therapy with lansoprazole, 30 mg daily, significantly raised the citric acid cough threshold relative to placebo [27], whereas 8 weeks of treatment with esomeprazole demonstrated no such effect [1]. Inhibition of citric acid threshold was noted, however, in a group of patients with GERD after laparoscopic fundoplication [26].

## Reflux and Bronchial Responsiveness

The instillation of acid into the esophagus has been shown to induce bronchoconstriction and/or airway neurogenic inflammation in a variety of animal models, including cat, dog, guinea pig and mouse [28, 29]. In humans, a variety of different methodological approaches and subject populations have been investigated to examine the role of acid reflux and its effect on bronchial responsiveness. Multiple studies in asthmatics have demonstrated that intraesophageal instillation of acid enhances bronchial responsiveness to methacholine [30–32]; associated bronchoconstriction was observed in most [30, 31] but not all [32] of these studies. Interestingly, another study of esophageal acidification in asthmatics demonstrated enhanced methacholine sensitivity only in the subgroup of subjects with documented reflux [33]. Other studies examining the relationship of reflux and bronchial responsiveness have demonstrated an association between number of reflux episodes and bronchial responsiveness to methacholine in asthmatics [34], as well as enhanced responsiveness to methacholine in non-asthmatic subjects with GERD compared with healthy volunteers [35]. In an interesting twist on the subject, two studies incorporating measurements of lower esophageal sphincter (LES) pressure and esophageal pH have demonstrated the *induction* of reflux episodes during methacholine-induced bronchoconstriction in subjects with asthma [36, 37].

The aforementioned studies incorporating bronchial challenge have used methacholine as the provocative agent. However, other studies using histamine as the challenge agent have also demonstrated enhanced bronchial responsiveness after esophageal acid instillation in asthmatics [38, 39] as well as in non-asthmatic subjects with GERD [40].

Negative mechanistic studies have also been published. In a group of stable asthmatics, pulmonary function and BHR to methacholine were not different between subjects with and without GERD [41]. A study of esophageal acid perfusion in subjects with mild persistent asthma demonstrated enhancement of cough reflex sensitivity to capsaicin, but no change in pulmonary function parameters [11]. In a group of poorly controlled asthmatics undergoing 24-h esophageal pH monitoring, no difference was noted in respiratory symptoms, medication use, pulmonary function parameters or methacholine responsiveness between subjects with and without proximal or distal reflux [42]. Similarly, no association was demonstrated between nocturnal GERD symptoms and lung function and bronchial responsiveness to methacholine in a prospectively followed group of non-asthmatic subjects [43].

A number of studies have evaluated the effect of treatment of GERD on bronchial responsiveness. In a randomized trial of 30 patients with asthma and GERD, those subjects treated for reflux with a regimen of daily omeprazole (20 mg) and domperidone (10 mg three times daily) for 6 weeks, in addition to asthma therapy, demonstrated improvement in pulmonary function parameters and inhibition of BHR to histamine, compared to subjects treated with asthma therapy alone [44]. Another study of patients with asthma and GERD receiving an 8-week course of therapy with lansoprazole (30 mg daily) documented inhibition of bronchial responsiveness to methacholine, though no significant improvement in pulmonary function parameters [45]. One study of asthmatic children with GERD, documented by esophageal pH monitoring, demonstrated inhibition of BHR to methacholine after prolonged anti-reflux therapy [46]. A study of non-pharmacological GERD therapy with Nissen fundoplication demonstrated, in a group of asthmatic and non-asthmatic subjects, a positive correlation between the severity of distal esophageal reflux and bronchial responsiveness to methacholine, as well as inhibition of BHR in asthmatic subjects after operative intervention [47]. Furthermore, in a study of patients with endoscopically documented esophagitis and no previous history of asthma, a 6-month course of therapy with pantoprazole, 40 mg daily, significantly inhibited bronchial responsiveness to methacholine [48].

In contrast, other studies have failed to demonstrate an effect of reflux therapy on BHR. In a randomized, double-blind, placebo-controlled study of 36 subjects with airway obstruction, severe airway hyperresponsiveness despite maintenance therapy with an inhaled corticosteroid, and GERD documented by 24-h esophageal pH measurement, a 3-month course of omeprazole, 40 mg twice daily, had no effect on pulmonary function parameters and degree of bronchial responsiveness to methacholine, despite a significant effect on acid reflux and reflux symptom scores [49]. In a study of 29 asthmatics with objectively documented reflux, a 12-day course of omeprazole (20 mg twice daily) inhibited cough reflex sensitivity to capsaicin, but had no effect on bronchial responsiveness to methacholine [16]. A recent study evaluating the effects of high-dose esomeprazole (40 mg twice daily) and of fundoplication in asthmatic and non-asthmatic subjects with GERD found no difference in pulmonary function parameters and airway responsiveness to methacholine after 3 months of pharmacological therapy, as well as 3 months after surgical intervention [50].

### Conclusion

A significant body of evidence documents the association of gastroesophageal reflux with enhanced cough reflex sensitivity and/or enhanced bronchial responsiveness. However, the presence of such hyperresponsiveness does not uniformly predict the presence of underlying pathology or presence of symptoms. Furthermore, treatment aimed at suppressing cough reflex sensitivity or bronchial responsiveness, even when successful, often fails to ameliorate associated symptoms. Thus, the relevance of acid and non-acid reflux to airway hypersensitivity is likely a heterogeneous phenomenon, varying from one condition or patient phenotype to another, and quite possibly varying from patient to patient within one diagnostic category.

## References

1. Faruqi S, Molyneux ID, Fathi H, Wright C, Thompson R, Morice AH. Chronic cough and esomeprazole: a double-blind placebo-controlled parallel study. Respirology. 2011;16:1150–6.
2. Shaheen NJ, Crockett SD, Bright SD, Madanick RD, Buckmire R, Couch M, et al. Randomised clinical trial: high-dose acid suppression for chronic cough-a double-blind, placebo-controlled study. Aliment Pharmacol Ther. 2011;33:225–34.
3. American Lung Association Asthma Clinical Research Centers, Mastronarde JG, Anthonisen NR, Castro M, Holbrook JT, Leone FT, Teague WG, et al. Efficacy of esomeprazole for treatment of poorly controlled asthma. N Engl J Med. 2009;360:1487–99.
4. Chan WW, Chiou E, Obstein KL, Tignor AS, Whitlock TL. The efficacy of proton pump inhibitors for the treatment of asthma in adults: a meta-analysis. Arch Intern Med. 2011;171:620–9.
5. Kiljander TO, Junghard O, Beckman O, Lind T. Effect of esomeprazole 40 mg once or twice daily on asthma: a randomized, placebo-controlled study. Am J Respir Crit Care Med. 2010;181:1042–8.
6. Smid SD, Page AJ, O'Donnell T, Langman J, Rowlan R, Blackshaw LA. Oesophagitis-induced changes in capsaicin-sensitive tachykininergic pathways in the ferret lower oesophageal sphincter. Neurogastroenterol Motil. 1998;10:403–11.
7. Zhang S, Liu Z, Heldsinger A, Owyang C, Yu S. Intraluminal acid activates esophageal nodose C fibers after mast cell activation. Am J Physiol Gastrointest Liver Physiol. 2014;306:G200–7.
8. Yu X, Hu Y, Yu S. Effects of acid on vagal nociceptive afferent subtypes in guinea pig esophagus. Am J Physiol Gastrointest Liver Physiol. 2014;307:G471–8.
9. Morice AH, Fontana GA, Belvisi MG, Birring SS, Chung KF, Dicpinigaitis PV, Kastelik JA, McGarvey LP, Smith JA, Tatar M, Widdicombe J. European Respiratory Society Task Force. ERS guidelines on the assessment of cough. Eur Respir J. 2007;29:1256–76.
10. Javorkova N, Varechova S, Pecova R, Tatar M, Balaz D, Demeter M, et al. Acidification of the esophagus acutely increases the cough sensitivity in patients with gastro-oesophageal reflux and chronic cough. Neurogastroenterol Motil. 2008;20:119–24.
11. Wu DN, Yamauchi K, Kobayashi H, Tanifuli Y, Kato C, Suzuki K, et al. Effects of esophageal acid perfusion on cough responsiveness in patients with bronchial asthma. Chest. 2002;122:505–9.
12. Ferrari M, Olivieri M, Sembenini C, Benini L, Zuccali V, Bardelli E, et al. Tussive effect of capsaicin in patients with gastroesophageal reflux without cough. Am J Respir Crit Care Med. 1995;151:557–61.
13. Qiu Z, Yu L, Xu S, Liu B, Zhao T, Lu H, et al. Cough reflex sensitivity and airway inflammation in patients with chronic cough due to non-acid gastro-esophageal reflux. Respirology. 2011;16:645–52.
14. Xu X, Yang Z, Chen Q, Yu L, Liang S, Lu H, et al. Comparison of clinical characteristics of chronic cough due to non-acid and acid gastroesophageal reflux. Clin Respir J. 2015;9:196–202.
15. Varechova S, Mikler J, Murgas D, Dragula M, Banovcin P, Hanacek J. Cough reflex sensitivity in children with suspected and confirmed gastroesophageal reflux disease. J Physiol Pharmacol. 2007;58(Suppl 5;Pt 2):717–27.
16. Ferrari M, Benini L, Brotto E, Locatelli F, De Iorio F, Bonella F, et al. Omeprazole reduces the response to capsaicin but not to methacholine in asthmatic patients with proximal reflux. Scand J Gastroenterol. 2007;42:299–307.
17. Benini L, Ferrari M, Sembenini C, Olivieri M, Micciolo R, Zuccali V, et al. Cough threshold in reflux oesophagitis: influence of acid and of laryngeal and oespophageal damage. Gut. 2000;46:762–7.
18. O'Connell F, Thomas VE, Pride NB, Fuller RW. Capsaicin cough sensitivity decreases with successful treatment of chronic cough. Am J Respir Crit Care Med. 1994;150:374–80.
19. Torrego A, Cimbollek S, Hew M, Chung KF. No effect of omeprazole on pH of exhaled breath condensate in cough associated with gastro-esophageal reflux. Cough. 2005;1:10.

20. Nieto L, de Diego A, Perpina M, Compte L, Garrigues V, Martinez E, et al. Cough reflex testing with inhaled capsaicin in the study of chronic cough. Respir Med. 2003;97:393–400.
21. Herrera-Lopez JA, Mejia-Rivas MA, Vargas-Vorachkova F, Valdovinos-Diaz MA. Capsaicin induction of esophageal symptoms in different phenotypes of gastroesophageal reflux disease. Rev Gastroenterol Mex. 2010;75:396–404.
22. Kindt S, Vos R, Blondeau K, Tack J. Influence of intra-oesophageal capsaicin instillation on heartburn induction and oesophageal sensitivity in man. Neurogastroenterol Motil. 2009;21:1032–e82.
23. Rodriguez-Stanley S, Collings KL, Robinson M, Owen W, Miner PB. The effects of capsaicin on reflux, gastric emptying and dyspepsia. Aliment Pharmacol Ther. 2000;14:129–34.
24. Grossi L, Cappello G, Marzio L. Effect of an acute intraluminal administration of capsaicin on oesophageal motor pattern in GORD patients with ineffective oesophageal motility. Neurogastroenterol Motil. 2006;18:632–6.
25. Dariusz Z, Wojciech J, Jozef D, Andrzej K, Jacek C, Jan C, et al. Assessment of cough threshold in patients with gastroesophageal reflux disease [article in Polish]. Pneumonol Alergol Pol. 2003;71:221–9.
26. Ziora D, Jarosz W, Dzielicki J, Ciekalski J, Krzywiecki A, Dworniczak S, et al. Citric acid cough threshold in patients with gastroesophageal reflux disease rises after laparoscopic fundoplication. Chest. 2005;128:2458–64.
27. Ebihara S, Ebihara T, Yamasaki M, Asada M, Yamanda S, Niu K, et al. Contribution of gastric acid in elderly nursing home patients with cough reflex hypersensitivity. J Am Geriatr Soc. 2007;55:1686–8.
28. Stein MR. Possible mechanisms of influence of esophageal acid on airway hyperresponsiveness. Am J Med. 2003;115(Suppl 3A):55S–9S.
29. Allen GB, Leclair TR, von Reyn J, Larrabee YC, Cloutier ME, Irvin CG, et al. Acid aspiration-induced airways hyperresponsiveness in mice. J Appl Physiol. 2009;107:1763–70.
30. Herve P, Denjean A, Jian R, Simonneau G, Duroux P. Intraesophageal perfusion of acid increases the bronchomotor response to methacholine and to isocapnic hyperventilation in asthmatic subjects. Am Rev Respir Dis. 1986;134:986–9.
31. Chakrabarti S, Singh K, Singh V, Nain CK, Jindal SK. Airway response to acid instillation in esophagus in bronchial asthma. Indian J Gastroenterol. 1995;14:44–7.
32. Wu DN, Tanifuji Y, Kobayashi H, Yamauchi K, Kato C, Suzuki K, et al. Effects of esophageal acid perfusion on airway hyperresponsiveness in patients with bronchial asthma. Chest. 2000;118(6):1553.
33. Dal Negro RW, Tognella S, Micheletto C, Sandri M, Guerriero M. A MCh test pre-post esophageal acidification in detecting GER-related asthma. J Asthma. 2009;46:351–5.
34. Vincent D, Cohen-Jonathan AM, Leport J, Merrouche M, Geronimi A, Pradalier A, et al. Gastro-oesophageal reflux prevalence and relationship with bronchial reactivity in asthma. Eur Respir J. 1997;10:2255–9.
35. Bagnato GF, Gulli S, Giacobbe O, De Pasquale R, Purello D'Ambrosio F. Bronchial hyperresponsiveness in subjects with gastroesophageal reflux. Respiration. 2000;67:507–9.
36. Moote DW, Lloyd DA, McCourtie DR, Wells GA. Increase in gastroesophageal reflux during methacholine-induced bronchospasm. J Allergy Clin Immunol. 1986;78:619–23.
37. Zerbib F, Guisset O, Lamouliatte H, Quinton A, Galmiche JP, Tunon-De-Lara JM. Effects of bronchial obstruction on lower esophageal sphincter motility and gastroesophageal reflux in patients with asthma. Am J Respir Crit Care Med. 2002;166:1206–11.
38. Ekstrom T, Tibbling L. Esophageal acid perfusion, airway function, and symptoms in asthmatic patients with marked bronchial hyperreactivity. Chest. 1989;96:995–8.
39. Singh V, Aggarwal V, Bansal S, Nijhawan S, Chaudhary N. Effect of intraesophageal acid instillation on airway reactivity in patients with asthma. J Assoc Physicians India. 2000;48:601–2.
40. Agarwal A, Rishi JP, Gupta AN, Bhandari VM. Histamine bronchoprovocation tests in subjects with gastro-oesophageal reflux disease. J Assoc Physicians India. 1990;38:159–61.
41. Compte L, Garrigues V, Perpina M, Ponce J. Prevalence of gastroesophageal reflux in asthma. J Asthma. 2000;37:175–82.

42. DiMango E, Holbrook JT, Simpson E, Reibman J, Richter J, Narula S, et al. Effects of asymptomatic proximal and distal gastroesophageal reflux on asthma severity. Am J Respir Crit Care Med. 2009;180:809–16.
43. Emilsson OI, Bengtsson A, Franklin KA, Toren K, Benediktsdottir B, Farkhoov A, et al. Nocturnal gastro-oesophageal reflux, asthma and symptoms of OSA: a longitudinal, general population study. Eur Respir J. 2013;41:1347–54.
44. Jiang SP, Liang RY, Zeng ZY, Liu QL, Liang YK, Li JG. Effects of antireflux treatment on bronchial hyper-responsiveness and lung function in asthmatic patients with gastroesophageal reflux disease. World J Gastroenterol. 2003;9(5):1123.
45. Sato A, Tanifuji Y, Kobayashi H, Inoue H. Effects of proton pump inhibitor on airway hyper-responsiveness in asthmatics with gastroesophageal reflux. Arerugi. 2006;55:641–6.
46. Khoshoo V, Mohnot S, Haydel R, Saturno E, Edell D, Kobernick A. Bronchial hyperreactivity in non-atopic children with asthma and reflux: effect of anti-reflux treatment. Pediatr Pulmonol. 2009;44:1070–4.
47. Kiljander TO, Salomaa ER, Hietanen EK, Ovaska J, Helenius H, Liippo K. Gastroesophageal reflux and bronchial responsiveness: correlation and the effect of fundoplication. Respiration. 2002;69:434–9.
48. Karbasi A, Ardestani ME, Ghanei M, Harandi AA. The association between reflux esophagitis and airway hyper-reactivity in patients with gastro-esophageal reflux. J Res Med Sci. 2013;18:473–6.
49. Boeree MJ, Peters FT, Postma DS, Kleibeuker JH. No effects of high-dose omeprazole in patients with severe airway hyperesponsiveness and (a)symptomatic gstro-oesophageal reflux. Eur Respir J. 1998;11:1070–4.
50. Kiljander T, Rantanen T, Kellokumpu I, Koobi T, Lammi L, Nieminen M, et al. Comparison of the effects of esomeprazole and fundoplication on airway responsiveness in patients with gastro-oesophageal reflux disease. Clin Respir J. 2013;7:281–7.

# Part II
# Diagnosis

# Questionnaire Diagnosis of Airways Reflux

7

Shoaib Faruqi

**Abstract**

Gastro-oesophageal reflux disease may present with extra-oesophageal symptoms. A wide assortment of questionnaires is available to use for the evaluation of different dimensions of the classical symptoms of gastro-oesophageal reflux disease. In contrast, there are very few validated questionnaires available which evaluate extra-oesophageal symptoms. In this review specific questionnaires which evaluate variously termed laryngopharyngeal, supra-oesophageal or airway reflux are described and discussed.

## Introduction

The classical symptoms of gastro-oesophageal reflux disease (GORD) are reported by up to a third of the population in the western world [1–3]. The most commonly reported symptoms of GORD are heart burn and regurgitation. However GORD may have a varied presentation. At a consensus meeting in Montreal, GORD was defined as "a condition that develops when the reflux of stomach contents causes troublesome symptoms and/or complications" [4]. This is a definition primarily based on symptoms. Even in the gastroenterology fraternity the atypical, or so termed "extra oesophageal", manifestations of GORD are increasingly being recognised. For instance in the Montreal Classification chronic cough and laryngitis, amongst others, are grouped amongst the extra oesophageal syndromes of GORD. In literature these symptoms have been variously described as "extraoesophageal",

---

S. Faruqi
Department of Respiratory Medicine, Hull York Medical School and the Hull and East Yorkshire Hospitals NHS Trust, Hull, UK
e-mail: shoaib.faruqi@hey.nhs.uk

© Springer International Publishing AG, part of Springer Nature 2018
A. H. Morice, P. W. Dettmar (eds.), *Reflux Aspiration and Lung Disease*,
https://doi.org/10.1007/978-3-319-90525-9_7

"laryngopharyngeal" "supraoesophageal" or "airway" reflux, with considerable overlap. The author's personal terminology of choice is airway reflux.

The characteristics of airway reflux are quite different from those of oesophageal reflux in many ways, including the clinical presentation. This is due to the composition of the refluxate being predominately gaseous and non or weakly acidic [5]. In fact, the typical dyspeptic symptoms of GORD are often absent in those presenting solely with airways reflux. Patients may present only with a cough, throat clearing, hoarseness of voice or globus sensation [6]. Factors such as association of symptoms with eating, phonation or change in posture may suggest airways reflux. Findings on laryngoscopic examination as codified by a "reflux finding score (RFS)" has been described, may also support the diagnosis of airway reflux [7]. However these findings are variable both between patients as well as between evaluators. Trial of treatment with acid suppressive therapy, an effective option in classic GORD, has limited utility in the management of airway reflux [8]. The above in conjunction with a lack of classic specific symptoms poses a diagnostic challenge, especially to those who do not assess patients presenting with airway reflux on a regular basis.

A diagnosis of GORD is made based on the combination of typical symptoms, response to acid suppressive therapy and objective investigations; the presence of symptoms being the key. However the correlation of symptoms with the various diagnostic modalities, including oesophago-gastro duodenoscopy (OGD), radiological investigations and 24-h pH study is poor [9–11]. A wide assortment of questionnaires has been used in the assessment of GORD. These assess disparate dimensions of GORD which include symptoms, diagnosis, response to treatment and disease-specific quality of life. A recent systematic review on this topic identified a total of 65 questionnaires [12]. Of these 3 were generic gastrointestinal and 33 addressed classic gastrointestinal symptoms of GORD. Since many of the symptoms of airways reflux are quite different from that of classical GORD, the diagnosis may not be straightforward if GORD specific questionnaires are used. There is also no specific objective gold-standard diagnostic test to detect airway reflux. Therefore an objective, simple, highly sensitive investigation to make a diagnosis of airway reflux is lacking. Hence there is a need for a standardised and validated questionnaire to aide in the diagnosis of airway reflux. In comparison to the plethora of questionnaires evaluating the classical oesophageal symptoms of GORD there are very few questionnaires pertaining specifically to airway reflux.

## Airway Reflux Questionnaires

As described above the literature is replete with questionnaires assessing the classical manifestations of GORD. On the contrary very few are available which evaluate airway reflux. Four specific questionnaires have been described which evaluate variously termed laryngopharayngeal, supraoesophageal or airway reflux. These 4 questionnaires assessing airway reflux are the Hull Airways Reflux Questionnaire, the Reflux Symptom Index, the Supraesophageal Reflux Questionnaire and the Pharyngeal Reflux Symptom Questionnaire [13–16]. These questionnaires are described in detail below.

## Reflux Symptom Index (RSI)

The Reflux Symptom Index (RSI) is a well established diagnostic tool. It has been validated in the context of patients with voice disorders and has been designed to assess the severity of laryngeal symptoms that may be secondary to laryngopharyngeal reflux (LPR) [14]. It comprises a nine-item self-administered questionnaire. The scale for each individual item in the questionnaire ranges from 0 (no problem) to 5 (severe problem), giving a maximum possible score of 45. The RSI asks the question "Within the last month, how did the following problems affect you?" with scoring as above. The specific questions are as below.

1. Hoarseness or a problem with your voice
2. Clearing your throat
3. Excess throat mucus or postnasal drip
4. Difficulty swallowing food, liquids or pills
5. Coughing after you ate or after lying down
6. Breathing difficulties or choking episodes
7. Troublesome or annoying cough
8. Sensations of something sticking to your throat or a lump in your throat
9. Heartburn, chest pain, indigestion, or stomach acid coming up

The validation cohort for the RSI comprised 25 patients with LPR, selected on the basis of the clinical diagnosis being confirmed by 24-h ambulatory pH recording. The questionnaire was repeated at a mean duration of 8 days and age and gender matched asymptomatic individuals without any evidence of LPR were used as controls. The RSI was shown to be both reproducible and responsive to treatment.

## Supraesophageal Reflux Questionnaire (SERQ)

The SERQ was developed and validated to evaluate the symptoms of supraesophageal reflux (SER). The rationale for developing the SERQ was that the RSI lacked content domains concerning frequency and duration of symptoms [15]. In the validation study for the SERQ the RSI was evaluated as well. This was because the RSI validation study analysed the overall reproducibility of the questionnaire but not that of the individual items themselves, leading to some uncertainty as to their validity. The SERQ was developed by incorporating questions to characterise symptoms commonly attributed to SER. Nine symptom domains (throat clearing, globus sensation, dry cough overall, nocturnal cough overall, sore throat overall, dysphagia overall, hoarseness overall, heartburn overall and acid regurgitation overall) were included with three questions per domain to detail symptom duration, frequency and severity. Additional items regarding medical conditions and medications were used to identify factors that might impact patients' symptoms.

Patients were recruited from unselected oesophageal and ENT Clinics. A group of patients completed both the SERQ and the RSI on two occasions, 2–21 days after the first, to evaluate reproducibility of the questionnaires. Two hundred and twenty four patients took part in either the concurrent validity or the reproducibility phases of the study. A weighted kappa statistic was used for assessment of validity and reproducibility; k values greater than 0.8 considered excellent and that greater than 0.6 good. The concurrent validity and reproducibility of both instruments was good to excellent for most items tested. On several parameters the SERQ was observed to be superior to the RSI; none of the RSI items had significantly better concurrent validity than the SERQ items. Not only does the study validate the SERQ but in addition independently validates the RSI. It is to be noted that the RSI was observed to be completed in a minute compared to 10 minutes it takes for the SERQ.

To evaluate predictive validity, or the ability to diagnose SER, the treating physicians overall impression of SER was used as the "gold standard". Both the RSI and the SERQ were evaluated in this manner. Logistic regression modelling indicated that chronic sinusitis and the use of over-the-counter (OTC) medications were associated significantly with physician impression of SER, after adjusting for all other covariates ($P = 0.04$ and $P < 0.001$, respectively). The estimated odds ratio (95% confidence intervals) for chronic sinusitis and OTC medications were 0.44 (0.2, 0.96) and 4.78 (2.22, 10.30) respectively. The SERQ, with the covariates of chronic sinusitis use and OTC acid suppression medication use, was shown to demonstrate better predictive value for SER than the RSI and the SERQ without these covariates.

## Pharyngeal Reflux Symptom Questionnaire (PRSQ)

The aim for the development of the PRSQ was to evaluate both frequency and severity of laryngopharyngeal reflux (LPR) symptoms, both parameters not being part of the RSI or the SERQ, in an attempt to improve the sensitivity of the instrument [16]. The PRSQ is self administered and in the initial version consisted of 24 items, including both frequency and severity aspects, within the following domains; Cough (9 questions), Voice/Hoarse (5 questions), Dysphagia (4 questions), Reflux (3 questions) and Chest (3 questions). Patient responses were on a six-point Likert scale for frequency and severity with a 4-week recall period. Frequency of symptoms ranged from "0" (never) to "5" (7 days a week). Severity of symptoms ranged from "0" (not at all/no bother) to "4" (very bothersome).

Patients who had symptoms thought to be commonly associated with LPR (hoarseness, chronic cough, globus or chronic throat clearing) and who had a two-level 24-h pH monitoring done were invited to participate in the study. In addition to the PRSQ, subjects completed the RSI, the Laryngopharyngeal Reflux Health Related Quality of Life questionnaire (LPR-HRQL) and the SF-36, a generic questionnaire to measure HRQL. Two hundred and twenty-eight subjects were included in the validation study. On an RSI score cut off of 13, 126 were classified as normal controls. Following evaluation of the initial PRSQ a total of seven items were excluded from the initial 24. This led to the final version of the PRSQ having 17 items in four domains ("Chest" being excluded), assessing frequency and severity. The 17 questions of the PRSQ are as below.

1. Coughed in day time
2. Coughed at night

3. Felt that your voice changed, sounded worse
 4. Had difficulties swallowing
 5. Had a "burning" sensation in the throat
 6. Coughed after meals
 7. Suffered from acid regurgitation
 8. Been hoarse
 9. Had phlegm in throat
10. Had pains when swallowing
11. Suffered from heart burn
12. Had a strained voice
13. Had a sore throat from talking
14. Been coughing when lying down
15. Been coughing when upright
16. Had a tired voice, felt speaking to be tiring
17. Had a lump in your throat

The PRSQ was well accepted by patients with satisfactory compliance and low missing item rates. Following the item reduction process the final construct achieved was with noscaling errors and high internal consistency (Cronbach's alpha coefficient 0.79–0.93). The PRSQ was evaluated in a cross-sectional design study and was not re-tested, which may limit generalizability. The responsiveness of the PRSQ to any intervention was also not evaluated in this validation study.

## Hull Airways Reflux Questionnaire (HARQ)

The authors of the HARQ hypothesised that patients with chronic cough represent a distinct entity consisting of chronic cough with cough hypersensitivity and termed it the Cough Hypersensitivity Syndrome [13]. The HARQ elicits the major symptoms of this clinical entity. Some questions analogous to the RSI were used in the HARQ, with permission from the authors of the RSI. The validated questionnaire consists of 14 questions with responses on a numeric response scale from 0 to 5. A score of "0" means that no problems are caused by the symptom and "5" implying severe/frequent problems. Thus the total score can range from 0 to 70. The HARQ is a self-administered questionnaire and is depicted below (Table 7.1).

The HARQ was validated in prospective patients presenting with chronic cough to a dedicated "Cough Clinic", the Hull Cough Clinic. Patients were requested to complete the questionnaire at the clinic review. Subsets of patients completed the questionnaire 4–8 weeks prior to the clinic review and 2 months after the clinic visit. Normal volunteers were used as controls. Therefore, validity of the questionnaire, reproducibility as well as response to treatment could be ascertained.

One hundred and eight-five patients and 70 volunteers were included in the validation study. All items in the scale significantly correlated positively with others in the scale and with the total score. Factor analysis did not produce clear or interpretable factors with either two or three factors. The questionnaire is best treated as having a single dimension. The Cronbach's alpha coefficient for the scale was observed to be 0.81. On repeatability testing in 96 subjects using Cohen's kappa

**Table 7.1** The Hull Airway Reflux Questionnaire. This is self-administered and has 14 items. Responses to each question can vary from 0 to 5

| Within the last *month*, how did the following problems affect you? 0 = no problem and 5 = severe/frequent problem | | | | | | |
|---|---|---|---|---|---|---|
| Hoarseness or a problem with your voice | 0 | 1 | 2 | 3 | 4 | 5 |
| Clearing your throat | 0 | 1 | 2 | 3 | 4 | 5 |
| Excess mucus in the throat, or drip down the back of your nose | 0 | 1 | 2 | 3 | 4 | 5 |
| Retching or vomiting when you cough | 0 | 1 | 2 | 3 | 4 | 5 |
| Cough on first lying down or bending over | 0 | 1 | 2 | 3 | 4 | 5 |
| Chest tightness or wheeze when coughing | 0 | 1 | 2 | 3 | 4 | 5 |
| Heartburn, indigestion, stomach acid coming up (or do you take medications for this, if yes score 5) | 0 | 1 | 2 | 3 | 4 | 5 |
| A tickle in your throat, or a lump in your throat | 0 | 1 | 2 | 3 | 4 | 5 |
| Cough with eating (during or soon after meals) | 0 | 1 | 2 | 3 | 4 | 5 |
| Cough with certain foods | 0 | 1 | 2 | 3 | 4 | 5 |
| Cough when you get out of bed in the morning | 0 | 1 | 2 | 3 | 4 | 5 |
| Cough brought on by singing or speaking (for example, on the telephone) | 0 | 1 | 2 | 3 | 4 | 5 |
| Coughing during the day rather than night | 0 | 1 | 2 | 3 | 4 | 5 |
| A strange taste in your mouth | 0 | 1 | 2 | 3 | 4 | 5 |
| Total score | __/70 | | | | | |

Copyright of the University of Hull and is available for use for free for research purposes, but requires a licence for commercial purposes. Version 5, July 2009

with quadratic weights, significant agreement was noted for all items of the questionnaire. Good agreement (kappa >0.6) was obtained for 11 items and moderate agreement (kappa between 0.4 and 0.6) for the remaining three. There was a tendency for the first score to be greater than the second score. The correlation coefficient between the scores was 0.78.

There was a marked difference in the HARQ scores between patients and normal volunteers with little overlap. Both direct estimation as well as mean ±2 SD yielded the best estimate of the upper limit of the 95% reference range to be 13. Using 13 as a as a cut-off point the estimated sensitivity and specificity of the HARQ was calculated to be 94.1% and 95% respectively. This led to the construction of a receiver operating characteristic curve which was very striking (Fig. 7.1). It was also shown that the HARQ was responsiveness to change; if cough improved the HARQ scores significantly decreased.

## Composite Questionnaires

There is both considerable overlap as well as differences between the symptomatology of GORD and that of airways or extraoesophageal reflux. There have been attempts to combine questionnaires assessing classical GORD with that of extraoesophageal reflux. One such is the Comprehensive Reflux Symptom Scale (CReSS) [17]. One of the commonly used questionnaires to asses classic GORD

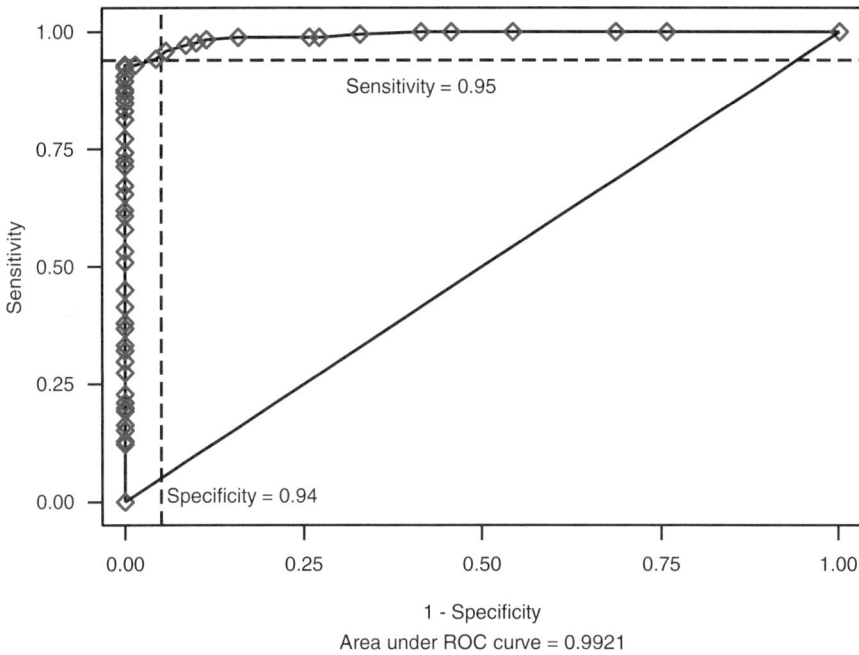

**Fig. 7.1** Receiver operating characteristics curve for the Hull Airways Reflux Questionnaire

is the Gastroesophgeal Symptoms Assessment Scale (GSAS) [18]. The CReSS combines the GSAS, as the original score described with 25 items, and the RSI resulting in a 34-item questionnaire. The CReSS uses a Likert scale to record symptoms as experienced in the preceding month. For individual questions scores range from 0 (no problem) to 5 (severe problem). Hence, the total score can range from 0 to 170 with higher scores indicating greater burden of symptoms. The CReSS was demonstrated to have good internal reliability with a Cronbach's alpha coefficient of 0.93. Three major, robust CReSS factors emerged; oesophageal, pharyngeal and upper airway.

## Discussion

The classic symptoms of GORD are well recognised. In someone presenting with these classic symptoms of GORD in conjunction with respiratory/airway symptoms one may argue that the diagnosis is rather easy to make with no need for any diagnostic questionnaires. However often patients may present only with the airway symptoms without the classic features of GORD. Here specific questionnaires to assess airways reflux are likely to have diagnostic utility, especially so to those physicians who do not see this patient group on a regular basis or are unaware of the significance of questions such as 'a funny taste in the mouth' or 'cough on rising'.

These standardised questionnaires are also useful from the research perspective, particularly in assessment of therapeutic efficacy.

Though both the SERQ and the PRSQ are validated questionnaires they are quite cumbersome to use. This limits their application in routine clinical practice. Similarly the CReSS suffers from the same limitation, but to a greater degree, making routine clinical use difficult. In contrast, both the HARQ and the RSI are relatively easy self administered tools conducive to use in the outpatient setting, as well in formal research studies. Both these validated questionnaires have been widely used in clinical practice. The RSI has been in use to aide in the diagnosis of LPR for over 15 years now. It has been independently validated by groups separate to the describing authors, again in the context of LPR. It is the most used questionnaire to aide in the diagnosis of LPR and has been validated in languages other than English such as French, Italian, Arabic, Filipino and Chinese [19–23]. The threshold for the cut-off to diagnose LPR has been described in the allergy patient population [24]. In the context of LPR it has been used to asses outcome in trials of medical as well as surgical therapies [25–28].

Validation of the HARQ was described in 2011. Similar to the RSI the HARQ has also been validated separately and in different languages as well [29, 30] (available on ISSC.info). The unique nature of the HARQ is that it is a diagnostic aide in those presenting with chronic cough rather than symptoms of LPR. Chronic cough without any associated obvious respiratory disease is one of the most common presentations to secondary care. As an underlying attribute, patients with chronic cough have afferent upper airways sensitivity to a wide variety of common irritants. The authors of the HARQ hypothesised, founded on their experience of evaluating patients with chronic cough, that these patients could be categorised as having a single syndrome based on their symptom complex. This was termed the "Cough Hypersensitivity Syndrome" and the HARQ was constructed to diagnose this.

The authors suggest that the major precipitant of this syndrome is airways reflux with phenotypes existing within this umbrella rubric. This airways reflux can be gaseous, non-acid and undetectable by currently available diagnostic methodologies. One may also hypothesise that in the context of airway hypersensitivity, normal or physiological reflux episodes may also lead to cough and the perpetuation of cough hypersensitivity. The HARQ was excellent at differentiating those with this syndrome as compared to normal volunteers with sensitivity and specificity of 94 and 95% respectively, using a cut-off score of 13. The striking ROC curve, with the area under the ROC curve of 0.99, yields outstanding ability to differentiate subjects from controls. The area under the ROC curve was exactly the same in the Swedish validation study [30]. This can be interpreted that for 99% of pairs of people (patients and controls), the patient would have the higher score.

Cough in many respiratory diseases is thought to be related to reflux. The HARQ has been used to evaluate underlying airways reflux in many chronic respiratory diseases including idiopathic pulmonary fibrosis, cystic fibrosis as well as non-cystic fibrosis bronchiectasis [31–33]. Similar to the RSI the HARQ has also been used to evaluate outcomes of medical and surgical interventions [8, 34–36]. In conclusion specific validated questionnaires have been shown to aide in the diagnosis of airway reflux. The RSI has been extensively used in the context of LPR. In the context of respiratory conditions, and in particular chronic cough, the HARQ has been commonly used. Hence the applicability of the above two questionnaires is in different clinical contexts. All questionnaires come with their own limitations and have to be interpreted in the clinical context of the patient. The use of the questionnaire itself doesn't "establish" a diagnosis but aids in making one; a diagnosis should be made in the clinical context.

## References

1. El-Serag HB, Sweet S, Winchester CC, Dent J. Update on the epidemiology of gastro-oesophageal reflux disease: a systematic review. Gut. 2014;63(6):871–80.
2. Moayyedi P, Axon AT. Review article: gastro-oesophageal reflux disease – the extent of the problem. Aliment Pharmacol Ther. 2005;22(Suppl 1):11–9.
3. Holtmann G. Reflux disease: the disorder of the third millennium. Eur J Gastroenterol Hepatol. 2001;13(Suppl 1):S5–11.
4. Vakil N, van Zanten SV, Kahrilas P, Dent J, Jones R, Global Consensus Group. The Montreal definition and classification of gastroesophageal reflux disease: a global evidence-based consensus. Am J Gastroenterol. 2006;101(8):1900–20.
5. Blondeau K, Dupont LJ, Mertens V, Tack J, Sifrim D. Improved diagnosis of gastro-oesophageal reflux in patients with unexplained chronic cough. Aliment Pharmacol Ther. 2007;25(6):723–32.
6. Everett CF, Morice AH. Clinical history in gastroesophageal cough. Respir Med. 2007;101(2):345–8.
7. Belafsky PC, Postma GN, Koufman JA. The validity and reliability of the reflux finding score (RFS). Laryngoscope. 2001;111(8):1313–7.
8. Faruqi S, Molyneux ID, Fathi H, Wright C, Thompson R, Morice AH. Chronic cough and esomeprazole: a double-blind placebo-controlled parallel study. Respirology. 2011;16(7):1150–6.
9. Badillo R, Francis D. Diagnosis and treatment of gastroesophageal reflux disease. World J Gastrointest Pharmacol Ther. 2014;5(3):105–12.
10. Madan K, Ahuja V, Gupta SD, Bal C, Kapoor A, Sharma MP. Impact of 24-h esophageal pH monitoring on the diagnosis of gastroesophageal reflux disease: defining the gold standard. Gastroenterol Hepatol. 2005;20(1):30–7.
11. Gawron AJ, Pandolfino JE. Ambulatory reflux monitoring in GERD – which test should be performed and should therapy be stopped? Curr Gastroenterol Rep. 2013;15(4):316.
12. Bolier EA, Kessing BF, Smout AJ, Bredenoord AJ. Systematic review: questionnaires for assessment of gastroesophageal reflux disease. Dis Esophagus. 2015;28(2):105–20.
13. Morice AH, Faruqi S, Wright CE, Thompson R, Bland JM. Cough hypersensitivity syndrome: a distinct clinical entity. Lung. 2011;189(1):73–9.
14. Belafsky PC, Postma GN, Koufman JA. Validity and reliability of the reflux symptom index (RSI). J Voice. 2002;16(2):274–7.
15. Dauer E, Thompson D, Zinsmeister AR, Dierkhising R, Harris A, Zais T, Alexander J, Murray JA, Wise JL, Lim K, Locke GR 3rd, Romero Y. Supraesophageal reflux: validation of a symptom questionnaire. Otolaryngol Head Neck Surg. 2006;134(1):73–80.
16. Andersson O, Rydén A, Ruth M, Möller RY, Finizia C. Development and validation of a laryngopharyngeal reflux questionnaire, the Pharyngeal Reflux Symptom Questionnaire. Scand J Gastroenterol. 2010;45(2):147–59.
17. Drinnan M, Powell J, Nikkar-Esfahani A, Heading RC, Doyle J, Griffin SM, Leslie P, Bradley PT, James P, Wilson JA. Gastroesophageal and extraesophageal reflux symptoms: similarities and differences. Laryngoscope. 2015;125(2):424–30.
18. Rothman M, Farup C, Stewart W, Helbers L, Zeldis J. Symptoms associated with gastroesophageal reflux disease: development of a questionnaire for use in clinical trials. Dig Dis Sci. 2001;46(7):1540–9.

19. Lechien JR, Huet K, Finck C, Khalife M, Fourneau AF, Delvaux V, Piccaluga M, Harmegnies B, Saussez S. Validity and reliability of a French version of reflux symptom index. J Voice. 2017;31(4):512.e1–7.
20. Schindler A, Mozzanica F, Ginocchio D, Peri A, Bottero A, Ottaviani F. Reliability and clinical validity of the Italian reflux symptom index. J Voice. 2010;24(3):354–8.
21. Farahat M, Malki KH, Mesallam TA. Development of the Arabic version of reflux symptom index. J Voice. 2012;26(6):814.e15–9.
22. Lapeña JFF Jr, Ambrocio GMC, Carrillo RJD. Validity and reliability of the Filipino reflux symptom index. J Voice. 2017;31(3):387.e11–6.
23. Li J, Zhang L, Zhang C, Cheng JY, Li J, Jeff Cheng CF. Linguistic adaptation, reliability, validation, and responsivity of the Chinese version of reflux symptom index. J Voice. 2016;30(1):104–8.
24. Brauer DL, Tse KY, Lin JC, Schatz MX, Simon RA. The utility of the reflux symptom index for diagnosis of laryngopharyngeal reflux in an allergy patient population. J Allergy Clin Immunol Pract. 2018;6:132–8.e1.
25. Lin RJ, Sridharan S, Smith LJ, Young VN, Rosen CA. Weaning of proton pump inhibitors in patients with suspected laryngopharyngeal reflux disease. Laryngoscope. 2018;128:133–7. https://doi.org/10.1002/lary.26696.
26. Zhang C, Hu ZW, Yan C, Wu Q, Wu JM, Du X, Liu DG, Luo T, Li F, Wang ZG. Nissen fundoplication vs proton pump inhibitors for laryngopharyngeal reflux based on pH-monitoring and symptom-scale. World J Gastroenterol. 2017;23(19):3546–55.
27. Catania RA, Kavic SM, Roth JS, Lee TH, Meyer T, Fantry GT, Castellanos PF, Park A. Laparoscopic Nissen fundoplication effectively relieves symptoms in patients with laryngopharyngeal reflux. J Gastrointest Surg. 2007;11(12):1579–87.
28. Kim SJ, Kim HY, Jeong JI, Hong SD, Chung SK, Dhong HJ. Changes in the reflux symptom index after multilevel surgery for obstructive sleep apnea. Clin Exp Otorhinolaryngol. 2017;10(3):259–64.
29. Huang Y, Yu L, Xu XH, Chen Q, Lyu HJ, Jin XY, Qiu ZM. Validation of the Chinese version of Hull airway reflux questionnaire and its application in the evaluation of chronic cough. Zhonghua Jie He He Hu Xi ZaZhi. 2016;39(5):355–61.
30. Johansson EL, Ternesten-Hasséus E. Reliability and validity of the Swedish version of the hull airway reflux questionnaire (HARQ-S). Lung. 2016;194(6):997–1005.
31. Fahim A, Dettmar PW, Morice AH, Hart SP. Gastroesophageal reflux and idiopathic pulmonary fibrosis: a prospective study. Medicina (Kaunas). 2011;47(4):200–5.
32. Zeybel GL, Pearson JP, Krishnan A, Bourke SJ, Doe S, Anderson A, Faruqi S, Morice AH, Jones R, McDonnell M, Zeybel M, Dettmar PW, Brodlie M, Ward C. Ivacaftor and symptoms of extra-oesophageal reflux in patients with cystic fibrosis and G551D mutation. J Cyst Fibros. 2017;16(1):124–31.
33. Mandal P, Morice AH, Chalmers JD, Hill AT. Symptoms of airway reflux predict exacerbations and quality of life in bronchiectasis. Respir Med. 2013;107(7):1008–13.
34. Faruqi S, Shiferaw D, Morice AH. Effect of ivacaftor on objective and subjective measures of cough in patients with cystic fibrosis. Open Respir Med J. 2016;10:105–8.
35. Smith JE, Morjaria JB, Morice AH. Dietary intervention in the treatment of patients with cough and symptoms suggestive of airways reflux as determined by Hull airways reflux questionnaire. Cough. 2013;9(1):27.
36. Faruqi S, Sedman P, Jackson W, Molyneux I, Morice AH. Fundoplication in chronic intractable cough. Cough. 2012;8(1):3.

# Pepsin Detection as a Diagnostic Test for Reflux Disease

Peter W. Dettmar, Rhianna K. Lenham, Adrian J. Parkinson, and Andrew D. Woodcock

### Abstract

*Background*: The history of pepsin dates back to 1836, when it was discovered by Theodor Schwann. In 1938 Herriott studied the conversion of pepsinogen to pepsin, which is now known to be most aggressive proteolytic enzyme in gastric refluxate. Pepsin has been identified as a biomarker of gastric reflux into the esophagus, the airways and the lungs. Peptest was developed as a non-invasive, sensitive and specific diagnostic test to rapidly identify reflux in patients presenting with a range of symptoms and introduced on to the UK market in August 2010.

*Methods*: Patients diagnosed with the symptoms of gastro esophageal reflux disease (GERD), extra esophageal reflux (EER), laryngopharyngeal reflux (LPR) and various respiratory diseases were tested for the presence of reflux by Peptest. The reflux diagnostic test is based on lateral flow technology and contains two unique anti-pepsin human monoclonal antibodies; one to detect and one to capture pepsin within a clinical sample. The intensity of the pepsin 'test' line within the window of the lateral flow device is measured using a Peptest cube reader and the intensity automatically converts to a concentration of pepsin (ng/ml).

*Results*: There are over 100 publications describing the reflux diagnostic activity of Peptest across upper gastrointestinal and airway/lung diseases. Compared to healthy asymptomatic control subjects patients presenting with heartburn were shown to have a significantly higher prevalence of salivary pepsin. There is growing evidence that pepsin is a major aetiological factor in LPR and Peptest is routinely used in many ENT clinics. Key respiratory centres in the UK and the Czech Republic demonstrated similar pepsin positivity in patients presenting with a range of respiratory diseases.

P. W. Dettmar (✉) · R. K. Lenham · A. J. Parkinson · A. D. Woodcock
RD Biomed Limited, Castle Hill Hospital, Cottingham, UK
e-mail: peter.dettmar@rdbiomed.com

*Conclusions*: Peptest as a marker of prior reflux improves the accuracy of reflux diagnosis in order to better tailor appropriate treatments in patients presenting across a range of upper gastrointestinal, airway and respiratory diseases. Therefore reducing the use and dependency on invasive and expensive diagnostic tests.

**Keywords**
Peptest · Reflux disease · Diagnostic tests · Salivary pepsin · Gastro-esophageal reflux disease · Laryngopharyngeal reflux · Respiratory diseases · Lateral flow teat · Unique pepsin monoclonal antibodies

## Introduction

### History of Reflux

The anatomy of reflux is illustrated in Fig. 8.1. The origin of reflux disease dates back to 1903—Coffin stated gas refluxed from the stomach was responsible for causing hoarseness and rhinorrhoea, often being misunderstood and classified as heartburn as described in Gelardi et al. [1]. Current research has led to the

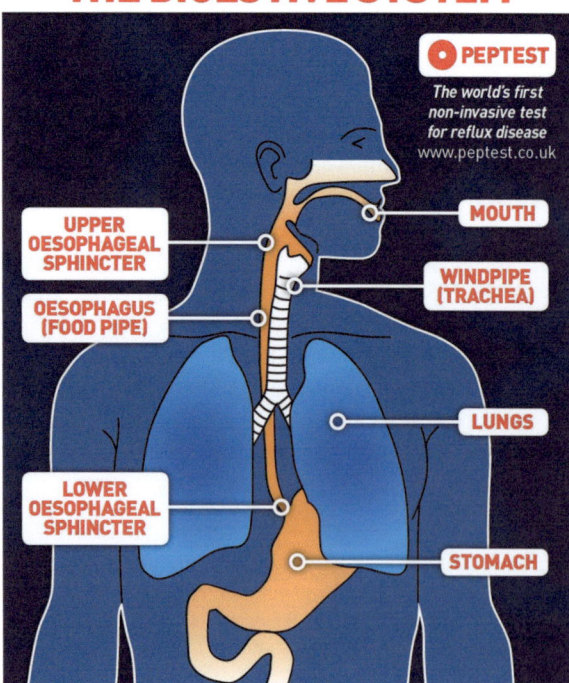

**Fig. 8.1** The anatomy of reflux

understanding and definition that reflux is 'an event that causes troublesome symptoms, mucosal injury in the oesophagus, or both of these' [2] causing a plethora of problematic painful symptoms for reflux disease sufferers including postnasal drip and regurgitation [3]. Within the growing population gastroesophageal reflux disease (GERD) is known to be affecting up to 20–40% of the adult population and extra esophageal reflux (EER) additionally affecting up to 20–30% [4, 5] with a full percentage breakdown presented in Fig. 8.2.

## History of Pepsin

The history of pepsin dates back to 1836 when Theodor Schwann made the remarkable discovery of the compound [6]. Studying digestion through mucus membranes, Schwann obtained a yellow-tinged filtrate and proceeded to note the effects of the filtrate were different to those of hydrochloric acid also present, subsequently naming the filtrate pepsin [7].

Northop crystallised porcine pepsin and his description allowed Herriott in 1938 [7] to discover and study the conversion of pepsinogen to pepsin. He concluded pepsin is secreted as its precursor pepsinogen and upon acidification pepsinogen is converted into the active form of pepsin. Now, after years of extensive research it is known that pepsin is the most aggressive proteolytic enzyme of the gastric contents, responsible for causing damage to internal tissues and organs including the esophagus (see Fig. 8.3).

**Fig. 8.2** Prevalence of reflux

**PREVALENCE OF REFLUX**

By Percentage Global Population

- GERD – 20%-40%
- EER –20%-30%
- Chronic diseases affecting all age groups
- A major clinical problem
- Can lead to more serious conditions

**PEPSIN**

- Major component of gastric refluxate
- Composed of a family of isoenzymes
- Pepsin 3 complex accounts for 80% of total pepsin
- Main activity pH 2 to pH 4
- Active up to pH 6.5
- Denatured pH 7.8
- Normal basal secretion
    o 123mg/hr
    o 0.9mg/ml

**Fig. 8.3** Key information about pepsin

The structure of human pepsin was determined using x-ray crystallography displaying the molecule to be composed of 2438 protein atoms, 102 water molecules and have a disulphide separation of 2.0 Å (see Fig. 8.4). Correlations were found when comparing the amino acid sequences of human and porcine pepsin, [8, 9] with the only true differences occurring at amino acids 8 and 18. At amino acid 8, human pepsin contains glutamine whereas lysine is present in porcine pepsin, similarly amino acid 18 in human pepsin is phenylalanine which is replaced by tyrosine in porcine pepsin [10]. This slight alteration results in subtle chemical differences between the two species of pepsin such as the pH they are denatured and their isoelectric point.

Luebke (2016) reports pepsin is irreversibly denatured at pH 8 due to the depletion of the molecule's secondary structure, however, the enzyme is dormant and stable up until pH 7.5, eventually resulting in consequences such as GERD [11]. This is due to re-acidification occurring, allowing the dormant pepsin to be re-activated and exposing its damaging effects. Furthermore, pepsin is maximally active over a wide range of pH values including 3.2 and 4.2, however the enzyme's optimal pH for digestion is 2 [12, 13]. This vast range of activity emphasises pepsin to be a major aggressive enzyme as the re-acidification process does not need to occur at a pH as low as the gastric juice (pH 1) but can happen through the consumption of an acidic drink [14].

In addition, pepsin is composed of a family of isoenzymes, all of which have slightly different characteristics and optimal pH values further embedding pepsin to be maximally active over a wide pH range. Human gastric juice contains isoforms 1, 3a, 3b, 3c and 5 with pepsin 3b being the most prominent [15] (see Fig. 8.3). The nomenclature for pepsin isoenzymes is due to their ability to mobilise in electrophoresis with isoenzyme 1 displaying the most movement [16].

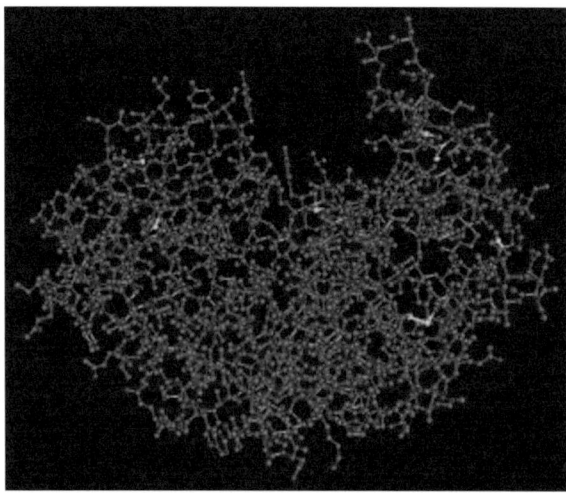

**Fig. 8.4** The structure of pepsin

| PEPSIN | |
|---|---|
| **Identified in** | **Detected in** |
| • GERD<br>• Extra Esophageal Reflux<br>• Laryngopharyngeal Reflux<br>• Chronic Cough<br>• Asthma<br>• Sinusitis<br>• Cystic fibrosis<br>• Lung Allograph Rejection<br>• Otitis Media with Effusion | • Saliva<br>• Sputum<br>• Tracheal Aspirate<br>• Exhaled Breath Condensate<br>• Broncho alveolar Lavage fluid<br>• Middle Ear Effusions<br>• Nasal Lavage Fluid<br>• Laryngeal Biopsy |

**Fig. 8.5** An extensive list of pepsin identification and detection

## Reflux Diagnostic Tests: Invasive and Non-invasive

Pepsin has been detected in saliva, sputum, and secretions from the trachea, lung, nose, sinus, middle ear and exhaled breath condensate (see Fig. 8.5) and pepsin detection has been proposed as a method for GERD diagnosis. In addition to GERD, pepsin has been identified in patients presenting with other upper gastrointestinal diseases listed in Fig. 8.5.

There are many mainly invasive diagnostic methods currently available to confirm or reject if a patient's symptoms are caused by reflux disease. However, these tests are not only invasive and expensive but also do not achieve high sensitivity and specificity. This includes empirical PPI treatment with a reported sensitivity of around 68% and a specificity as low as 44% [17, 18] specific questionnaires [19] (63% sensitivity and 67% specificity), endoscopy with only 30% [20] sensitivity for diagnosing reflux disease and pHmetry with sensitivity in the region of 60% [17]. The reflux disease diagnostic tests available are listed in Fig. 8.6.

The current chapter describes the use of the non-invasive reflux test Peptest, which detects pepsin [21] as a biomarker for reflux in a clinical sample.

## Methods

### Patient Recruitment

Previously diagnosed patients were recruited from gastroenterology clinics, ENT clinics and various respiratory disease clinics throughout the UK and Europe. All patients recruited provided saliva samples into collection tubes containing 0.5 ml of 0.01M citric acid which were analysed for pepsin content within 7 days of collection using Peptest (RD Biomed Limited, UK).

**Fig. 8.6** Current reflux diagnostic tests

---
**CURRENT DIAGNOSTIC TESTS FOR REFLUX DISEASE**

*Depending on the severity of symptoms:*
- History, advice and medication
- Questionnaires

*Invasive Procedures:*
- Upper gastrointestinal endoscopy
- 24 hour oh monitoring or BRAVO
- pH + Impedance
- X-ray procedure – barium swallow radiography
- High-resolution manometry (HRM)
- Videofluroscopic swallow study (VFSS or VSS)

*No-invasive Procedures:*
- Laboratory based assays for pepsin – ELISA
- Peptest™ – rapid pepsin analysis
---

## Sample Collection

Each patient provided three saliva samples at specific time points. The first of the samples was provided in the morning on waking before eating and cleaning teeth. The second and third samples were provided post-prandial; (pp) 60 min after finishing a meal and in some studies the third sample was provided 15 min after experiencing symptoms. All the saliva samples were stored in a fridge at 4 °C before being analysed for the presence of pepsin using Peptest (RD Biomed Limited, UK). Patients were informed not to take any medication during the study period and not to consume caffeinated or carbonated drinks 60 min prior to providing a sample.

## Pepsin Analysis

Saliva collection tubes were centrifuged at 4000 rpm for 5 min until a clear supernatant layer was visible. 80 μL from the surface layer of the centrifuged sample was drawn up into an automated pipette. The 80 μL sample was transferred to a screw-top microtube containing 240 μL of Migration Buffer solution. The sample was mixed with a vortex mixer for 10 s. A second pipette was used to transfer 80 μL of the sample to the circular well of a Lateral Flow Device (LFD) (Fig. 8.7) containing two unique human monoclonal antibodies; one to detect and the other to capture pepsin in the saliva sample (Fig. 8.8) (Peptest, RD Biomed Limited, UK). A 'C' (control) line is produced if the test was successful and a 'T' (test) line was generated if the sample is pepsin positive due to the monoclonal antibody capturing pepsin.

Each device was read by the Peptest Cube (Fig. 8.9), measuring the intensity of the 'T' line before automatically converting to a concentration pepsin in ng/ml within the clinical sample.

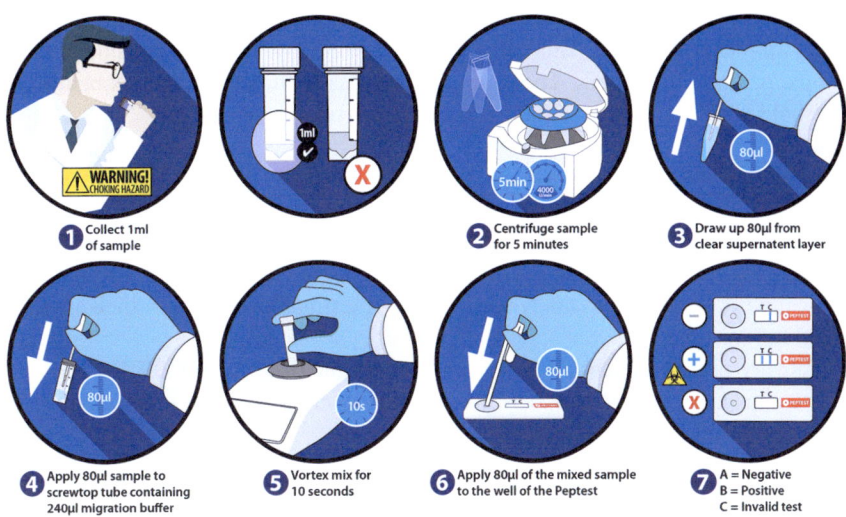

**Fig. 8.7** Schematic procedure of Peptest from sample collection to sample analysis

**Fig. 8.8** A representation of two monoclonal antibodies detecting and capturing pepsin in a positive pepsin sample

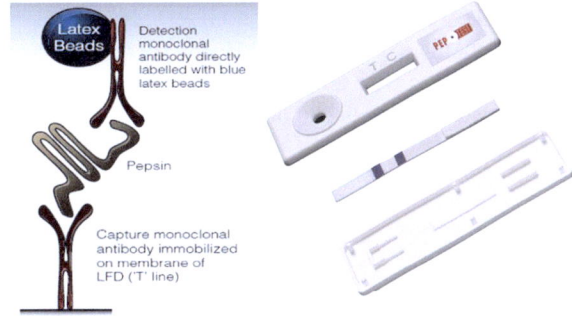

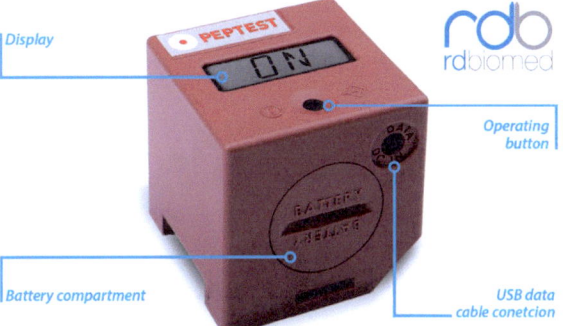

**Fig. 8.9** Annotated Peptest cube

The lower limit for accurate detection of pepsin (as determined by the manufacturer) was set at 16 ng/ml. This value was used as a cut-off point to consider a saliva sample positive for pepsin. Therefore, all samples with determinations below this threshold were considered to have 0 ng/ml in the results.

## Results

Peptest is a non-invasive and rapid test for diagnosing reflux disease and has been clinically evaluated across many upper gastro intestinal disciplines, which are illustrated in Fig. 8.10.

Salivary pepsin was tested as a biomarker for the diagnosis of GERD, LPR and various respiratory diseases across a series of clinical studies, which will be described in the following sections.

Some of the key clinical studies in both GERD and NERD patients are illustrated in Fig. 8.11.

It was interesting that the percentage Peptest (pepsin) positivity was similar across all studies [22, 23]. In the first of the studies conducted, Peptest was compared across a symptomatic patient population with asymptomatic healthy controls [24]. The study recruited a total of 111 patients from the Centre for Digestive Diseases, Barts and the London School of Medicine and Dentistry, UK. Of these patients 58 were diagnosed with GERD, 26 with Hypersensitive Esophagus (HE) and 27 patients with Functional Heartburn (FH) and compared to 87 asymptomatic healthy subjects who served as the control population [23]. In total, 33/87 healthy asymptomatic subjects had one or more saliva samples positive with a low level of

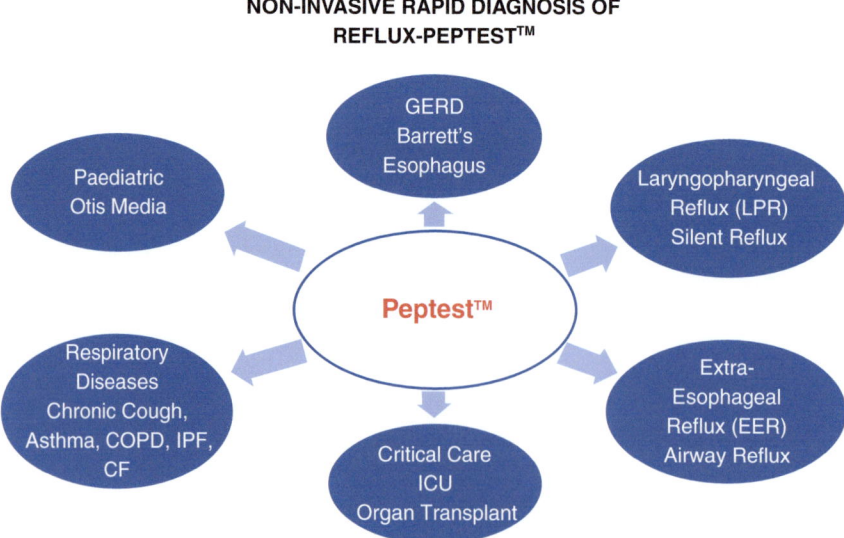

**Fig. 8.10** Disciplines where Peptest has analysed the presence of pepsin

pepsin. Compared to the healthy control subjects, patients with heartburn had a significantly higher prevalence of salivary pepsin [23]. In patients with GERD, 45/58 subjects had one or more samples pepsin positive. Similarly a high prevalence of positive pepsin was observed in HE patients 21/26. By contrast patients with FH had a significantly lower prevalence of pepsin detection (9/27). This was significantly different to those patients presenting with GERD ($p < 0.0002$) or patients presenting with HE ($p < 0.0008$). Interestingly the prevalence of pepsin detection was similar between FH patients and asymptomatic controls [23].

There is growing evidence that pepsin is a major aetiological factor in Laryngopharyngeal reflux (LPR) and the value of the salivary pepsin test (Peptest) has become an important diagnostic test for LPR [25]. Figure 8.12 shows pepsin detection (ng/ml) in patients presenting with LPR in five UK ENT clinics. There was a total of 865 patients recruited into this series of clinical studies. There was a mean pepsin concentration of 150 ng/ml in the 2475 salivary pepsin samples analysed and in all five clinics there was a similar level of pepsin positivity observed. In

**COMPARATIVE PEPTEST STUDIES GASTRO-ESOPHAGEAL REFLUX DISEASE**

| Patients presenting with | % Peptest Positive | n= |
|---|---|---|
| GERD and Hypersensitive Esophagus Sifrim, London, UK | 79% | 84 |
| GERD. Bardhan, Rotherham, UK | 80% | 59 |
| GERD. Jackson, Hull, UK | 81% | 80 |
| GERD. Bor, Izmir, Turkey | 73% | 10 |
| NERD. De Bortoli, Italy | 93% | 38 |
| Functional Heartburn- Sifrim, London, UK | 30% | 27 |

**Fig. 8.11** Key Peptest clinical studies displaying the percentage pepsin positivity

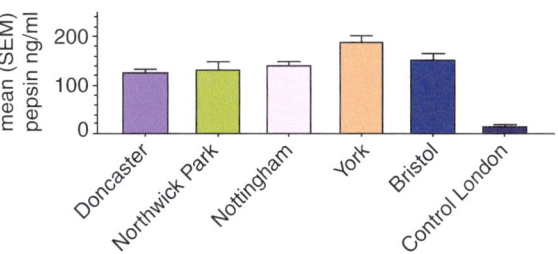

**Fig. 8.12** Pepsin concentration (ng/ml) detected in patients with LPR in five different UK ENT clinics

865 patients and 2475 saliva samples with a mean pepsin concentration of 150 ng/mL (median pepsin concentration 54 ng/mL)

the study conducted at Doncaster Royal Infirmary, 100 consecutive patients presenting with upper aerodigestive track symptoms were recruited and each patient provided three salivary samples at specific time points as described in the method section and these were analysed for pepsin [26]. All patients had a clinical diagnosis and the pepsin analysis was correlated with the clinical findings by an independent clinician. Of the 100 patients (287 salivary samples) 78 patients were confirmed with LPR and 22 patients without LPR. In this study the salivary pepsin assay gave 81% sensitivity and a 100% specificity in diagnosing LPR. The positive predictive value (PPV) of the test was 100% and the negative predictive value (NPV) was 60% (see Fig. 8.13) [26].

There is evidence that reflux into the airways (lower and upper and lungs) is responsible for the aetiology and the exacerbation of a range of respiratory conditions. Peptest/pepsin detection has become a quick and easy routine diagnostic test to identify airway reflux in patients with respiratory disease [27]. Peptest was used in routine clinical practise in patients presenting with a range of respiratory/pulmonary diseases in UK clinics and in the department of Pneumology and Physiology, Charles University, Plzen, Czech Republic (see Fig. 8.14). There were large groups of patients presenting with bronchial asthma, chronic cough, idiopathic pulmonary fibrosis, progressive sarcoidosis, exogenic allergic alveolitis, chronic obstructive pulmonary disease and cystic fibrosis [28]. It was interesting to compare the

LPR ROUTINE TESTING

- Patients provided 3 saliva samples for pepsin analysis

*Breakdown*

- 100 patients and 287 saliva samples analysed

- Used to rule out and reflux in complex patients and confirm reflux in those suspected of LPR

- 78 patients confirmed with LPR
  - 81% LPR patients pepsin positive

- 22 patients without LPR (other diagnostic)

- Sensitivity 81% Specificity 100%
  - 0% non-LPR pepsin positive

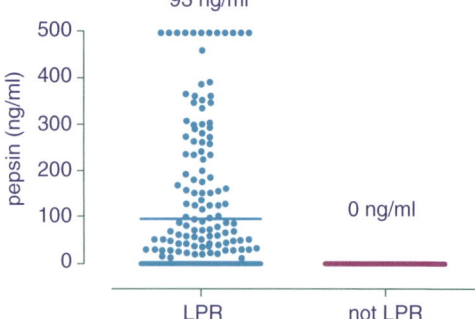

**Fig. 8.13** Breakdown of LPR testing using Peptest, displaying sensitivity and specificity

percentage Peptest positivity and strong similarities between the UK centres and the centre in the Czech Republic across the range of respiratory diseases [29].

In the routine testing of chronic cough reflux is a substantial but as yet undefined component in the aetiology of cough hypersensitivity syndrome. Routinely, Peptest was used in outpatients attending a major world renowned cough clinic based at Castle Hill Hospital (Cottingham, UK). Patients were instructed to provide three expectorated saliva/sputum samples into sample collection tubes (containing 0.01M citric acid) immediately after three spontaneous coughing episodes.

In patients with airway hypersensitivity only small amounts of reflux may be sufficient to induce a cough. Over a period of 4 months, 93 patients provided 262 evaluable samples for pepsin analysis by Peptest. Eighty patients had at least one pepsin positive sample (86%) resulting in a mean pepsin concentration of 104 ng/ml (see Fig. 8.15) [30].

**COMPARATIVE PEPSIN STUDIES UK VERSUS OVERSEAS RESPIRATORY CENTRES**

| Patients presenting with | % Peptest Positive | |
|---|---|---|
| | UK | Non-UK |
| Idiopathic Pulmonary Fibrosis (IPF) | 79% (n=29) | 89% (n=55)<br>68% (n=38) |
| Chronic Obstructive Pulmonary Disease (COPD) | 67% (n=12) | 78% (n=37) |
| Chronic Cough | 86% (n=94) | 77% (n=78) |
| Cystic Fibrosis (CF) | 83% (n=24) | 86% (n=7) |
| Progressive Asthma | - | 81% (n=102) |
| Progressive/symptomatic sarcoidosis | - | 74% (n=46) |
| Exogenic Allergic Alveolitis | - | 78% (n=27) |
| Chronic Rhinosinusitis | 83% (n=25) | - |

**Fig. 8.14** UK and overseas results for percentage pepsin positivity over a range of respiratory diseases

**Fig. 8.15** Routine testing for chronic cough using Peptest

**CHRONIC COUGH ROUTINE TESTING**

- Routine sequential testing of patients attending chronic cough clinic
- Patients provided 3 saliva samples during coughing episodes for pepsin analysis
- Used to confirm reflux in those patients suspected of airway reflux
- In patients with airway hypersensitivity only small amount of reflux may be sufficient to induce cough

*Breakdown*
- n=93 cough patients
- 262 samples
- 38 male: 55 female
- 58.4 years mean age
- 5.6 years mean duration of cough
- 32 mean HARQ score
- 86% patients pepsin positive
- Mean [pepsin] 104 ng/ml

## Discussion

Clinicians are frequently faced with the dilemma as to whether a patient's symptoms are due to reflux. This is particularly important for patients presenting with the atypical symptoms of extra esophageal reflux or due to other reasons for example infections, allergies, smoking and medications. Clinicians frequently turn to the use of invasive diagnostic tests to diagnose the presence of reflux disease for example 24 h pHmetry, endoscopy and impedance + pHmetry. However, these tests are not only invasive but also expensive and often there are long waiting lists to have the diagnosis carried out. More importantly the sensitivity and specificity is questionable. This has led to the development of Peptest: a non-invasive, rapid and inexpensive test with good sensitivity and specificity for diagnosing reflux disease, thus making Peptest an attractive alternative for clinicians and health professionals to use instead of the current invasive tests. Furthermore, another advantage of Peptest is that pepsin is able to be detected even in those patients prescribed PPI medication which clearly influences acid secretion but not the reflux of pepsin. This is especially important in those patients presenting with extra esophageal reflux/LPR and respiratory disease symptoms. Reflux above the upper esophageal sphincter and into the airways may not always be causative of these conditions but the presence of damaging pepsin will certainly be a negative influence, which can lead to an increase in disease severity and a reduction in the impact of treatment.

Peptest and the salivary pepsin assay had excellent specificity and positive predictive value (PPV) in diagnosing LPR and has proved to be an excellent diagnostic tool for diagnosing reflux in this difficult group of patients. It was also interesting to observe that patients presenting with the symptoms of LPR were more likely to have a higher concentration of pepsin present in their early morning saliva sample compared to patients diagnosed with GERD, NERD and hypersensitive esophagus. The determination of pepsin in saliva in these patients was considered to be an inexpensive method for confirming or excluding the diagnosis of GERD and generally the higher the concentration of pepsin in the saliva was reflected in patients presenting with more severe symptoms.

Across all patient groups studied with Peptest, we observed a high prevalence of pepsin positivity in patients with conditions linked with reflux for example GERD, EER, LPR, chronic cough and respiratory disorders. These high pepsin concentrations were considered to be pathological. Of particular interest was the low prevalence and concentration of pepsin in healthy control subjects, where in well controlled studies around 30% of subjects were found to have low physiological levels of pepsin present. Therefore, in terms of pepsin as a biomarker there is a clear differentiation between healthy asymptomatic individuals and patients presenting with the symptoms of reflux.

### Conclusion

Peptest was first introduced onto the market in the UK in 2010 and is now commercially available in over 24 countries. Peptest contains two unique anti-human pepsin monoclonal antibodies to detect and capture pepsin. This enables the rapid detection of pepsin in saliva or other sources of refluxate to improve the accuracy of reflux diagnosis in order to better tailor appropriate treatments. Peptest/pepsin analysis can also complement the use of questionnaires and office based reflux diagnosis, lessening the use and dependency on invasive and expensive diagnostic tests.

## References

1. Gelardi M, Eplite A, Mezzina A, Taliente S, Plantone F, Dettmar PW, Quaranta N. Clinical-diagnostic correlations in laryngopharyngeal reflux (LPR). The role of peptest. Int J Open Access Otolarymgol. 2017;1:1–8.
2. Bredenoord AJ, Pandolfino JE, Smout AJPM. Gastro-oesophageal reflux disease. Lancet. 2013;381:1933–42.
3. Eren E, Arslanoğlu S, Aktaş A, Kopar A, Ciğer E, Önal K, Katilmiş H. Factors confusing the diagnosis of laryngopharyngeal reflux: the role of allergic rhinitis and inter-rater variability of laryngeal findings. Eur Arch Otorhinolayngol. 2014;271:743–7.
4. Lowden M, McGlashan JA, Steel A, Strugala V, Dettmar PW. Prevalence of symptoms suggestive of extra-oesophageal reflux in a general practice population in the UK. Logoped Phoniatr Vocol. 2009;34:32–5.
5. Reulbach TR, Belafsky PC, Blalock PD, Koufman JA, Postma GN. Occultlaryngeal pathology in a community-based cohort. Otolaryngol Head Neck Surg. 2001;124:448–50.
6. Fruton JS. A history of pepsin and related enzymes. Q Rev Biol. 2002;77:127–47.
7. Fruton JS. Aspartyl proteinases. In: Neuberger A, Brocklehurst K, editors. Hydrolytic enzymes. New York: Elsevier; 1988. p. 1–37.
8. Taylor WH. The proteolytic activity of human gastric juice and pig and calf gastric mucosal extracts below pH 5, studies on gastric proteolysis. Biochem J. 1959;71:73–83.
9. Taylor WH. The nature of the enzyme-substrate interaction responsible for gastric Proteolytic pH-activity curves with two maxima, studies on gastric proteolysis. Biochem J. 1959;71(2):373–83.
10. Fujinaga M, Chernaia MM, Tarasova NI, Mosimann SC, James MNG. Crystal structure of human pepsin and its complex with pepstatin. Protein Sci. 1995;4:960–72.
11. Luebke KE, Samuels TL, Johnston N. The role of pepsin in LPR: will it change our diagnostic and therapeutic approaches to the disease. Curr Otorhinolaryngol Rep. 2016;4:55–62.
12. Taylor WH. Proteinases of the stomach in health and disease. Physiol Rev. 1962;42:519–53.
13. Roberts NB. Human pepsins – their multiplicity, function and role in reflux disease. Aliment Pharmacol Ther. 2006;24(Suppl. 2):2–9.
14. Strugala V, Avis J, Jolliffe IG, Johnstone LM, Dettmar PW. The role of an alginate suspension on pepsin and bile acids – key aggressors in the gastric refluxate. Does this have implications for the treatment of gastro-oesophageal reflux disease? J Pharm Pharmacol. 2009;61:1021–8.
15. Strugala V, Pearson JP, Panetti M, Koufman JA, Dettmar PW. Considering the still potent enzymatic activity of gastric juice at high pH values, what should be the threshold to consider above the UES? In: Giuli R, Scarpignato C, Collard J-M, Richter JE, editors. The duodenogastroesophageal reflux. Paris: Pub John Libbey; 2006. p. 181.
16. Etherington DJ, Taylor WH. Nomenclature of the pepsins. Nature. 1967;216:219–80.
17. Dent J, Vakil N, Jones R, et al. Accuracy of the diagnosis of GORD by questionnaire, physicians and a trial of proton pump inhibitor treatment: the diamond study. Gut. 2010;59:714–21.
18. Bytzer P, Jones R, Vakil N, et al. Limited ability of the proton-pump inhibitor test to identify patients with gastroesophageal reflux disease. Clin Gastroenterol. 2012;10:1360–6.
19. Vakil NB, Halling K, Becher A, et al. Systematic review of patient-reported outcome instruments for gastroesophageal reflux disease symptoms. Eur J Gastroenterol Hepatol. 2013;25:2–14.

20. Savarino E, Zentilin P, Masracci L, et al. Microscopic esophagitis distinguishes patients with non-erosive reflux disease from those with functional heartburn. J Gastroenterol. 2013;48:473–82.
21. Bardhan KD, Strugala V, Dettmar PW. Reflux revisited: advancing the role of pepsin. Int J Otolaryngol. 2012;2012:646901. https://doi.org/10.1155/2012/646901.
22. Bortoli N, Savarino E, Furnari M, Matrinucci I, Zentilin P, Bertani L, Franchi R, Bellini M, Savarino V, Marchi S. Use of a non-invasive pepsin diagnostic test to detect GERD: correlation with MII-pH evaluation in a series of suspected NERD patients. A pilot study. Gastroenterology. 2013;144(5 Suppl 1):S118.
23. Hayat JO, Gabieta-Somnez S, Yazaki E, Kang J-Y, Woodcock A, Dettmar P, Mabary J, Knowles CH, Sifrim D. Pepsin in saliva for the diagnosis of gastro-oesophageal reflux disease. Gut. 2015;64:373–80.
24. Hayat JO, Gabieta S, Woodcock A, Dettmar PW, Mabary J, Yazaki E, Kang J-Y, Sifrim D. Postprandial pepsin saliva in healthy subjects and patients with GERD. Relationship with postprandial reflux. Gastroenterology. 2014;146(5 Suppl 1):S751.
25. Barona-Lleo L, Duval C, Barona-de Guzman R. Salivary pepsin test: useful and simple tool for the laryngopharangeal reflux diagnosis. Acta Otorrinolaringol Esp. 2018;69(2):80–5.
26. Stapleton E, Watson M, Strugala V, Dettmar P. Salivary pepsin assay as a diagnostic test for laryngopharyngeal reflux. In: 15th British Academic Conference in Otolaryngology and ENT Expo; 2015.
27. Strugala V, Dettmar PW, Bittenglova R, Fremundova L, Pešek M. Use of pepsin detection to identify airways reflux in a range of pulmonary diseases. Clin Respir J. 2017;11(5):666–7.
28. Pesek M, Fremundova L, Bittenglova R, Turkova-Sedlackova T, Dettmar PW. Report on the first results of pepsin positivity in upper airway secretions in patients with chronic bronchial and lung diseases. Stud Pneumol Phthiseol. 2014;74(4):143–9.
29. Pesek M, Bittenglova R, Fremundova L, Turkova-Sedlackova T, Dettmar PW. Detection of pepsin in airway secretions in interstitial lung disease. Stud Pneumol Phthiseol. 2014;74(5):168–73.
30. Strugala V, Woodcock AD, Dettmar PW, Faruqi S, Morice AH. Detection of pepsin in sputum: a rapid and objective measure of airways reflux. Eur Respir J. 2016;47(1):339–41.

# Imaging Reflux

9

Luca Marciani

## Abstract

Diagnostic imaging methods allow evaluating morphology and function of the upper gastrointestinal tract and have been used to evaluate reflux and its complications. In this chapter the main whole-body imaging techniques used to image reflux are described briefly, including their advantages and limitations. X-ray and video fluoroscopy in conjunction with oral barium contrast media can document reflux and a range of morphological changes such as hiatal hernia. Whist X-ray methods are well established, generally available and relatively cheap, they involve giving a dose of ionizing radiation to the patients. Nuclear medicine techniques exploit the sensitivity to small amounts of radiolabels to form images that can evaluate gastroesophageal reflux disease. This sensitivity allows demonstrating postprandial pulmonary aspiration of the ingested radiolabel by showing increased counts in the lung fields. Two and three dimensional nuclear medicine techniques used to image lung delivery of inhaled pharmacological agents could provide a promising technology to investigate airway reflux. More recently a role for MRI has emerged. MRI fluoroscopy is capable to image directly reflux, swallowing and bolus passage in the esophagus. MRI has the advantages of using non ionizing radiation, multi-planar capability, good spatial resolution and good soft tissue contrast. Sensitivity however is low.

## Introduction

Diagnostic testing for the evaluation of gastroesophageal reflux disease (GERD) and its complications has been based over the years on well established techniques including endoscopy, pH and impedance monitoring and radiological methods

---

L. Marciani
Gastrointestinal MRI, Nottingham Digestive Diseases Centre, School of Medicine,
The University of Nottingham, Nottingham, UK
e-mail: Luca.Marciani@nottingham.ac.uk

[1–3]. Until recently the imaging methods have focused mostly on evaluation of morphological changes rather than function. Imaging of orogastric function and in particular direct imaging of the reflux events has become the focus of increased attention in recent years [4]. A particular imaging challenge is presented by extraesophageal manifestations [5], when the reflux extends to the pharynx and larynx, as in laryngopharyngeal reflux (LPR) [6], or into the airways, as in airway reflux [7, 8]. In this Chapter the main, non-endoscopic, whole-body imaging techniques used to image reflux will be described; their ability to image airways reflux contamination will be considered together with their advantages and limitations.

## X-ray

Conventional radiological X-ray techniques form an image of the body based on a beam of X-rays travelling in straight lines through the body of the patient. Detection of the beam occurs on the other side of the patient, opposite to the X-rays source. Detection methods have evolved from the old scintillators converting the beam into light for film capture to digital capture plates and panels. Different body tissues attenuate the X-rays beam differently; hence the beam carries spatial absorption information that generates the contrast in the image. Highly absorbing contrast media such as barium-containing drinks are used to fill the gastrointestinal lumen and provide additional contrast to aid diagnosis.

The diagnostic evaluation of gastroesophageal reflux disease (GERD) and its complications has primarily been carried out using the barium esophagram [3, 9]. The main aims of the barium esophagram are to document morphological changes such as reflux esophagitis, scarring and strictures together with assessing esophageal emptying, the presence of hiatal hernia or reflux (Fig. 9.1) [11]. The exam usually comprises multiple steps. These may include double-contrast views of the esophagus, whereby the patient ingests an effervescent preparation and also a high density barium suspension, followed by an evaluation of motility and reflux using a low density barium suspension [10, 11]. Reflux events that are spontaneous or follow provocative maneuvers can be visualized with fluoroscopic techniques (Fig. 9.2) [10, 12].

X-ray methods are well established; they have been developed and used for over 100 years. They are generally widely available, quick to use and relatively cheap. They have good spatial resolution. One of the main limitations of X-rays is the radiation dose given to the patients. X-rays carry enough energy to ionize atoms and molecules, which in simple words means that they can knock out an electron from an atom shell therefore altering bonds and producing reactive ions, which in turn induces biological damage. The effective radiation dose from a single X-ray exam is relatively low (order of a fraction of mSv) but this is much higher for a fluoroscopy exam. Another limitation is that the X-ray image is a two-dimensional projection through the whole body of the patient hence the image contains unwanted organs and tissues superimposed within the region of interest. The literature reports a marked variation in GERD detection rates for the barium esophagram compared

# 9 Imaging Reflux

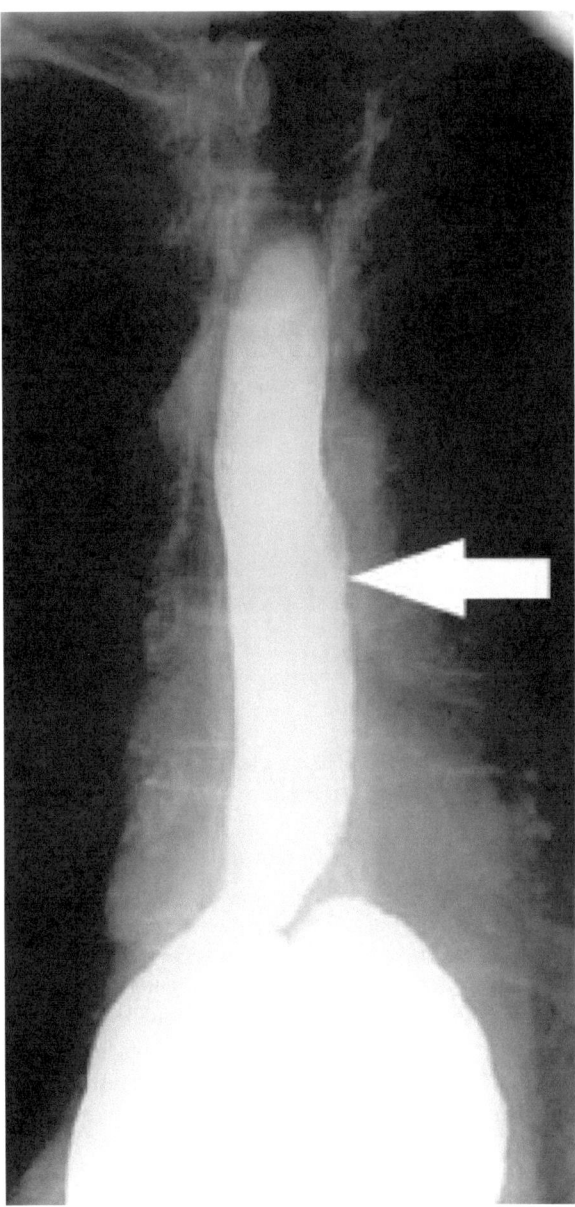

**Fig. 9.1** Supine anteroposterior esophagram in a patient with a large hiatal hernia. The image shows the reflux identification phase of the exam. A spontaneous, high-volume reflux (arrow) can be seen. Reproduced with permission from [10]

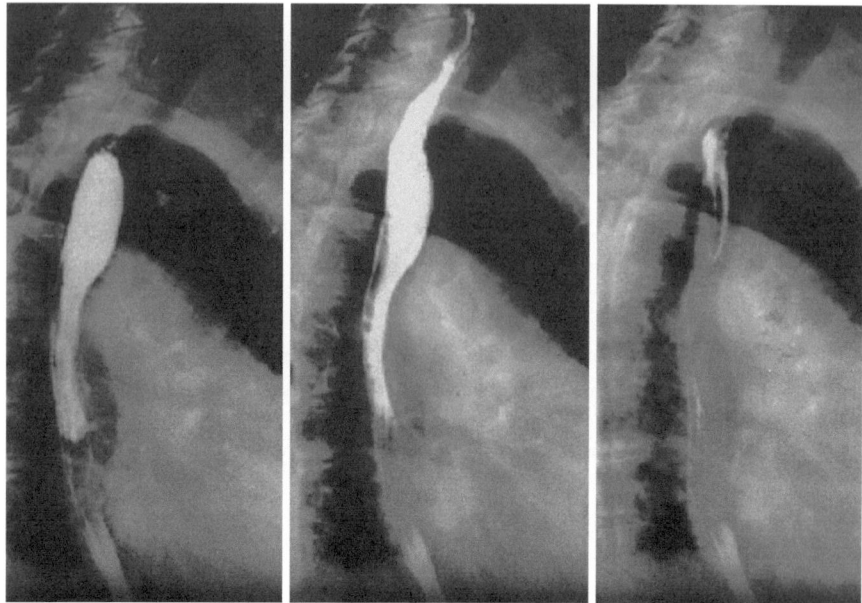

**Fig. 9.2** Example of an esophagopharyngeal reflux of barium recorded during a videofluoroscopic swallowing study. Reproduced with permission from [12]

to pH and impedance monitoring and its diagnostic value is debated [13–15]. Recent guidelines recommend not to perform barium radiographs to diagnose GERD [2].

## Nuclear Medicine

By contrast with the X-ray methods described above, nuclear medicine techniques form an image by administering radiolabelled compounds to the inside the body of the patient and detecting the radiation emitted through the body using external detectors. Gamma emitting tracers and arrays of detectors are used in gamma scintigraphy to locate the source of the radiation inside the patient and to reconstruct an image. Gamma scintigraphy yields a two-dimensional, planar image. Three-dimensional imaging is achieved using a higher degree of sophistication in the detectors array and image reconstruction as used in single photon emission computed tomography (SPECT) and positron emission tomography or PET.

Gamma scintigraphy has long been used to evaluate GERD [16]. The radionuclide of choice is technetium-99m ($^{99m}$Tc) usually added to the solid phase of a meal; in addition, indium-113m ($^{113m}$In) is sometimes used as a dual label for the liquid phase of a meal. Anterior and posterior images are usually acquired for several seconds at pre-defined intervals during gastric emptying of the meal. Radioactive markers are placed on the subjects to allow spatial alignment of the time series. Various methods have been used to maximize the chance of detecting reflux events. These vary from using refluxogenic meals [17] to positioning of the patient [18] and physiological maneuvers [19]. [18]F-Fluorodeoxyglucose (FDG) positron emission tomography (PET) findings on esophageal inflammation have been shown to correlate with endoscopic findings and symptoms in GERD [20].

Imaging lung aspiration of refluxate is a challenge but nuclear medicine techniques offer a better chance due to the high sensitivity to the radioactive tracers and therefore the small quantities of tracer needed for detection. There has been renewed interest [21] in the use of scintigraphy to demonstrate pulmonary aspiration in the postprandial period in GERD-related respiratory disease [22]. The scans can clearly demonstrate aspiration of the radiolabel as increased counts in the lung fields (Fig. 9.3). The use of the technique to evaluate pharyngeal contamination in LPR [23] and lung aspiration [24] is promising. In particular, refluxate may not necessarily be in liquid form but can consist of an aerosol/mist [25]; this makes it more difficult

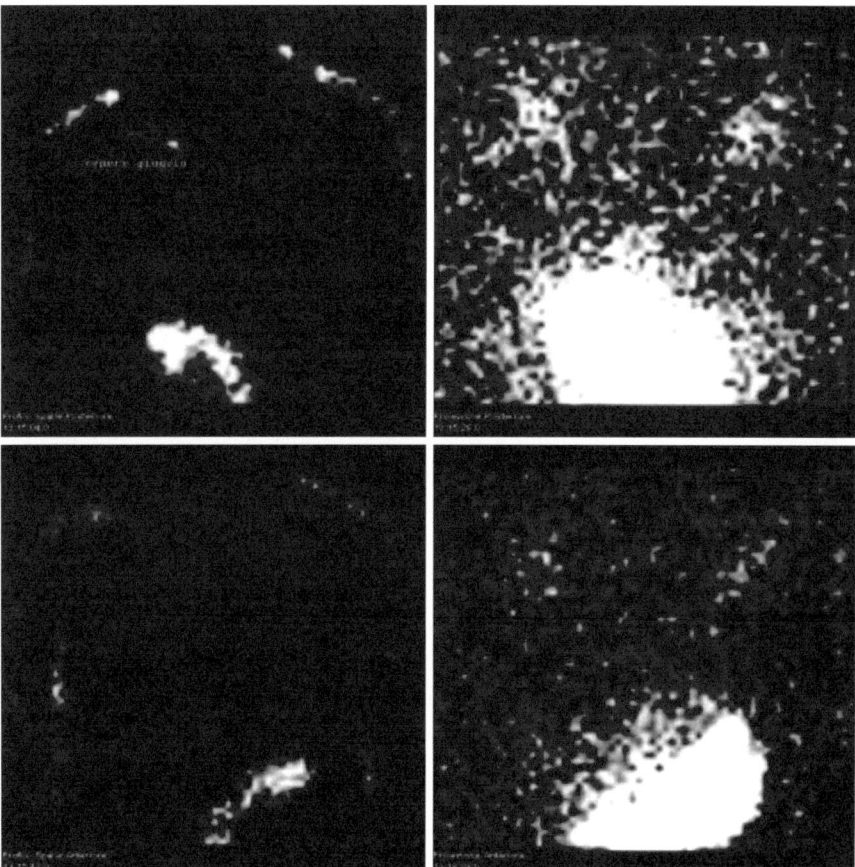

**Fig. 9.3** Overnight [99]Tc scintigraphic scan showing pulmonary aspiration of gastroesophageal reflux. The left panel shows jugular markings and the shoulder and trunk (the anterior projection is shown at the top and the posterior projection at the bottom). The right panel shows zoomed images. The presence of radioactivity is detected within both lung fields indicating bilateral pulmonary aspiration. Reproduced with permission from [21]

to image but the sensitivity of nuclear medicine techniques has been proven to be able to image lung delivery of inhaled aerosol doses for a variety of respiratory medicine indications [26–28]. Two and three dimensional methods are used to image successfully lung regional drug deposition [26] and such methods are promising for the imaging of airway reflux.

As already mentioned, sensitivity is one of the advantages of nuclear medicine techniques, only small concentrations of tracers are administered so the radiation dose is generally not high. The emission images can contain information on activity, function and location. Limitations of scintigraphy are the low temporal and spatial resolution and the relatively sparse availability of units, with the need for large infrastructure or an external supply of radiolabelled tracers. A limitation within the context of reflux is that concomitant pH monitoring studies have shown acid reflux without an increase in gamma counts [17], suggesting that gastric acid secretion can reflux without having mixed with the radioisotope-labeled food and therefore some reflux events are invisible to the gamma camera [29]. Small ambulatory gamma detectors worn over the esophagus have also been used in a research setting to overcome the limitation of restricting the patients to the static gamma camera unit [17]. The literature shows a wide variation of results; this is mostly due to differences in the methods used, from test meals to data acquisition and analysis.

## Magnetic Resonance Imaging

The MRI imaging technique is inherently different from the X-ray and nuclear medicine techniques. When placed in a strong magnetic field the nuclei of hydrogen atoms inside the body of a patient can receive a radiofrequency signal at a given frequency and, in turn, transmit a signal back. Spatial encoding of this process allows reconstructing images from the received radio signal. The signal itself contains information on the physicochemical environment of those hydrogen atoms, which generates the contrast in the images. The skilled operator can tune the imaging to highlight particular characteristics of the tissues or luminal contents. The lack of ionizing radiation allows serial imaging without concerns for a radiation dose, making the technique particularly suited to image gastrointestinal function [30].

Reflux events can be imaged directly by MRI (Fig. 9.4) [31, 32] using MRI fluoroscopy [33] using a positive oral contrast medium. Dynamic swallowing studies investigated the physiology of normal swallowing [34], bolus passage [35] and possible applications to 'MR esophagography' [36]. Both morphology and function could be investigated in such studies, with findings on reflux, motility, hiatal hernias, effects of surgery and cancer [36–40]. MRI has allowed unprecedented insights into the biomechanics of the gastroesophageal junction as a reflux barrier [41, 42]. MRI showed that GERD patients have wider insertion angle of the esophagus into the stomach [43]. This morphological change may alter the function of the 'flap valve' of the sphincter complex; the opening of the esophagogastric junction was

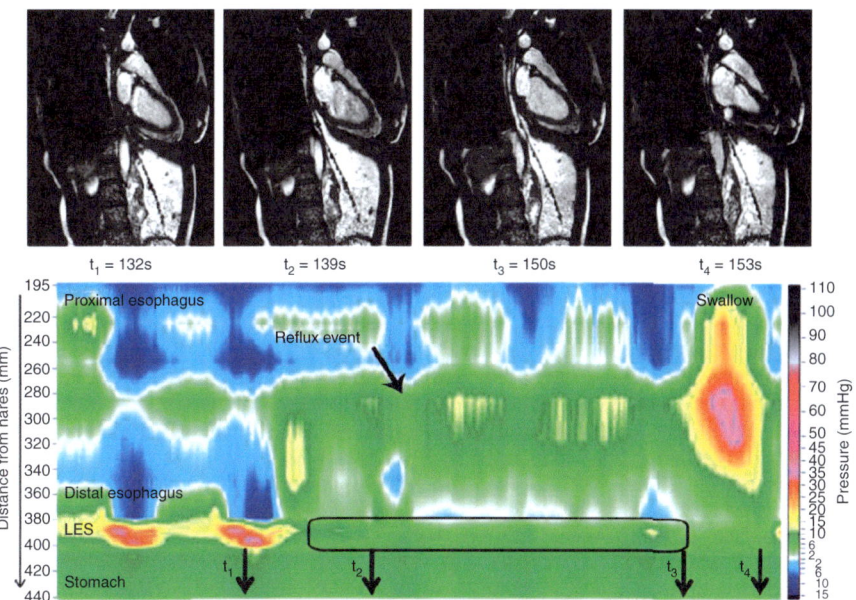

**Fig. 9.4** Concurrent magnetic resonance imaging and high-resolution manometry detection of a gastroesophageal reflux event. Note that shortening of the esophagus in the dynamic MR images appears to draw the proximal stomach upwards relative to the catheter. Reproduced with permission from [31]

also larger in GERD patients compared to control [43] and demonstrated an effect of baclofen treatment on the esophagogastric junction 'functional anatomy' [44].

MRI has various advantages including the lack of ionizing radiation, the multiplanar capability, good spatial resolution and soft tissue contrast. MRI scanners are nowadays widely available. MRI has various limitations. One is the low sensitivity. Imaging can be carried out only in the horizontal position due to the standard configuration of the scanners. It is expensive compared to X-rays. MRI is also contraindicated for patients with certain metal implants in the body such as cardiac pacemakers. Particularly large patients may not fit in the bore of the scanners.

### Conclusions

Reflux is an imaging challenge. The existing whole-body imaging techniques provide information on morphology and function of the upper gastrointestinal tract. Whilst the barium radiographs are currently not recommended to diagnose GERD, a role for MRI is emerging although this is still in its infancy. Nuclear medicine methods can provide information from the orophaynx and lungs, regions of the body that are not accessible to other conventional techniques such as pH and impedance probes. As such they hold promise for the imaging investigation of airway reflux.

## References

1. DeVault KR, Castell DO. Updated guidelines for the diagnosis and treatment of Gastroesophageal reflux disease. Am J Gastroenterol. 2005;100(1):190–200. https://doi.org/10.1111/j.1572-0241.2005.41217.x.
2. Katz PO, Gerson LB, Vela MF. Guidelines for the diagnosis and management of gastroesophageal reflux disease. Am J Gastroenterol. 2013;108(3):308–28. https://doi.org/10.1038/ajg.2012.444.
3. Younes Z, Johnson DA. Diagnostic evaluation in gastroesophageal reflux disease. Gastroenterol Clin N Am. 1999;28(4):809–30. https://doi.org/10.1016/s0889-8553(05)70091-1.
4. Neumann H, Neurath MF, Vieth M, Lever FM, Meijer GJ, Lips IM, McMahon BP, Ruurda JP, van Hillegersberg R, Siersema P, Levine MS, Scharitzer M, Pokieser P, Zerbib F, Savarino V, Zentilin P, Savarino E, Chan WW. Innovative techniques in evaluating the esophagus; imaging of esophageal morphology and function; and drugs for esophageal disease. Ann N Y Acad Sci. 2013;1300:11–28. https://doi.org/10.1111/nyas.12233.
5. Poelmans J, Tack J. Extraoesophageal manifestations of gastrooesophageal reflux. Gut. 2005;54(10):1492–9. https://doi.org/10.1136/gut.2004.053025.
6. Spyridoulias A, Lillie S, Vyas A, Fowler SJ. Detecting laryngopharyngeal reflux in patients with upper airways symptoms: symptoms, signs or salivary pepsin? Respir Med. 2015;109(8):963–9. https://doi.org/10.1016/j.rmed.2015.05.019.
7. Mandal P, Morice AH, Chalmers JD, Hill AT. Symptoms of airway reflux predict exacerbations and quality of life in bronchiectasis. Respir Med. 2013;107(7):1008–13. https://doi.org/10.1016/j.rmed.2013.04.006.
8. Morice AH. Review article: reflux in cough and airway disease. Aliment Pharmacol Ther. 2011;33:48–52.
9. Levine MS, Rubesin SE, Laufer I. Barium esophagography: a study for all seasons. Clin Gastroenterol Hepatol. 2008;6(1):11–25. https://doi.org/10.1016/j.cgh.2007.10.029.
10. Baker ME, Einstein DM, Herts BR, Remer EM, Motta-Ramirez GA, Ehrenwald E, Rice TW, Richter JE. Gastroesophageal reflux disease: integrating the barium esophagram before and after antireflux surgery. Radiology. 2007;243(2):329–39. https://doi.org/10.1148/radiol.2432050057.
11. Levine MS, Rubesin SE. Diseases of the esophagus: diagnosis with esophagography. Radiology. 2005;237(2):414–27. https://doi.org/10.1148/radiol.2372050199.
12. Torrico S, Corazziari E, Habib FI. Barium studies for detecting esophagopharyngeal reflux events. Am J Med. 2003;115:124S–9S. https://doi.org/10.1016/s0002-9343(03)00210-9.
13. Pan JJ, Levine MS, Redfern RO, Rubesin SE, Laufer I, Katzka DA. Gastroesophageal reflux: comparison of barium studies with 24-h pH monitoring. Eur J Radiol. 2003;47(2):149–53. https://doi.org/10.1016/s0720-048x(02)00150-x.
14. Saleh CMG, Smout AJPM, Bredenoord AJ. The diagnosis of gastro-esophageal reflux disease cannot be made with barium esophagograms. Neurogastroenterol Motil. 2015;27(2):195–200. https://doi.org/10.1111/nmo.12457.
15. Thompson JK, Koehler RE, Richter JE. Detection of gastroesophageal reflux - value of barium studies compared with 24-h pH monitoring. Am J Roentgenol. 1994;162(3):621–6.
16. Kaul B, Petersen H, Grette K, Erichsen H, Myrvold HE. Scintigraphy, pH measurement, and radiography in the evaluation of gastroesophageal reflux. Scand J Gastroenterol. 1985;20(3):289–94. https://doi.org/10.3109/00365528509091652.
17. Washington N, Moss HA, Washington C, Greaves JL, Steele RJC, Wilson CG. Noninvasive detection of gastroesophageal reflux using an ambulatory system. Gut. 1993;34(11):1482–6. https://doi.org/10.1136/gut.34.11.1482.
18. Asakura Y, Imai Y, Ota S, Fujiwara K, Miyamae T. Usefulness of gastroesophageal reflux scintigraphy using the knee-chest position for the diagnosis of gastroesophageal reflux disease. Ann Nucl Med. 2005;19(4):291–6. https://doi.org/10.1007/bf02984621.

19. Yapici O, Basoglu T, Canbaz F, Sever A. The role of coughing as a gastroesophageal-reflux provoking maneuver: the scintigraphical evaluation. Nucl Med Commun. 2009;30(6):440–4. https://doi.org/10.1097/MNM.0b013e3283298f90.
20. Wu Y-W, Tseng P-H, Lee Y-C, Wang S-Y, Chiu H-M, Tu C-H, Wang H-P, Lin J-T, Wu M-S, Yang W-S. Association of esophageal Inflammation, obesity and gastroesophageal reflux disease: from FDG PET/CT perspective. PLoS One. 2014;9(3):e92001. https://doi.org/10.1371/journal.pone.0092001.
21. Ravelli AM, Panarotto MB, Verdoni L, Consolati V, Bolognini S. Pulmonary aspiration shown by scintigraphy in gastroesophageal reflux-related respiratory disease. Chest. 2006;130(5):1520–6. https://doi.org/10.1378/chest.130.5.1520.
22. Ruth M, Carlsson S, Mansson I, Bengtsson U, Sandberg N. Scintigraphic detection of gastropulmonary aspiration in patients with respiratory disorders. Clin Physiol. 1993;13(1):19–33. https://doi.org/10.1111/j.1475-097X.1993.tb00314.x.
23. Falk GL, Beattie J, Ing A, Falk SE, Magee M, Burton L, Van der Wall H. Scintigraphy in laryngopharyngeal and gastroesophageal reflux disease: a definitive diagnostic test? World J Gastroenterol. 2015;21(12):3619–27. https://doi.org/10.3748/wjg.v21.i12.3619.
24. Falk M, Van der Wall H, Falk GL. Differences between scintigraphic reflux studies in gastrointestinal reflux disease and laryngopharyngeal reflux disease and correlation with symptoms. Nucl Med Commun. 2015;36(6):625–30. https://doi.org/10.1097/mnm.0000000000000289.
25. Morice AH. Airway reflux as a cause of respiratory disease. Breathe. 2013;9(4):257–66.
26. Conway J. Lung imaging—two dimensional gamma scintigraphy, SPECT, CT and PET. Adv Drug Deliv Rev. 2012;64(4):357–68. https://doi.org/10.1016/j.addr.2012.01.013.
27. Conway J, Fleming J, Majoral C, Katz I, Perchet D, Peebles C, Tossici-Bolt L, Collier L, Caillibotte G, Pichelin M, Sauret-Jackson V, Martonen T, Apiou-Sbirlea G, Muellinger B, Kroneberg P, Gleske J, Scheuch G, Texereau J, Martin A, Montesantos S, Bennett M. Controlled, parametric, individualized, 2-D and 3-D imaging measurements of aerosol deposition in the respiratory tract of healthy human subjects for model validation. J Aerosol Sci. 2012;52:1–17. https://doi.org/10.1016/j.jaerosci.2012.04.006.
28. Corcoran TE. Imaging in aerosol medicine. Respir Care. 2015;60(6):850–5. https://doi.org/10.4187/respcare.03537.
29. Shay SS, Eggli D, Johnson LF. Simultaneous esophageal pH monitoring and scintigraphy during the postprandial period in patients with severe reflux esophagitis. Dig Dis Sci. 1991;36(5):558–64. https://doi.org/10.1007/bf01297019.
30. Marciani L. Assessment of gastrointestinal motor functions by MRI: a comprehensive review. Neurogastroenterol Motil. 2011;23(5):399–407. https://doi.org/10.1111/j.1365-2982.2011.01670.x.
31. Sweis R, Kaufman E, Anggiansah A, Wong T, Dettmar P, Fried M, Schwizer W, Avvari RK, Pal A, Fox M. Post-prandial reflux suppression by a raft-forming alginate (Gaviscon advance) compared to a simple antacid documented by magnetic resonance imaging and pH-impedance monitoring: mechanistic assessment in healthy volunteers and randomised, controlled, double-blind study in reflux patients. Aliment Pharmacol Ther. 2013;37(11):1093–102. https://doi.org/10.1111/apt.12318.
32. Manabe T, Kawamitsu H, Higashino T, Shirasaka D, Aoyama N, Sugimura K. Observation of gastro-esophageal reflux by MRI: a feasibility study. Abdom Imaging. 2009;34(4):419–23. https://doi.org/10.1007/s00261-006-9093-0.
33. Manabe T, Kawamitsu H, Higashino T, Lee H, Fujjj M, Hoshi H, Sugimura K. Esophageal magnetic resonance fluoroscopy optimization of the sequence. J Comput Assist Tomogr. 2004;28(5):697–703. https://doi.org/10.1097/01.rct.0000136863.71871.bb.
34. Zhang S, Olthoff A, Frahm J. Real-time magnetic resonance imaging of normal swallowing. J Magn Reson Imaging. 2012;35(6):1372–9. https://doi.org/10.1002/jmri.23591.
35. Kulinna-Cosentini C, Schima W, Cosentini EP. Dynamic MR imaging of the gastroesophageal junction in healthy volunteers during bolus passage. J Magn Reson Imaging. 2007;25(4):749–54. https://doi.org/10.1002/jmri.20868.

36. Zhang J, Hu W, Zang L, Yao Y, Tang Y, Qian Z, Gao P, Wu X, Li S, Xie Z, Yuan X. Clinical investigation on application of water swallowing to MR esophagography. Eur J Radiol. 2012;81(9):1980–5. https://doi.org/10.1016/j.ejrad.2011.05.010.
37. Baumann T, Kuesters S, Grueneberger J, Marjanovic G, Zimmermann L, Schaefer A-O, Hopt UT, Langer M, Karcz WK. Time-resolved MRI after ingestion of liquids reveals motility changes after laparoscopic sleeve gastrectomy: preliminary results. Obes Surg. 2011;21(1):95–101. https://doi.org/10.1007/s11695-010-0317-6.
38. Kulinna-Cosentini C, Schima W, Ba-Ssalamah A, Cosentini EP. MRI patterns of Nissen fundoplication: normal appearance and mechanisms of failure. Eur Radiol. 2014;24(9):2137–45. https://doi.org/10.1007/s00330-014-3267-x.
39. Kulinna-Cosentini C, Schima W, Lenglinger J, Riegler M, Koelblinger C, Ba-Ssalamah A, Bischof G, Weber M, Kleinhansl P, Cosentini EP. Is there a role for dynamic swallowing MRI in the assessment of gastroesophageal reflux disease and oesophageal motility disorders? Eur Radiol. 2012;22(2):364–70. https://doi.org/10.1007/s00330-011-2258-4.
40. Miyazaki Y, Nakajima K, Sumikawa M, Yamasaki M, Takahashi T, Miyata H, Takiguchi S, Kurokawa Y, Tomiyama N, Mori M, Doki Y. Magnetic resonance imaging for simultaneous morphological and functional evaluation of esophageal motility disorders. Surg Today. 2014;44(4):668–76. https://doi.org/10.1007/s00595-013-0617-2.
41. Curcic J, Fox M, Kaufman E, Forras-Kaufman Z, Hebbard GS, Roy S, Pal A, Schwizer W, Fried M, Treier R, Boesiger P. Gastroesophageal junction: structure and function as assessed by MR imaging. Radiology. 2010;257(1):115–24.
42. Roy S, Fox MR, Curcic J, Schwizer W, Pal A. The gastro-esophageal reflux barrier: biophysical analysis on 3D models of anatomy from magnetic resonance imaging. Neurogastroenterol Motil. 2012;24(7):616–25. https://doi.org/10.1111/j.1365-2982.2012.01909.x.
43. Curcic J, Roy S, Schwizer A, Kaufman E, Forras-Kaufman ZA, Menne D, Hebbard GS, Treier R, Boesiger P, Steingoetter A, Fried M, Schwizer W, Pal A, Fox M. Abnormal structure and function of the esophagogastric junction and proximal stomach in gastroesophageal reflux disease. Am J Gastroenterol. 2014;109(5):658–67. https://doi.org/10.1038/ajg.2014.25.
44. Curcic J, Schwizer A, Kaufman E, Forras-Kaufman Z, Banerjee S, Pal A, Hebbard GS, Boesiger P, Fried M, Steingoetter A, Schwizer W, Fox M. Effects of baclofen on the functional anatomy of the oesophago-gastric junction and proximal stomach in healthy volunteers and patients with GERD assessed by magnetic resonance imaging and high-resolution manometry: a randomised controlled double-blind study. Aliment Pharmacol Ther. 2014;40(10):1230–40. https://doi.org/10.1111/apt.12956.

# High Resolution Oesophageal Manometry in the Investigation of Unexplained Cough

**10**

Jennifer Burke and Warren Jackson

## Introduction

Abnormal motor activity in the oesophagus can result in oesophageal dysmotility, leading to a variety of complaints such as difficulty swallowing, chest pain and acid reflux [1]. Until recent technological advances in the arena of clinical gastrointestinal measurement, oesophageal motility has been investigated using conventional manometry systems. Conventional oesophageal manometry involves the trans-nasal passage of a pressure sensitive catheter in to the stomach. Pressure sensitivity is achieved with this system by using a series of transducers located either within, or fixed directly to the catheter as shown in Fig. 10.1. This enables motor function assessment of the upper oesophageal sphincter (UOS), oesophageal body and lower oesophageal sphincter (LOS).

In recent years an association between oesophageal dysmotility and cough has been demonstrated [2–4]. Although this relationship is poorly understood, there are a number of mechanisms by which it is suspected that abnormal oesophageal motility could elicit a cough response; these will be discussed later in the chapter.

The association between respiratory complaints and oesophageal motor abnormalities identified using conventional manometry was first explored by Fouad et al. [2] who compared patients presenting exclusively with heartburn to a group of chronic cough patients. Comparison of the manometric profiles of the groups demonstrated that ineffective oesophageal motility was a common abnormality in both cohorts; however, weak or failed peristalsis was significantly more prevalent in patients with chronic cough. Kastelik et al. [3] also examined the oesophageal motility of patients with unexplained cough.

---

J. Burke (✉) · W. Jackson
Hull & East Yorkshire Hospitals NHS Trust, Hull, UK
e-mail: Jennifer.burke@hey.nhs.uk; Warren.jackson@hey.nhs.uk

© Springer International Publishing AG, part of Springer Nature 2018
A. H. Morice, P. W. Dettmar (eds.), *Reflux Aspiration and Lung Disease*,
https://doi.org/10.1007/978-3-319-90525-9_10

Comparably to Fouad et al., these authors also revealed a high incidence of oesophageal dysmotility, revealing suboptimal peristalsis in one-third of the cohort.

Although historical studies point to a previously undiscovered association between cough and oesophageal dysmotility, study participants have routinely been investigated using conventional manometry. For several decades conventional oesophageal manometry has been the test of choice to assess motor function, however, the accuracy of this manometric system with as few as three pressure sensors is limited by several factors. Firstly, the poor spatial resolution between pressure recording sites results in a loss of contractile data from sections of the oesophageal body. Secondly, the scarcity of pressure recording sites necessitates a separate assessment for each section of the oesophagus. Consequently, the sheer volume of line graphs produced can be time-consuming and complicated to interpret. Outcomes of the investigations have also been thwarted by a lack of a standardised process in performing the study and thus defining oesophageal motility disorders.

## Conventional Manometry

During conventional oesophageal manometry, each of the pressure sensors illustrated in Fig. 10.1 record the amplitude of the contraction of the muscle layers as the peristaltic sequence passes through the oesophageal body. The pressure generated by the contraction of the muscle layers distorts the transducer membrane which alters the electrical resistance across the sensor. The changes in the electrical signal for each particular sensor are then modified and converted in to a real time individual line graph as demonstrated in Fig. 10.1.

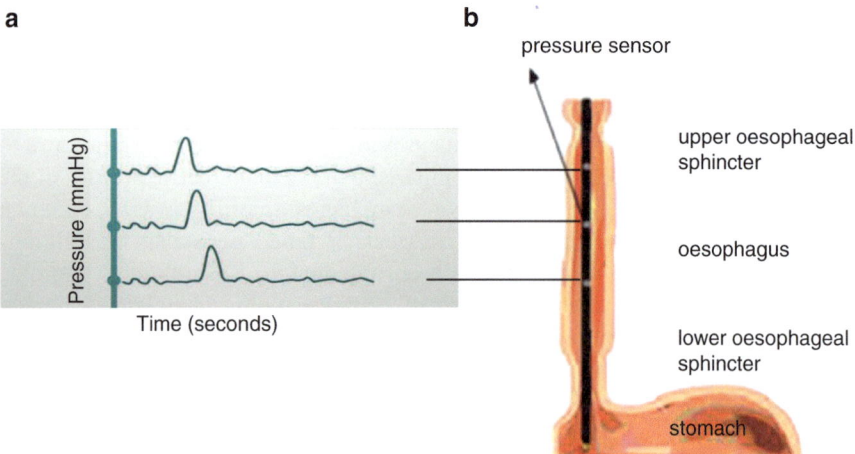

**Fig. 10.1** (**a**) shows a simplified conventional manometry trace of a peristaltic contraction. (**b**) Indicates the positioning of three pressure sensors along the length of the manometry catheter

## High Resolution Manometry: How Does it Work?

The relatively recent introduction of high resolution oesophageal manometry (HRM) has transformed the contractile data available from the oesophagus by vastly increasing the number of pressure transducers. HRM catheters can offer up to 36 closely spaced pressure recording sites allowing a simultaneous examination of the pressure profile throughout the entire length of the oesophagus. A fundamental advantage of HRM is that it enables the valuable addition of colour topography. Colour contour plots (topography) are derived from the intraluminal pressure data enabling operators of the system to be led by picture recognition resulting in faster and more accurate analysis.

The technical theory of HRM topography can be illustrated using pressure graphs from a conventional manometry trace during a peristaltic contraction.

Firstly, each unit of pressure is assigned a colour, creating a 'colour bar' which can be observed at the top of Fig. 10.2.

The software converts the pressure trace from each of the 36 sensors in to individual colour bars (Fig. 10.3).

Gaps in the data between each of the 36 pressure sensors are interpolated resulting in the final contour plot, Fig. 10.4. Interpolation describes the process by which algorithms provide estimated pressures between actual sensor data which gives the appearance of continuous pressure information along the entire length of the luminal axis as demonstrated in Fig. 10.4.

## Improved Detection of Transient Lower Oesophageal Sphincter Relaxations

HRM can effortlessly highlight previously elusive changes at the level of the LOS such as transient lower oesophageal sphincter relaxations (TLOSR). A TLOSR describes the spontaneous relaxation of the LOS and inhibition of the

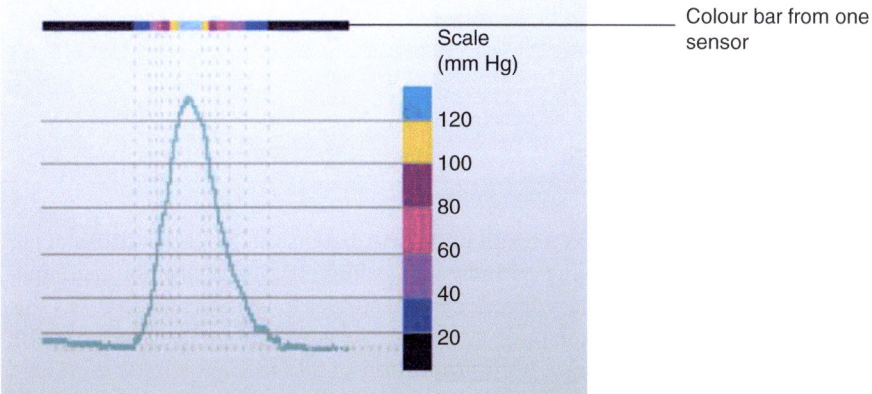

**Fig. 10.2** A recording from one pressure sensor within the oesophagus during a peristaltic contraction. Image used with permission of MMS International

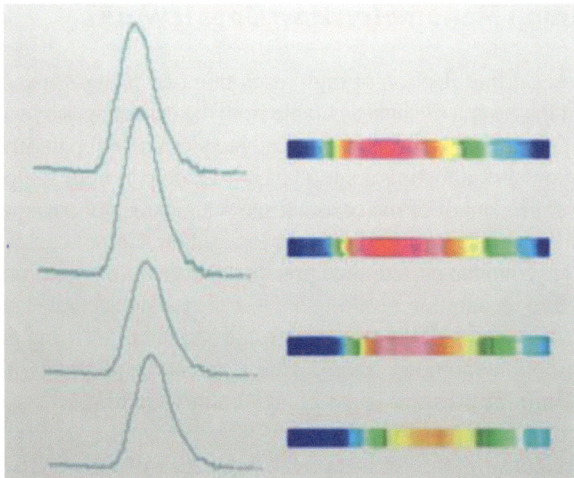

**Fig. 10.3** Pressure traces from 4 of the 36 pressure sensors during a peristaltic wave sequence and their corresponding colour bar. Image used with permission of MMS International

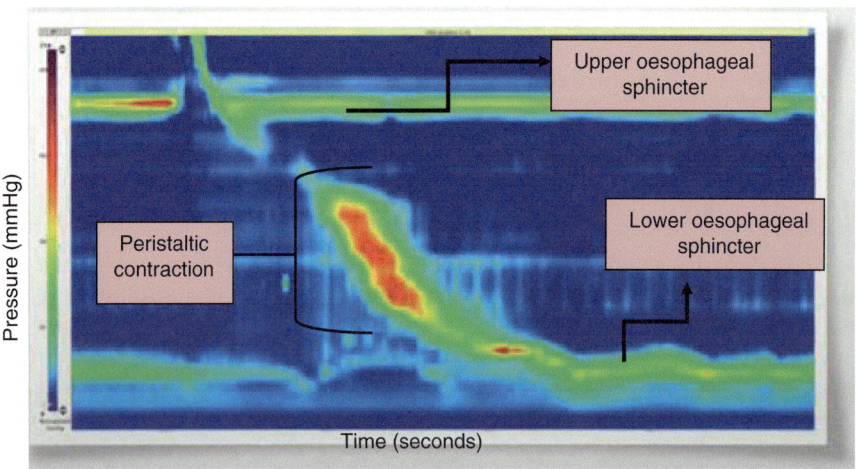

**Fig. 10.4** Final colour plot

crural diaphragm usually as a result of gastric distension [5]. Relaxations occur independently of swallowing as indicated in Fig. 10.5, and are not accompanied by peristalsis. In the last decade several studies have indicated that TLOSR represent the main mechanism of all types of gastro-oesophageal reflux, with the majority demonstrating a high proportion of TLOSR associated with acid reflux in gastro-oesophageal reflux disease patients as opposed to controls [6–9].

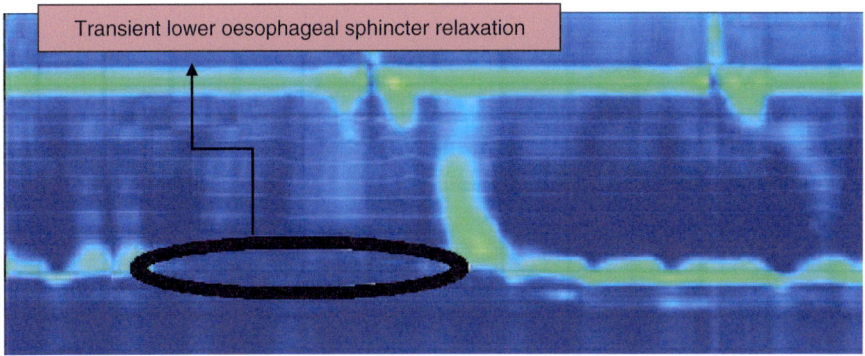

**Fig. 10.5** Spontaneous relaxation of the LOS during HRM. Image used with the permission of Wang et al. [10]

## Gastro-Oesophageal Pressure Gradients

Transient relaxations of the LOS pose a significant risk in respiratory diseases that exhibit hyperinflation due to the effect that this type of breathing has on the inspiratory gastro-oesophageal pressure gradient (GOPG). The GOPG refers to the gradient produced by the pressure profiles of the thorax and abdomen and their subsequent effect on oesophageal and gastric pressures. The gradient represents the difference between the intragastric and the intraoesophageal pressure and is generated by calculating the abdominal pressure minus the thoracic pressure. These figures are readily available and easy to identify using HRM as demonstrated in Fig. 10.6.

Pauwels et al. [11] revealed a significantly lower intraoesophageal pressure in the inspiratory phase of respiration in a small cohort of cystic fibrosis (CF) patients compared to healthy controls. As such, an increased inspiratory GOPG was found in the CF group. Since transient relaxations represent the most prevalent mechanism for reflux, an increased inspiratory GOPG during a TLOSR can promote reflux in this type of patient, since the usual protective barrier to reflux offered by the LOS and crural diaphragm are lost during a transient relaxation. This notion is supported by the fact that participants of the CF group in the study carried out by Pauwels and colleagues showed significantly more reflux episodes that started during inspiration than in expiration, whereas in healthy subjects, reflux occurred equally in both respiratory phases.

Using HRM, we [12] recently compared the inspiratory GOPG and oesophageal motility of a group of 61 patients with unexplained respiratory symptoms such as cough and breathlessness to an age and sex matched group of patients with typical dyspeptic symptoms. These findings demonstrated a significantly higher inspiratory GOPG in the respiratory group as well as a significantly higher prevalence of oesophageal dysmotility compared to the dyspeptic group.

## Performing HRM

Patients should remain nil-by-mouth for 4 h prior to the investigation. If the patient is undergoing HRM only, and on the instruction the referring physician, medications influencing esophageal motility should be stopped 72 h prior to the procedure. These include:

- Calcium antagonists
- Erythromycin
- Nitrates
- Prokinetics

The Association of Gastrointestinal Physiologists Guidelines for performing HRM are as follows:

- 10 × 5 ml swallows of water (each 5 ml water bolus separated by 20–30 s to allow evaluation of each peristaltic sequence).
- 30 s of tidal breathing to assess the resting tone of the lower oesophageal sphincter (uninterrupted by factors which may influence LOS tone such as swallowing, coughing and belching).
- A multiple rapid swallow consisting of 5 × 2 ml swallows of water (in rapid succession, allowing time to observe the peristaltic reserve).
- 5 single swallows of bread separated by a 20–30 s intervals to allow evaluation of the peristaltic sequence following a bread bolus.

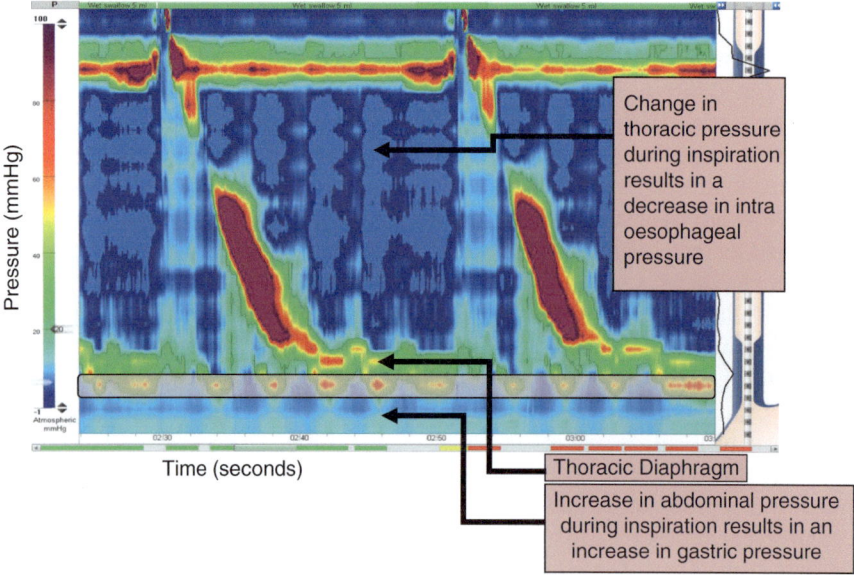

**Fig. 10.6** Demonstration of intragastric and intra oesophageal pressure fluctuations during tidal breathing

## Recent Developments in Physiological Measurement

Currently, the most comprehensive method of measuring oesophageal motility is HRM combined with impedance technology (HRIM). Impedance technology is a useful addition to HRM, employing a series of paired electrical components alongside the existing pressure transducers of the manometry catheter. The resistance to the electrical current passing between each pair of electrical components is derived depending on the conductivity of the matter passing over the sensors at any given time. The more conductive the matter between the paired components, the lower the resistance and thus the impedance, measured in Ohms ($\Omega$). Conversely, a high level of impedance is produced by poor conductivity between the components. As a result, it is possible to determine the direction and composition of a bolus as shown in Fig. 10.7. In oesophageal manometry, this is particularly beneficial since it enables investigators to examine the efficiency of the clearance following a peristaltic contraction after a swallowed bolus (as demonstrated in Fig. 10.8).

Almansa et al. [4] are the most recent investigators to employ both HRIM and 24-h impedance pH-metry in the study of chronic cough. This group concluded that one-third of their study population, comprised of chronic cough patients, exhibited weak peristalsis with large breaks. Using HRIM alongside ambulatory impedance pH-metry, this group demonstrated that chronic cough patients with suboptimal peristalsis categorised by weak peristalsis were associated with a significant delay in clearance of both reflux events and the clearance of swallowed boluses.

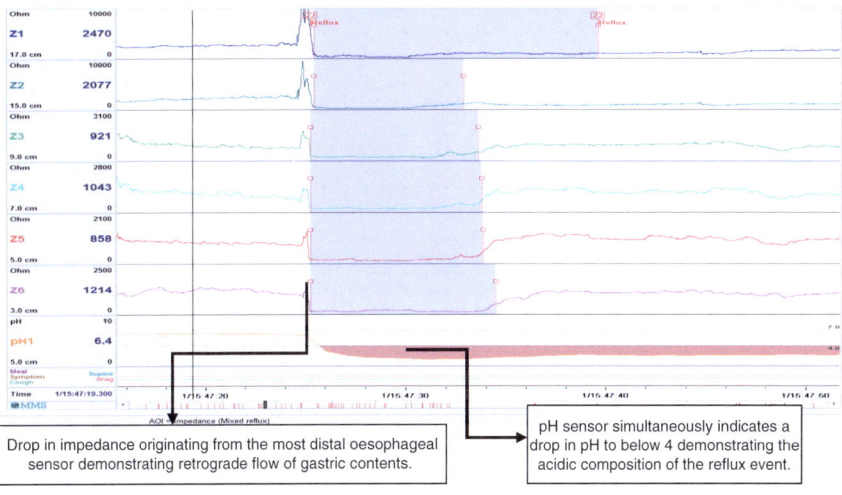

**Fig. 10.7** Impedance pH trace

## Oesophageal Dysmotility and the Mechanism of Cough

Microaspiration is one of several theories postulated in the mechanism of unexplained cough. Oesophageal dysmotility could be significant in this process since it is possible that physiological volumes of gastro-oesophageal reflux inadequately returned to the stomach could remain in the oesophagus and be encouraged upwards to the airways over a period of time. However, in one study [13] the gastric enzyme pepsin was used as a marker to explore the theory of microaspiration in chronic cough. These authors compared the amount of pepsin in the lungs of a group of unselected chronic cough patients, and a control group of healthy volunteers and found that patients with chronic cough did not have significant amounts of reflux into their proximal oesophagus or a significant amount of pepsin in their airways, despite having more reflux when compared with healthy volunteers. Furthermore, patients with abnormal levels of reflux had no more pepsin in the airways compared with those with physiological levels of reflux.

Another likely mechanism of unexplained cough is stimulation of the oesophageal-bronchial reflex. Convergence of afferents of the vagus nerve from the respiratory tract and oesophagus in the same part of the brain stem suggest the existence of an oesophageal-bronchial reflex, with preliminary evidence showing that a transcription factor is expressed in the distal oesophagus [14]. Oesophageal dysmotility could be a key factor in the activation of this reflex since poor clearance of

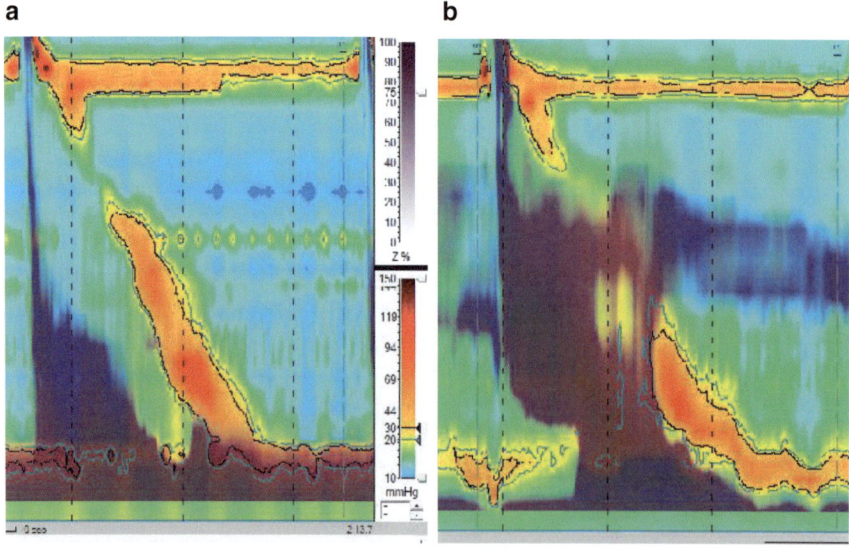

**Fig. 10.8** HRIM trace. (**a**) A normal peristaltic contraction of adequate amplitude showing sufficient clearance of the purple overlay denoting the low impedance associated with a liquid bolus. (**b**) A peristaltic contraction with a large break in the upper oesophagus. Impedance technology indicates poor clearance of the swallowed bolus with visual escape of liquid which remains in the proximal oesophagus. Image used with the permission of the Functional Gut Clinic, London, UK

swallowed food and liquids could lead to prolonged exposure thus triggering significant respiratory symptoms. It is possible that reflux events could elicit the same response. Ing et al. [15, 16] supported this theory by conducting a study in which acid was infused in to the oesophagus of patients with chronic cough to determine the response of the oesophageal-bronchial reflex. This group of authors found that infusion of acid in to the distal oesophagus resulted in an increased frequency of coughing when compared to infusions of normal saline. In addition, Rosztocy et al. [17] found that individuals with an oesophageal-bronchial response to acid exposure were more likely to have an acid-sensitive oesophagus. This may indicate hypersensitivity to physiological levels of gastro-oesophageal reflux deemed to be normal by 24 h pH-metry.

Along with other outcome based studies [18], Ziora et al. [19] demonstrated an increased threshold for cough in patients that had undergone laparoscopic fundoplication which the authors theorize is as a result of a weakening of the oesophageal-bronchial reflex. This assumption could explain why some patients who had failed PPI therapy had marked improvement following a Nissen's fundoplication [20].

Oesophageal function tests have become increasingly popular in the assessment of unexplained respiratory symptoms. As technological advances such as HRIM and impedance pH-metry facilitate the exploration of the association between respiratory disease and disorders of oesophageal motility, it is hoped that we can further our understanding of this complex relationship and ultimately develop resolutions for these troubling, unexplained symptoms.

## References

1. Daum C, Sweis R, Kaufman E, Fuellemann A, Anggiansah A, Fried M, Fox M. Failure to respond to physiologic challenge characterizes esophageal motility in erosive gastro-esophageal reflux disease. Neurogastroenterol Motil. 2011;23:517–e200.
2. Fouad YM, Katz PO, Hatlebakk JG, et al. Ineffective esophageal motility: the most common motility abnormality in patients with GERD- associated respiratory symptoms. Am J Gastroenterol. 1999;94:1464–7.
3. Kastelik JA, Redington AE, Aziz I, Buckton GK, Smith CM, Dakkak M, Morice AH. Abnormal oesophageal motility in patients with chronic cough. Thorax. 2003;58:699–702.
4. Almansa C, Smith JA, Morris J. Weak peristalsis with large breaks in chronic cough: association with poor esophageal clearance. Neurogastroenterol Motil. 2015;27(3):431–42.
5. Pickering M, Jones JF. The diaphragm: two physiological muscles in one. J Anat. 2002;201:305–12.
6. Sifrim D, Holloway R, Silny J, Tack J, Lerut A, Janssens J. Composition of the postprandial refluxate in patients with gastroesophageal reflux disease. Am J Gastroenterol. 2001;96:647–55.
7. Trudgill NJ, Riley SA. Transient lower esophageal sphincter relaxations are no more frequent in patients with gastroesophageal reflux disease than in asymptomatic volunteers. Am J Gastroenterol. 2001;96:2569–74.
8. Sifrim D, Holloway R. Transient lower esophageal sphincter relaxations: how many or how harmful? Am J Gastroenterol. 2001;96:2529–32.
9. Schoeman MN, Tippett MD, Akkermans LM, Dent J, Holloway RH. Mechanisms of gastro-esophageal reflux in ambulant healthy human subjects. Gastroenterology. 1995;108:83–91.
10. Wang YT, Yazaki E, Sifrim D. High-resolution manometry: esophageal disorders not addressed by the "Chicago Classification". J Neurogastroenterol Motil. 2012;18(4):365–72. https://doi.org/10.5056/jnm.2012.18.4.365.

11. Pauwels A, Blondeau K, Dupont L, Sifrim D. Mechanisms of increased gastroesophageal reflux in patients with cystic fibrosis. Am J Gastroenterol. 2012;107(9):1346–53.
12. Burke J, Jackson W, Faruqi S, Morice A. High incidence of oesophageal dysmotility in unexplained respiratory symptoms. Eur Respir J. 2015;46(suppl 59). https://doi.org/10.1183/13993003.congress-2015.PA45.
13. Decalmer S, Stovold R, Houghton LA, Pearson J, Ward C, Kelsall A, Jones H, Mcguinness K, Woodcock A, Smith JA. Chronic cough: relationship between microaspiration, gastroesophageal reflux, and cough frequency. Chest. 2012;142:958–64.
14. Crisera CA, et al. TTF-1 and HNF-3beta in the developing tracheoesophageal fistula: further evidence for the respiratory origin of the distal esophagus. J Pediatr Surg. 1999;34:1322–6.
15. Ing AJ, Ngu MC, Rosen R, Johnston N, Hart K, Khatwa U, Nurko S. The presence of pepsin in the lung and its relationship to pathologic gastro-esophageal reflux. Neurogastroenterol Motil. 2012;24:129–33. e84–5
16. Breslin AB. Pathogenesis of chronic persistent cough associated with gastroesophageal reflux. Am J Respir Crit Care Med. 1994;149:160–7.
17. Rosztóczy A, Makk L, Izbéki F, Róka R, Somfay A, Wittmann T. Asthma and gastroesophageal reflux: clinical evaluation of esophago-bronchial reflex and proximal reflux. Digestion. 2008;77(3–4):218–24.
18. Novitsky YW, Zawacki JK, Irwin RS, French CT, Hussey VM, Callery MP. Chronic cough due to gastroesophageal reflux disease: efficacy of antireflux surgery. Surg Endosc. 2002;16:567–71.
19. Ziora D, Jarosz W, Dzielicki J, Ciekalski J, Krzywiecki A, Dworniczak S, Kozielski J. Citric acid cough threshold in patients with gastroesophageal reflux disease rises after laparoscopic fundoplication. Chest. 2005;128:2458–64.
20. Irwin RS, Zawacki JK, Wilson MM, et al. Chronic cough due to gastroesophageal reflux disease: failure to resolve despite total/near-total elimination of esophageal acid. Chest. 2002;121:1132–40.

# Cough Monitoring in Reflux Lung Disease

**11**

Aakash K. Pandya, Joanne E. Kavanagh, and Surinder S. Birring

## Introduction

Gastro-oesophageal reflux (GOR) is a common cause of chronic cough and its assessment is a key component of cough management guidelines [1]. GOR may be suspected in a patient complaining of heartburn but it is often unclear if GOR and cough are causally linked since GOR is prevalent in the general population. Furthermore, typical symptoms of GOR may be absent and cough may be the only manifestation. The assessment of patients may therefore require objective demonstration of GOR and its relationship with cough. The most widely used tools are oesophageal pH and impedance monitors and manometry. Cough is usually recorded by the patient with an event marker or detected during oesophageal manometry from increases in oesophageal pressure. A can then be calculated to determine if cough and GOR are temporally related [2]. This involves calculating the probability that the observed association between reflux and cough occurred by chance with the Fisher exact test.

The investigation of GOR in patients with cough is challenging for a number of reasons. First, the presence of GOR is a poor predictor of a response to therapy [3] and so many clinicians resort to trials of anti-reflux therapy rather than pursue investigations. This may involve high-dose drug therapy for a prolonged duration, which is not ideal given it may be ineffective, delay alternative investigations or treatments for the patient's cough and expose them to potential side effects. Second, although the demonstration of a temporal relationship between cough and GOR is thought to

---

A. K. Pandya · J. E. Kavanagh
King's College London, Respiratory Medicine, Division of Asthma, Allergy and Lung Biology, London, UK

S. S. Birring (✉)
Centre for Human and Applied Physiological Sciences, School of Basic and Medical Biosciences, Faculty of Life Sciences and Medicine, King's College London, London, UK
e-mail: surinder.birring@nhs.net

© Springer International Publishing AG, part of Springer Nature 2018
A. H. Morice, P. W. Dettmar (eds.), *Reflux Aspiration and Lung Disease*, https://doi.org/10.1007/978-3-319-90525-9_11

be more important than the presence of GOR, it has been hampered by the inaccuracy of cough detection associated with subjective reporting. Recently, there have been significant advances in the assessment of cough severity, and a number of validated tools are now available. The development of objective cough monitoring tools has allowed an in-depth investigation of the relationship between GOR and cough events. This chapter reviews the utility of cough monitoring in reflux lung disease, particularly in patients with chronic cough in whom most studies have been conducted. The review will discuss the relationship between the type and site of GOR and cough frequency, the temporal relationship between cough and GOR, and the use of cough monitors to evaluate the efficacy of therapy.

## Limitations of Current Methodology Used to Assess Cough During GOR Investigations

A typical patient with chronic cough will cough on average 500 times per 24-h (these are single events, whether occurring singly or in bouts recorded during 24-h cough monitoring). This is significantly higher than a healthy subject, who on average will cough 25 times per 24-h [4–6].

Cough is commonly assessed during 24-h oesophageal monitoring with either a patient-triggered event marker or detection from simultaneous oesophageal manometry, however, both of these methods are inaccurate for detecting cough frequency. The poor relationship between subjective and objective measures of cough has been well documented [7]. The true rates of coughing are 6–18 times more than those reported in studies using patient reported cough [8]. Oesophageal manometry is likely to miss low-intensity coughs, and is also likely to be associated with significant false-positives. The true rates of cough are likely to be 2–3 times greater than those reported from oesophageal manometry studies [7]. This is likely to impact the accuracy of the SAP index reported in oesophageal studies. There is clearly a need for accurate methods of quantifying cough in future studies. Another important consideration is that the presence of an oesophageal catheter has a significant impact on the frequency of cough, reducing it by 33% compared to subjects without a catheter [9]. It is not known whether this impacts the temporal relationship between GOR and cough.

## Validated Tools to Assess the Severity of Cough

A comprehensive assessment of cough involves the assessment of its severity, frequency and intensity and its impact on health related quality of life. There are a number of validated patient reported outcome tools available [10]. Cough severity can be assessed with a 100mms visual analogue scale, which is perhaps the simplest and most practical tool [11]. Cough severity can also be assessed with a Cough Severity Diary, a seven-item questionnaire [12]. The impact of cough on health-related quality of life can be assessed with either the Leicester Cough Questionnaire

(LCQ) or the Cough-specific Quality of Life Questionnaire (CQLQ); both have been well validated [13, 14]. The LCQ is a 19-item questionnaire and the CQLQ comprises 28 items. The objective assessment of cough intensity is possible in the laboratory with physiological measures such as cough flow [15], but the subjective assessment of cough intensity has seldom been studied. Recent advances in digital recording devices and improved battery life have facilitated the development of validated cough frequency monitors. Cough frequency monitoring has emerged as a key objective outcome measure in trials of anti-tussive therapy. Its advantage over subjective end-points is that it is not influenced by the mood of the patient or their perception of symptoms, and more accurately reflects the degree of coughing. The ideal assessment of patients is one that includes both subjective and objective measures to capture the frequency and intensity of cough and its impact on the individual.

## Cough Monitoring

Cough detection is possible in the patient's own environment with ambulatory cough monitors. They detect cough from sound recordings; an example of a cough sound is illustrated in Fig. 11.1. The two most widely used cough monitors are the Leicester Cough Monitor (LCM) and the VitaloJak [4, 16] and both have been validated for cough detection. The LCM comprises a portable MP3 recorder that can record for up to 4 days and a free-field microphone. The recording is processed by automated software. The LCM detects cough using an approach based on Hidden Marker Models that are commonly used in speech recognition software. An example of 24-h cough frequency report from a patient with cough and GOR is shown in Fig. 11.2. The LCM has been utilised in clinical trials of Gabapentin, Pregabalin and Erythromycin in patients with cough [17–19]. The VitaloJak monitor comprises a recorder and two microphones; skin contact and free-field types [16]. The recording is processed through software that eliminates segments containing low-level noise or no sound. The condensed recording is then manually analysed by a trained observer, who listens to the sound in conjunction with the visual sound signal. The

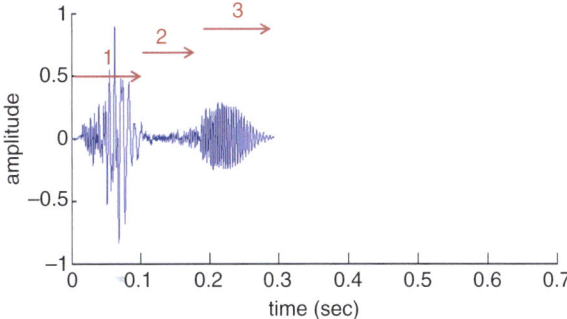

**Fig. 11.1** A cough sound. Cough sound with 3 phases: (1) explosive, (2) intermediate and (3) voiced

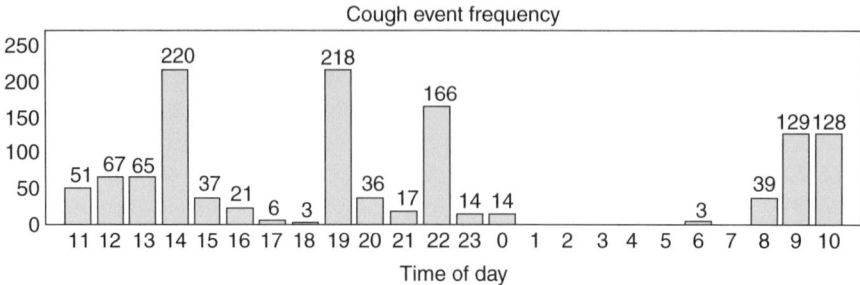

**Fig. 11.2** 24-h objective cough frequency in a patient with gastro-oesophageal reflux and cough. Note reduced or absent cough at night during sleep (physiological diurnal variation in cough frequency). The peaks of cough frequency corresponded to the meal times

VitaloJak has been used in clinical trials of a P2X3 inhibitor, Codeine and Transient Receptor Potential Vanilloid-1 (TRPV1) antagonist [20–22].

Cough frequency is subject to diurnal variation, with most coughing occuring when a subject is awake. Female subjects cough more frequently than males, consistent with gender differences in other cough outcome measures such as cough reflex sensitivity and quality of life. Cough frequency, is a repeatable and responsive measure, and therefore ideal to assess the efficacy of therapy. An advantage of cough monitoring tools over other objective measures such as cough reflex sensitivity challenge tests is their ability to discriminate subjects with cough from healthy controls. Cough monitoring tools are largely used in research and clinical trials to assess cough objectively; in the clinic, physicians prefer patient-reported measures of cough severity because they are the more clinically relevant from the patient's perspective and easier to administer.

## The Relationship Between the Type and Site of GOR and Cough Frequency

The ability to combine oesophageal studies with 24-h cough monitoring in a research setting has enabled an insight into the temporal relationship between the type of reflux and cough. Decalmer et al. investigated 100 unselected patients with chronic cough with 24-h oesophageal impendence/pH monitoring and cough monitoring [23]. They also assessed the concentration of pepsin, a potential marker of aspiration, in sputum and bronchoalveolar lavage (BAL) samples. They compared this group with 32 healthy controls. The median number of all reflux events in patients with chronic cough was 63 per 24 h and this was similar to healthy subjects, who had 59 reflux events per 24 h. Most reflux events occurred in the distal (80%) rather than proximal oesophagus. The distal oesophageal reflux events predicted 26% of the variance in 24-h cough frequency, whereas the proximal oesophageal reflux events did not predict cough frequency. There was no increase in detectable pepsin in the airways of the chronic cough patients. Therefore, distal oesophageal reflux events seem to be more important compared to proximal oesophageal reflux or micro-aspirations. This study is an excellent example of the use of cough monitoring in combination with oesophageal tests to understand the mechanism of disease. The findings of this study suggest that the number of reflux events in patients with chronic cough, acid or non-acid, are similar to healthy subjects and that microaspiration is not a common cause of cough. Could a temporal association between reflux and cough be more important than the number of reflux events?

## The Temporal Association Between Reflux and Cough Events

An example of the temporal association between GOR and cough events is shown in Fig. 11.3. The optimal conditions to conduct such a study are not known but it seems appropriate that the patient is studied when symptomatic and off proton pump inhibitors and other GOR treatments. Two studies have investigated the temporal association between reflux and cough events with objective cough sound monitoring. The study by Smith et al. is the most comprehensive [24]. This study investigated 71 unselected patients with chronic cough who had typical causes reflecting a specialist cough clinic, such as rhinitis, asthma, gastro-oesophageal reflux. Patients underwent combined and synchronised studies of oesophageal pH/impedance and 24-h cough monitoring. They also underwent assessment of cough reflex sensitivity with a citric acid cough challenge test. A temporal relationship was established if a cough event occurred within 2 minutes of a reflux event (with reflux

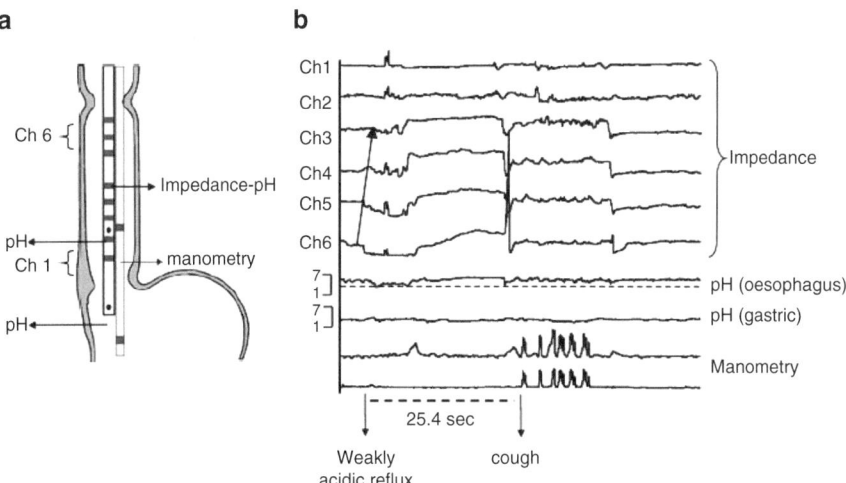

**Fig. 11.3** An example of a temporal association between gastro-oesophageal reflux and cough [2]. (**a**) An example of impedance-pH and manometry catheters positioned in the oesophagus. (**b**) An example of a tracing of impedance-pH and manometry monitoring—a weakly acid reflux preceding a cough event. With permission from Professor Daniel Sifrim [2]

preceding cough). A Symptom Association Probability Index was calculated for the temporal association, and this was based on the probability of the distribution of data occurring by chance alone. Smith et al. also assessed the temporal relationship when cough preceded reflux events, also using a 2-minute time window.

Most bouts of cough in the Smith study were not preceded by reflux events; only 33% were preceded by reflux events. There was a positive SAP for reflux causing (preceding) cough in 48% of subjects, but this was not related to the underlying aetiology of cough. The findings of Smith et al. raise the possibility that a positive SAP for reflux-cough may not be predictive of the response to reflux therapy since many patients would have undergone a trial of GOR therapy. The findings also suggest that reflux may be a co-factor important in many aetiologies of cough, such as cough-variant asthma and upper airways cough syndrome. The study findings require caution because the study was not designed to investigate the aetiology or therapeutic response and furthermore, the number of subjects with established reflux aetiology was small. A similar number of subjects (56%) had a positive SAP for cough preceding reflux events. Hence, it seems that reflux events are equally likely to follow cough when they are temporally associated. An interesting finding in this study was that patients with a positive SAP for reflux-cough had a heightened cough reflex, compared to those with a negative SAP for reflux-cough. This suggests central neuronal sensitisation may be the basis for the association between reflux and cough. These findings require confirmation in further studies.

Kunsch et al. also investigated the temporal relationship between cough and reflux events [25]. They investigated 25 patients with reflux who also reported respiratory symptoms and 20 healthy subjects with combined pH and biliary reflux measurements (Bilitec measurement). In contrast to the study by Smith et al., the cough monitor used by Kunsch et al., Lung Sound Monitoring Device has been less validated and reported in the literature. The monitor was used in a non-ambulatory setting at night time only and the analysis of cough was done manually. A 2-minute time window was also used to determine a temporal relationship between cough and reflux events. 21 of the 25 patients reporting symptoms of reflux had objective evidence of reflux on pH monitoring and spectrophotometer assessment of bilirubin, a marker of biliary reflux. In 43% of cough events, reflux events preceded cough, and were temporally related. The reflux events were more likely to be biliary in nature than acidic. In 49% of cough events, cough preceded reflux. It is difficult to compare the findings of Kunsch et al. with the Smith et al. study because they used different methods to assess both cough and reflux. A limitation of the Kunsch study is that the recordings were limited to night time, when the frequency of cough is markedly reduced in comparison to day-time. Patients in the Kunsch study were likely to have presented with typical reflux symptoms, hence the applicability of their findings to patients presenting with chronic cough is not known. Nevertheless, the Kunsch study does offer insights into the relationship between reflux and cough, and their findings also suggest that some cough events are temporally related to reflux but cough was equally as likely to precede reflux as to follow reflux.

The studies by Smith et al. and Kunsch et al. have provided a wealth of information into the relationship between cough and reflux events, and also highlight the difficulty in assessing patients. A number of challenges need to be addressed to improve the assessment of cough associated with reflux. The assessment of the temporal relationship involves using two devices; a combined device is likely to be more practical and easier to synchronise. Oesophageal and cough monitoring require manual analysis which is time-consuming and expensive; there is clearly a need for automation. There is considerable uncertainty over the optimal time window between reflux and cough events used to determine a temporal relationship. At present, a 2-min time window is used. A longer duration time window increases the statistical likelihood of a temporal relationship by chance, but conversely transient reflux events may lead to a prolonged sensitisation of the cough reflex and therefore episodes of cough may occur for some time after the reflux event. It is not known if the temporal relationship between reflux and cough predicts the response to treatment. This is a critical issue for the future success of these techniques and their further development. Future studies also need to investigate the temporal association with reflux into the larynx and pharynx.

## Are Cough Sounds Diagnostic for Reflux Cough?

There is considerable variability in the spectral and audio profile of cough sounds. Cough sounds differ between gender, individuals, and possibly aetiology. In a recent study, Abeyratne et al. have reported a cough sound analysis algorithm that is able to distinguish patients with pneumonia from other acute respiratory illnesses [26]. It is not known if the spectral profile of cough due to gastro-oesophageal reflux is distinct from other causes. In the author's experience, the auditory and spectral sound profile of reflux cough does not appear to differ from other categories of cough, such as asthma, rhinitis and idiopathic cough. A comparative study of the spectral profile of cough in a range of aetiologies is needed.

## Assessment of the Efficacy of Anti-Tussive Therapy with Cough Monitoring

Cough monitoring tools are being used more frequently to assess the efficacy of anti-tussive medications. Their main advantage is they provide an objective assessment. It is important to note they should always be used in combination with subjective assessments that include severity and impact on quality of life. The anti-tussive effects of anti-reflux treatments should also be evaluated with cough monitoring tools. Previous randomised controlled trials of proton pump inhibitor (PPI) treatments for unexplained chronic cough have only assessed cough with subjective outcome measures [8, 27]. There was a significant improvement in cough with PPI therapy, but a similar improvement was also observed with placebo. Hence the overall conclusion was PPIs were no better than placebo. The inclusion of cough monitoring in future studies may lead to a better understanding of the mechanism of action of active and placebo interventions.

We are only aware of one study that has evaluated the anti-tussive efficacy of anti-reflux therapy with objective cough monitoring. Kilduff et al. evaluated proton pump inhibitor therapy for patients with idiopathic pulmonary fibrosis and cough in an uncontrolled trial [28]. Eighteen subjects with idiopathic pulmonary fibrosis underwent therapy with either Omeprazole, 40 mg twice daily or Lansoprazole, 30 mg twice daily for 2 months. There was no change in cough frequency following therapy with proton pump inhibitors. As expected, there was a significant decrease in the number of acid reflux events.

### Conclusion

Cough can be assessed objectively with ambulatory cough frequency monitors. They should be used to assess the efficacy of anti-reflux therapy for patients with reflux-related respiratory symptoms. It is possible to combine cough monitoring with oesophageal monitors. Further studies are required to determine if a temporal relationship between reflux and cough events is predictive of a response to anti-reflux therapy. Further work is also required to develop combined oesophageal and cough monitoring devices, so they are automated and practical for clinical use. The relationship between laryngeal reflux and cough events has not been studied and deserves investigation.

## References

1. Morice AH, McGarvey L, Pavord I. Recommendations for the management of cough in adults. Thorax. 2006;61(Suppl 1):i1–i24.
2. Blondeau K, Dupont LJ, Mertens V, Tack J, Sifrim D. Improved diagnosis of gastro-oesophageal reflux in patients with unexplained chronic cough. Aliment Pharmacol Ther. 2007;25(6):723–32.
3. Patterson RN, Johnston BT, MacMahon J, Heaney LG, McGarvey LP. Oesophageal pH monitoring is of limited value in the diagnosis of "reflux-cough". Eur Respir J. 2004;24(5):724–7.
4. Birring SS, Fleming T, Matos S, Raj AA, Evans DH, Pavord ID. The Leicester cough monitor: preliminary validation of an automated cough detection system in chronic cough. Eur Respir J. 2008;31(5):1013–8.
5. Yousaf N, Monteiro W, Matos S, Birring SS, Pavord ID. Cough frequency in health and disease. Eur Respir J. 2013;41(1):241–3.
6. Sumner H, Woodcock A, Kolsum U, Dockry R, Lazaar AL, Singh D, et al. Predictors of objective cough frequency in chronic obstructive pulmonary disease. Am J Respir Crit Care Med. 2013;187(9):943–9.
7. Kahrilas PJ. Chronic cough and gastro-oesophageal reflux disease: new twists to the Riddle Editorial. Gastroenterology. 2010;139(3):716–8.
8. Faruqi S, Molyneux ID, Fathi H, Wright C, Thompson R, Morice AH. Chronic cough and esomeprazole: a double blind placebo-controlled parallel study. Respirology. 2011;16(7):1150–6.
9. Kelsall A, Houghton LA, Jones H, Decalmer S, McGuinness K, Smith JA. A novel approach to studying the relationship between subjective and objective measures of cough. Chest. 2011;139(3):569–75.

10. Birring SS, Spinou A. How best to measure cough clinically. Curr Opin Pharmacol. 2015;22:37–40.
11. Spinou A, Birring SS. An update on measurement and monitoring of cough: what are the important study endpoints? J Thorac Dis. 2014;6(Suppl 7):S728–34.
12. Vernon M, Kline LN, Nacson A, Nelsen L. Measuring cough severity: development and pilot testing of a new seven-item cough severity patient-reported outcome measure. Ther Adv Respir Dis. 2010;4(4):199–208.
13. Birring SS, Prudon B, Carr AJ, Singh SJ, Morgan MD, Pavord ID. Development of a symptom specific health status measure for patients with chronic cough: Leicester Cough Questionnaire (LCQ). Thorax. 2003;58(4):339–43.
14. French CT, Irwin RS, Fletcher KE, Adams TM. Evaluation of a cough-specific quality-of-life questionnaire. Chest. 2002;121(4):1123–31.
15. Lee KK, Ward K, Rafferty GF, Moxham J, Birring SS. The intensity of voluntary, induced and spontaneous cough. Chest. 2015;148(5):1259–67.
16. Barton A, Gaydecki P, Holt K, Smith JA. Data reduction for cough studies using distribution of audio frequency content. Cough. 2012;8(1):12.
17. Ryan NM, Birring SS, Gibson PG. Gabapentin for refractory chronic cough: a randomised, double-blind, placebo-controlled trial. Lancet. 2012;380(9853):1583–9.
18. Yousaf N, Monteiro W, Parker D, Matos S, Birring S, Pavord ID. Long-term low-dose erythromycin in patients with unexplained chronic cough: a double-blind placebo controlled trial. Thorax. 2010;65(12):1107–10.
19. Vertigan AE, Kapela SL, Ryan NM, Birring SS, McElduff P, Gibson PG. Pregabalin and speech pathology combination therapy for refractory chronic cough: a randomised control trial. Chest. 2016;149(3):639–48.
20. Abdulqawi R, Dockry R, Holt K, Layton G, McCarthy BG, Ford AP, Smith JA. P2X3 receptor antagonist (AF-219) in refractory chronic cough: a randomised, double-blind, placebo-controlled phase 2 study. Lancet. 2015;385(9974):1198–205.
21. Khalid S, Murdoch R, Newlands A, Smart K, Kelsall A, Holt K, Dockry R, Woodcock A, Smith JA. Transient receptor potential vanilloid 1 (TRPV1) antagonism in patients with refractory chronic cough: a double-blind randomised controlled trial. J Allergy Clin Immunol. 2014;134(1):56–62.
22. Smith J, Owen E, Earis J, Woodcock A. Effect of codeine on objective measurement of cough in chronic obstructive pulmonary disease. J Allergy Clin Immunol. 2006;117(4):831–5.
23. Decalmer S, Stovold R, Houghton LA, Pearson J, Ward C, Kelsall A, et al. Chronic cough: relationship between microaspiration, gastroesophageal reflux, and cough frequency. Chest. 2012;142(4):958–64.
24. Smith JA, Decalmer S, Kelsall A, McGuinness K, Jones H, Galloway S, et al. Acoustic cough-reflux associations in chronic cough: potential triggers and mechanisms. Gastroenterology. 2010;139(3):754–62.
25. Lenniger P, Gross V, Kunsch S, Nell C, Nolte JE, Sohrabi AK. Koehler U. Nocturnal long-term monitoring of lung sounds in patients with gastro-oesophageal reflux disease. Pneumologie. April. 2010;64(4):255–8.
26. Kosasih K, Abeyratne UR, Swarnkar V, Triasih R. Wavelet augmented cough analysis for rapid childhood pneumonia diagnosis. IEEE Trans Biomed Eng. 2015;62(4):1185–94.
27. Shaheen NJ, Crockett SD, Bright SD, Madanick RD, Buckmire R, Couch M, et al. Randomised clinical trial: high-dose acid suppression for chronic cough - a double-blind, placebo-controlled study. Aliment Pharmacol Ther. 2011;33(2):225–34.
28. Kilduff CE, Counter MJ, Thomas GA, Harrison NK, Hope-Gill BD. Effect of acid suppression therapy on gastroesophageal reflux and cough in idiopathic pulmonary fibrosis: an intervention study. Cough. 2014;10:4. https://doi.org/10.1186/1745-9974-10-4.eCollection.

# Part III

# Reflux Aspiration in Specific Lung Diseases

# The Relationship Between Asthma and Gastro-Esophageal Reflux

**12**

Adalberto Pacheco

## Abstract

The relationship between asthma and gastro-esophageal reflux has been the subject of many epidemiological studies over the past decades. But the mechanisms underlying this relationship remain obscure, principally for two reasons: first, the lack of studies with sufficient statistical power assessing the physiology of extra-esophageal reflux and the gastro-esophageal junction; and second, the need to understand the development of a vicious circle between the two entities. Comorbidities in asthma patients such as obesity, rhinitis and obstructive sleep apnea probably also intervene in the control of asthma, the link between them being the reflux material. The end result is that asthma and gastro-esophageal reflux are multifactorial entities with many points of contact, meaning that their study requires the participation of at least three specialties—Pulmonology, ENT and Gastroenterology—to thoroughly explore each asthma patient and thus to optimize therapy.

## Background

Over a century ago, William Osler observed that in asthma patients "severe paroxysms may be induced by overloading the stomach" [1]. Gastro-esophageal reflux disease (GERD) is habitual in human beings. This is because, during our evolutionary development to enable speech, the descent of the larynx joined together at a lower junction two pathways which had previously been separate, the respiratory tract and the digestive tract; this alteration in the position meant that the reflux could

A. Pacheco
Hospital Ramón y Cajal, Madrid, Spain
e-mail: adalberto.pacheco@salud.madrid.org

easily reach the upper airway [2]. The other reason for higher levels of reflux in humans than in animals is bipedalism and the consequence of the formation of a complex but imperfect gastro-esophageal junction as a barrier to avoid reflux.

The recent publication on GERD at the consensus meeting in Montreal concluded that this condition may be an "aggravating factor" in asthma [3]. Indeed, one large population-based epidemiological study found that subjects with the combination of asthma and GERD had a higher prevalence of asthma and respiratory symptoms than patients without reflux [4]. However, the mutual dependence of the two entities means that the relationship between them is highly complex; the creation of a vicious circle between the two makes each one the cause and also the effect of the other.

If we consider airway hyper-responsiveness (AHR) as the principal hallmark of asthma, there are three mechanisms that are implicitly involved in the influence that reflux exerts over this condition: (1) microaspiration, which may not only cause direct tissue injury but may also trigger vagal reflexes, (2) acid infusion of the esophagus in humans, which has been shown to result in vagally mediated reflexes leading to bronchoconstriction, and (3) neuroinflammatory reflexes, which have been found to play a role in airway responses through the release of neuropeptides [5]. But conversely, asthma as an obstructive problem of the airway may affect the ability of the gastro-esophageal barrier to prevent reflux; this is suggested by the finding of an increase in airway responsiveness in asthma patients who have documented GERD [6].

In asthma therapy, it is becoming increasingly apparent that more than 50% of asthma patients managed in accordance with standard guidelines are not well controlled or are refractory to treatment [7]. The acknowledged comorbidities in asthma are GERD, allergic rhinitis, obesity, depression, diabetes mellitus and cardiovascular disease. Of these comorbidities, above all GERD and rhinitis are either directly or indirectly related to asthma. It has not yet been established whether they form part of the natural history of asthma or are distinct events, a conceptual problem also encountered in patients with COPD [8]. What is more, their prevalence in asthma patients varies tremendously from study to study [9].

A new vision of airflow obstruction suggests that the coexistence of two or more inflammatory stimuli in the airway is a key factor in the development of more severe airway disease [10]. The effects of multiple inflammatory stimuli in asthma may merely be additive or synergistic. The net result of different inflammatory stimuli will then depend on whether the stimulus is acute or chronic, on variations in the host response to the stimuli, and on the degree to which the stimulus triggers an eosinophil- or neutrophil-dominated inflammatory response. But we should also consider the possibility that the inflammatory responses to different stimuli interacts in a synergistic fashion. This may occur at an early stage in the evolution of these responses. For example, smoking increases the risk of sensitization to a variety of occupational high- and low-molecular weight sensitizers [11], and exposure to smoke or endotoxin has been associated with an increased risk of infection. Nevertheless, the authors proposing this theory make no mention of the possible role of reflux material on reaching the lower third of the esophagus, where it may cause more AHR, or on reaching the laryngeal tissue, where it may render the tissue dysfunctional and cause more frequent aspiration; nor do they mention the toxic action or reflex mechanisms action caused by the reflux (hydrochloric acid, pepsin and bile salts etc.) in the bronchial or bronchiolar epithelium from the stomach to the upper and lower airways. Therefore, a classification of asthma is needed based on the pathophysiological mechanism or endotype, and bearing in mind the presence of multiple impacts, including reflux material, on the inflammatory process in the airway and thus on the clinical course of the disease.

In clinical terms, in asthma patients whose symptoms worsen after meals and those who do not respond to anti-asthma therapy the association with GERD should be suspected. Similarly, patients who present GERD symptoms before the onset of asthma symptoms should be taken to have reflux-induced asthma [12]. However, since both asthma and GERD are multifactorial entities, assessing the relationship from the perspective of a single medical specialty is very often insufficient. Most epidemiological studies that link the two entities tend to be confusing, either because they do not present a functional definition of asthma or, more frequently, because they do not objectively specify the presence of typical esophageal reflux (with heartburn and regurgitation) or atypical extra-esophageal reflux (with laryngeal or extra-esophageal symptoms such as irritation, precipitation by posture, dysphagia or aphonia). Another problem inherent in the study of the asthma-GERD relationship is the frequent absence of any attempt to identify the possible interactions of other entities in a specific patient, something that should be mandatory not just in epidemiological studies but in clinical studies as well. For example, obstructive sleep apnea (OSA), asthma and GERD are potentially linked at several levels. The pathophysiology of these conditions seems to overlap significantly given that airway obstruction, inflammation, obesity, and several other factors are implicated in the development of all three.

An extensive bibliography is available on the relationship between asthma and GERD. There is now a need for a thorough update of the studies of the trajectory of the reflux from the stomach, examining it at all the stages of its journey towards the airway and exploring the possible relationships with asthma in both directions. In a recent study of the trajectory of reflux material from the stomach to the airways and the appearance of asthma, Cheng et al. demonstrated that in a guinea pig model, direct acidification to the lower esophagus and subsequent micro-aspiration in the respiratory tract leads to airway hyper-responsiveness and overactive bronchial smooth muscle [13]. We should therefore abandon our conception of asthma and other airflow obstructions as closed compartments or exclusive phenotypes, and should instead consider that the altered physiology of the lung may be due to multiple causes in the same patient, possibly interconnected, as in the multiple origin of atheroma, for example, the direct influence of reflux material on a new or previously existing bronchial asthmatic inflammation, either eosinophilic or neutrophilic. On this premise, here we present the current state of our knowledge on the toxic trajectory of gastric material ascending to the upper and lower airways and on the interactions at the inflammatory level in the airway which lead to alterations in pulmonary function and the appearance of symptoms.

## Epidemiology

Clinically, GERD affects 12% of the adult population at least once a week [14], and the prevalence of asthma continues to rise: from 3.1% in 1980 to 8.4% in 2010 [15]. A recent systematic review of 28 epidemiological studies identified GERD in 59.2% of asthmatics and in 38.1% of controls [16]. Other studies have found this association in as many as 80% of well-established asthma [17]. The disparity is probably due to patient selection.

One of the largest epidemiological studies linking GERD and asthma is the Nord-Trøndelag health survey. Persons with heavy and wheezy breathing, daily cough, daily productive cough, or chronic cough showed a twofold to threefold statistically significant increase in risk of reflux symptoms [18]. Interestingly, in the cross-sectional Busselton health survey, the relationship between GERD and respiratory symptoms was independent of Body Mass Index, high risk of OSA or AHR, and the authors suggested that reflux contributes directly to respiratory symptoms [19].

A topical epidemiological study of the relationship between GERD and other symptoms is the follow-up analysis of individuals exposed to the destruction of the World Trade Center. Symptoms of GERD and OSA were significantly associated with poor or very poor control of the asthma diagnosed subsequent to 9/11 [20]. Aerodigestive tract inflammatory syndromes have now been documented in occupational groups exposed to the disaster, and syndrome incidence has been linked to the intensity of exposure to airborne pollutants. Interestingly, the hypothesis of a simultaneous aerodigestive impairment caused by dust suggests a dysfunction of the neurological vagal network common to both systems.

A recent epidemiological analysis of the relationship between asthma and GERD in the UK stressed the need for a high rate of initial suspicion in an asthma patient. The authors reported that during the first year after diagnosis patients with asthma are at a significantly increased risk of developing GERD [21].

## Basic Mechanisms of the Relationship Between Asthma and GERD. The Two Theories: Reflux Versus Reflex

In the pathophysiology of the extra-esophageal syndromes, of which asthma may be one, two main mechanisms have been proposed: the reflux theory and the reflex theory. According to the reflux theory, the refluxate leads to direct respiratory mucosal injury caused by the gastroduodenal contents, leading to extra-esophageal symptoms, asthma, sinusitis and laryngitis. Direct aspiration into the lung causes chronic inflammation, which can lead to impaired gas exchange and airway obstruction [22]. It should also be borne in mind that aspiration may be favoured by the inability of the larynx-pharynx to function as "the guardian to the lower airway" after suffering the action of the gastric juices. In the reflex theory, GERD causes the esophageal-bronchial reflex in the distal third of the esophagus, without the need to reach the upper airway [23].

Recent publications have stressed the central role of transient lower esophageal sphincter relaxations (tLESRs) in the genesis of reflux [24]. While the evidence suggests that tLESRs are no more frequent in GERD patients than in asymptomatic volunteers, the likelihood that GERD patients will reflux during the period of sphincter relaxation is almost twice as high [25]. Other theories are based on the likelihood that increased frequency of acid reflux during tLESRs may be a more important contributor to the genesis of extra-esophageal symptoms than an increased frequency of the events themselves. Further functional studies have suggested that the ascent of retrograde waves of peristalsis towards the esophagus appears to be propagated by the occurrence of tLESRs which may act to further increase aspiration events [24]. Assessments of gastrointestinal motility have also suggested that the position of the "acid pocket" (i.e., secreted gastric juice that sits above the meal bolus) in relation to the diaphragm may drive reflux [26]. Nonetheless, in a classical study, the prevalence of ineffective peristalsis motility (a feature that often remains unexplored in epidemiological studies) was identified as the most common motility abnormality in patients with GERD-associated respiratory symptoms [27].

Another key factor in the upward movement of the reflux is intragastric pressure, which is controlled by a complex array of neurohumoral pathways that govern lower esophageal and pyloric sphincter tone, gastric compliance, gastric secretion volume and gastric motility. Alongside vagal innervation, hormonal drives may govern all these factors [28]. Cholecystokinin release from the duodenal cells is a major driver for reduced gastric emptying, while gastrin release from gastric G cells increases gastric mixing. Both of these factors may increase intragastric pressure. At the same time, motilin release from intestinal enteroendocrine cells acts to increase the rates of gastric emptying, and would thus be expected to decrease intragastric pressure. Previous reviews have noted the potential of these agents and their receptors as targets for reflux therapy [28].

In asthma, non-eosinophilic forms are increasingly being recognized as important inflammatory subtypes [29, 30]. Potential triggers of neutrophilic inflammation include infection, which can cause an acute neutrophilic bronchitis, rhinosinusitis, and also GERD with aspiration. Recently, a novel clinical pattern of neutrophilic asthma was distinguished from paucigranulocytic and eosinophilic asthma, with evidence of abnormal upper airway responses and a higher presence of rhinosinusitis and GERD [31]. The need to contemplate asthma from a broader perspective—that is, not as a condition affecting exclusively the lower airway—appears to

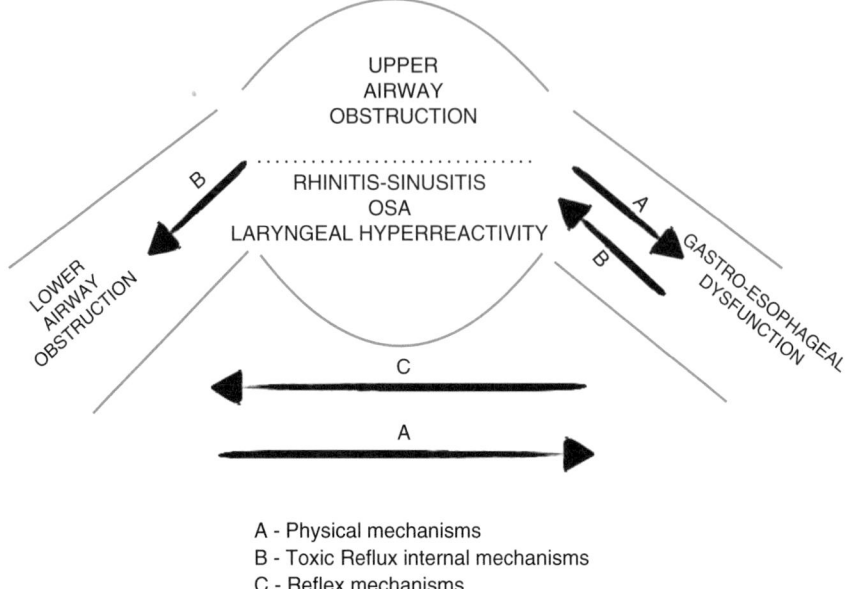

**Fig. 12.1** Gastroesophagical reflux and potential relations depending on anatomical areas

be clear in the light of the influence of other agents such as reflux material, which may not only act as aggravants but also as inducers of the inflammatory process in asthma (Fig. 12.1).

## Asthma and GERD: Cause or Effect

A causal relationship between silent or overt GERD and asthma is difficult to establish since we must accept that either condition can induce the other [32, 33]. The association has been described conceptually as a vicious circle, without a clear beginning or end. Although the presence of asthma is not more prevalent among individuals with GERD than in the normal population, the presence of reflex-mediated cough and upper airway symptoms is clearly very frequent; however, reversible airway obstruction if one defines asthma as such, does not appear to be as common. Upper airway conditions associated with GERD include chronic cough, wheezing, stridor, recurrent croup, sinusitis, laryngomalacia, and subglottic stenosis [34, 35]. However, despite the enormous volume of literature on the subject, Haveman et al. noted the paucity of data on the direction of the temporal sequence of the asthma-GERD association [16]. It often remains unclear whether GERD exacerbates lower airways disease like asthma through the reflux or reflex mechanism (an issue that has been widely studied), or whether, on the other hand, asthma patients develop pathologic GERD. There are two principles of physics that explain how airway obstruction, both upper and lower, might lead to GERD, and indeed many existing disease associations seem to lend support to this theory.

## Asthma Caused by GERD

The pathophysiology of GERD is not fully understood. However, like asthma it is now recognized to be a multifactorial disease. Among the factors that have been shown to be involved in the provocation or increase of reflux are sliding hiatus hernia, decreased lower esophageal sphincter pressure, transient lower esophageal sphincter relaxation, the acid pocket, obesity, increased distensibility of the gastro-esophageal junction, prolonged esophageal clearance, and delayed gastric emptying [36].

There is increasing evidence that asthma can be considered as a disease linked to extra-esophageal reflux. The interplay between asthma and GERD is complicated. Heartburn and regurgitation, the typically defined peptic esophageal symptoms, affect 35–40% of the adult population in the western world but GERD also presents extra-esophageal symptoms [37, 38]. Diagnosing extra-esophageal GERD can be difficult in the absence of heartburn or regurgitation, which are not present in 40–60% of asthma patients with GERD [39]. In a study using 24-h esophageal pH monitoring Kiljander et al. found that 35% of asthma patients had reflux but did not present typical symptoms such as heartburn and regurgitation; therefore, reflux is likely even if patients do not report such symptoms [40]. A careful history of non acid airway reflux such as that from the HARQ questionnaire [41] and physical examination is important in the evaluation of patients with asthma in which GERD is suspected to play a role.

However, a universal problem that persists with the problem of the asthma-GERD relationship is that current diagnostic testing for reflux in patients with asthma has sub-optimal sensitivity and/or specificity and often does not predict response to treatment. Esophageal impedance pH monitoring, for instance, is unreliable for assessing reflux that reach the upper airway. In the esophagus, the baseline impedance level remains stable because the impedance rings remain in contact with the esophageal mucosa. The pharynx, however, is an air-filled cavity and so the baseline impedance level fluctuates depending on whether the impedance rings are in contact with the moist mucosa or the air. Finally, subjective scoring systems for documenting apparent laryngo-pharyngeal reflux (LPR) reaching the upper airway have been used but have largely been discredited since inter-observer agreement is poor [42]. However, the assessment of the influence of reflux on pulmonary physiopathology is gaining ground. An interesting study of proximal and distal refluxes simultaneous to oxygen desaturations in peripheral blood found that nearly three quarters of GERD patients with predominance of respiratory symptoms had oxygen desaturations associated with esophageal acid exposure, compared with less than one third of those with predominance of typical reflux symptoms. Perhaps most importantly, successful anti-reflux surgery reduced the number of reflux-associated desaturations to values comparable to those in normal controls [43]. In another study, Mise et al. [44] evaluated the impact of reflux on pulmonary physiology by means of direct measurement of pH in the lung in patients who had recently been diagnosed with GERD but were otherwise healthy. Compared with normal controls, patients with GERD had lower pH in the peripheral alveolar branches (pH 5.13 vs 6.08, $p = 0.001$) and higher levels of LDH in broncho-alveolar aspirates, a sign of tissue damage.

## GERD Caused by Asthma

Asthma is a dynamic disease of the respiratory system, viewed as a set of interacting subsystems, inflammatory, immunological, but also mechanical. There is increasing evidence that upper or lower airway obstruction leads to GERD. Recent investigations stress that physical mechanisms such as Boyle's Law and Bernoulli's Principle can help to explain how airway obstruction might predispose to GERD [45]. Boyle's Law predicts that the increased negative inspiratory pressure required to overcome airway obstruction might result in positive abdominal pressure which compromises the anti-reflux barrier from below. Bernoulli's Principle predicts that upper airway obstruction might cause air to shunt into the esophagus and compromise the anti-reflux barrier from above, either through pressure swings within the esophagus or through gastric distension with air, both of which may affect the lower esophageal sphincter tone. Once GERD develops, the potential for asthma exacerbation exists. A recent epidemiological review of COPD, a disease with the same physiopathological basis as asthma (that is, chronic airway obstruction), evaluated the relationship between gastro-esophageal reflux disease and COPD in a large cohort of patients over a 5-year period. Patients with GERD did not have a higher risk of being diagnosed with COPD than controls, but patients with COPD were more likely to be diagnosed with GERD (OR, 1.46; 95% CI, 1.19–1.78). The authors concluded that COPD appears to predispose patients to GERD rather than vice versa, and it is possible that GERD may worsen pre-existing COPD. This may well be the case with asthma as well: a vicious circle that begins with airway obstruction [46].

In one of the few studies to suggest that asthma might be the precipitating factor in the GERD-asthma relationship, Moote et al. [47] conducted a methacholine challenge and simultaneous pH probe in 15 patients with mild asthma and 15 controls with no asthma. During bronchospasm, the patients with asthma had more episodes of reflux and lower esophageal pH than the control subjects who had no evidence of bronchospasm with methacholine. In 2002 Zerbib et al. replicated these findings and also provided evidence that the tLESRs represent the mechanism through which bronchospasm-induced GERD occurred [6]. Perhaps, then, the reason why antacid treatment with PPIs has not obtained a dramatic improvement in asthma symptoms is that we are not really addressing the underlying cause of the reflux: that is, the breach of the anti-reflux barrier formed by physical structures at the junction of the esophagus and diaphragm, esophageal motor function and acid clearance, the upper esophageal sphincter, and pharyngeal and laryngeal mucosal resistance. Sequential failure of all four barriers is necessary to produce extra-esophageal reflux [2]. Another problem regarding the action of the antacid therapy on the interrelation between asthma and GERD is that numerous studies have shown that it is other components of the gastric fluid, rather than the acid, which mediate in the bronchial response. Therefore, the failure of antacid medication to control the asthma cannot be taken to indicate that GERD does not affect asthma evolution.

## The Interface Between Esophageal Dysfunction and Extra-Esophageal Involvement: Reflux in the Upper Airway and Aspiration

The first issue to resolve in the investigation of the asthma-GERD association is whether the GERD is typical or atypical. The concept of atypical GERD is still not addressed by many pulmonologists, and it is more studied in the field of ENT; this may be the reason for the notable differences in the frequency of GERD in the studies that assess asthma and GERD simultaneously. The prevalence of asymptomatic or silent acid reflux in patients with asthma varies between 10% and 62% according to the underlying severity of the asthma and the measure used to identify symptoms [48–50]. Two problems emerge in the study of these asthma-GERD patients, one clinical and the other technical. The clinical difficulty in patients with GERD is due in many cases to the low presence of symptoms. For example, a population-based study from Sweden found that up to 36.8% of patients with erosive esophagitis presented no symptoms [51]. Furthermore, studies of the asthma-GERD relationship present shortcomings above all due to the low sensitivity and specificity achieved by tests for detecting GERD at various stages along its path towards the airways, probably due to the neglect of the non-acid reflux and the nature of the reflux material, which may be liquid or gas.

To assess distal acidification, ambulatory pH monitoring can be combined with symptom-reflux indices to help determine whether low pH values are causing pathological signs of GERD. Tools to quantify the relationship between symptoms and reflux include the Symptom Index (SI), the Symptom Sensitivity Index (SSI), the Symptom Association Probability (SAP) and the Binomial Symptom Index [52]. This relationship has been studied in chronic cough but has been assessed far less frequently in asthma, among other things because there is no clear symptom to establish a relationship with reflux episodes, as there is in the case of chronic cough and its monitoring [53]. Thus, given the low predictive value of pH testing, the lack of reliability of SAP and the temporal association, which may not be causal, pH testing in patients with chronic cough or asthma is likely to be misleading and therefore not routinely recommended.

To determine whether proximal or distal esophageal reflux is associated with asthma severity, symptoms, physiology, or functional status in patients with poorly controlled asthma, DiMango et al. [54] analysed 304 patients with minimal or no GERD symptoms using probe recordings. They found that 53% had reflux and 38% had proximal reflux. Patients with proximal reflux reported significantly worse asthma and health-related quality of life. The concordance between distal esophageal reflux and upper proximal reflux was only moderate; 25% of subjects had one without the other. The authors concluded that the evaluation of GERD using ambulatory pH probes in individuals with poorly controlled asthma without reflux symptoms is not usually warranted unless atypical symptoms, such as cough or unexplained chest symptoms, might suggest the diagnosis.

However, most patients with extra-esophageal symptoms were not found to exhibit increased proximal esophageal acid reflux compared with patients with typical esophageal symptoms of GERD [55] although this study did not take into consideration the role of the aerosolized droplet component in the reflux material. Oropharyngeal pH monitoring with the ResTech pH probe is another method for assessing reflux using a nasopharyngeal catheter to measure pH in either liquid or aerosolized droplets, since in short reflux episodes the gastric aspirate may not damage the respiratory mucosa sufficiently to trigger cough and the aspiration of aerosolized gastric contents may also harm the airway. In any case, while it would not deliver the same volume of gastric contents to the airways, it is believed that aerosolized vapor may act to coat the airway mucosa [56, 57]. However, many studies have compared Restech pH probe with concurrent esophageal pH monitoring or impedance monitoring and present inconsistent results, ranging from the oropharyngeal probe registering lower pH values during sleep and a higher rate of false positives and non-correlating pharyngeal events [58]. Therefore, further controlled outcome-driven studies are needed to assess the future role of this new device in these patients who are particularly difficult to diagnose and manage.

## Involvement of Reflux in the Upper Airway

Over a short time scale, gastric aspirate may not be damaging enough to the airway mucosa to provoke a relevant clearance response such as cough. As previously discussed, aspiration of aerosolized gastric contents may also cause damaging material to enter the airways. In chronic cough patients, after ruling out eosinophilic airway inflammation (asthmatic or non-asthmatic eosinophilic bronchitis which may be caused by such aerosolized reflux) there is growing evidence that the most important etiology is a sensory disorder of the laryngeal branches of the vagus nerve. In these cases LPR is often concurrently diagnosed [59]. This is no surprise, since the vagus nerve supplies the entire aerodigestive tract, including the upper and lower respiratory tracts and the digestive tract [60]. Phua et al. have suggested an elevated threshold for laryngo-pharyngeal sensitivity in refluxers with chronic cough [61, 62]. The same authors also demonstrated that patients with GERD exhibited diminished glottal closure in response to laryngeal puffs of air (the laryngeal adductor reflex) and patients have exaggerated pharyngeal reflexes compared with controls. This suggest that their laryngeal responses, but not their pharyngeal responses, may be impaired, with the resulting risk of microaspiration, and may therefore trigger asthma or worsen asthma that has already initiated [63].

In chronic cough the number of proximal refluxes in the esophagus do not present differences in relation to healthy controls [64]. In asthma, however, few studies have analysed this issue. One such study recently demonstrated that reflux can reach the upper airway either in liquid or in gas form and may cause aspiration even though conventional pH-metry is negative. Komatsu et al. recently studied the technical and methodological problems deriving from exposure to reflux in the proximal area of the esophagus and hypopharynx; in their cases with abnormal reflux at this level, the asthma responded positively to anti-reflux surgery [65].

In an interesting study of chronic cough and laryngeal dysfunction assessed by measuring laryngeal hyper-responsiveness, the degree of improvement in cough reflex sensitivity correlated with the improvement in extra-thoracic airway hyper-responsiveness, an entity that has only rarely been recognized in asthma patients [66]. Reflux material is probably one of the inducers of laryngeal irritation, since there is increasing evidence that a significant proportion of patients display statistical associations between reflux and cough events, in the absence of an excessive number of reflux events either inside or outside the esophagus [67]. Surprisingly, upper airway dysfunction mimicking resistant asthma or coexisting with asthma has not been comprehensively investigated, and despite numerous reports of upper airway dysfunction masquerading as difficult-to-treat asthma, it has been largely ignored as an alternative or coexisting diagnosis. A clear laryngeal dysfunction such as vocal cord dysfunction (VCD) has repeatedly been misdiagnosed as asthma; however, the relationship between asthma and VCD remains elusive. Mechanistically, it raises the possibility that asthma and laryngeal dysfunction are interrelated conditions and that laryngeal hyper-responsiveness is an intrinsic and unsuspected characteristic of asthma itself. Vocal cord movement abnormality may also occur intermittently, and therefore inspection of flow-volume loops in spirometry may produce false negative results. Although a psychological origin for VCD has been claimed, reflux material, nonspecific airway irritants, and exercise have also been associated with intermittent laryngeal obstruction, dyspnea and noisy breathing. But it should also be remembered that Bernoulli's Principle predicts that upper airway obstruction (laryngeal hyper-responsiveness, rhinitis-sinusitis or OSA) may cause air to shunt into the esophagus and compromise the anti-reflux barrier from above through the dysfunction of the lower esophageal sphincter.

Although in the analysis of asthma the associated GERD phenotype has not been systematically considered, this phenomenon was recently addressed in a study which used bronchoscopy in asthmatics, on the grounds that gastro-esophageal reflux may produce extra-esophageal manifestations such as LPR that can be measured during examination via the index of endoscopic findings. The group with LPR had good response control after treatment for reflux using fundoplication [68]. However, in a critical analysis of the literature between 1977 and 2008 Kotby et al. concluded that there is no "gold standard" diagnostic test for LPR [69]. This was recently confirmed by a study of LPR diagnosed by the reflux finding score and the reflux symptom index in which impedance monitoring confirmed GERD diagnosis in fewer than 40% of patients, probably due to the low specificity of laryngoscopic findings. As a result, the study stressed the usefulness of impedance in determining the association between GERD and LPR [42]. However, research in the field of ENT has reported new methods for diagnosing LPR such as laryngeal biopsy in refluxers. In a prospective translational research study, detectable levels of pepsin remained in the laryngeal epithelia after a reflux event. Pepsin bound there would be enzymatically inactive because the mean pH of the laryngo-pharynx was 6.8. Significantly, pepsin could remain in a form that would be reactivated by a subsequent decrease in pH, as would occur during an acidic reflux event or possibly after uptake into intracellular compartments of lower pH [70].

In another recent study, this time using laryngeal 320-slice CT technology in patients with difficult-to-treat asthma, vocal cord movement abnormality was detected in 50% of all patients. Albeit guardedly, the authors suggested that asthma and VCD may share similar mechanisms (airway inflammation and hyperresponsiveness); therefore, they may both be integral components of an "asthma syndrome" reflecting a "united airway" [71]. Some caution is in order, since there is a strong possibility that a number of the subjects with abnormal laryngeal movement had VCD rather than difficult-to-treat asthma. Nonetheless, the significant number of asthma patients with associated VCD indicates that some relationship exists between the conditions. However, whether upper airway dysfunction and VCD is the cause or the result of difficult-to-treat asthma remains to be established.

There is a clear need for a more profound and effective analysis of the connection between the involvement of the upper airway and aspiration as a potential mechanism of the origin or worsening of asthma. Asthma may develop either by an alteration in swallowing, a direct mechanism, or via aspiration of contents from the esophagus, that is, through an indirect mechanism. In the former case Terada et al. found a relationship between the number of exacerbations of COPD, another obstructive airway disorder, and altered swallowing. Abnormal swallowing reflexes frequently occurred in subjects with COPD and predisposed them to exacerbations; conceivably, these abnormalities might be affected by the presence of GERD, and may also cause bacterial colonization in the lower airway [72]. As for the influence and interrelation of GERD and asthma via the indirect mechanism, that is, through aspiration of the reflux content, in a recent study comparing different asthma phenotypes Gibson et al. found that the FIF50 tended to be lowest in patients with neutrophilic asthma, and that there was a significant inverse correlation between sputum neutrophils and FIF50% predicted with Spearman's rho $-0.326$, $p < 0.015$ [31]. GERD was common in neutrophilic asthma (73%) and the likelihood of the presence of GERD in patients with neutrophilic asthma was 4.6 times higher than in those with eosinophilic asthma and 2.9 times higher than in those with paucigranulocytic asthma. However, two criticisms of this study merit comment: (1) the diagnosis of GERD was based on a questionnaire on typical GERD devised by gastroenterologists, and so it did not include symptoms of extra-esophageal GERD; and (2) although the presence of typical GERD was more frequent in the neutrophilic asthma group, the possibility of combined phenotypes—for example, eosinophilia and GERD and sinusitis—was not mentioned. Achieving groups that are exclusive and not mixed is a universal problem in studies of obstructive airway disorders.

## Aspiration

Gastric fluid may also be an inducer of asthma. This has been demonstrated in murine models in which the aspiration of gastric fluid altered the bronchial hypersensitivity response [73]. The risk of food or refluxate entering the airway is likely to be a delicate balance between the complex reflex responses that have evolved to protect the airway and pathological processes that increase pharyngeal/laryngeal exposure to food and refluxate, such as impaired co-ordination of swallowing, excessive laryngo-pharyngeal reflux and esophageal dysmotility [74]. Two mechanisms have been proposed to explain the association of asthma and aspiration in the lower airway. Firstly, homogenized and partially hydrolysed foods may act as a more amenable substrate to bacterial species already occurring within the airways; secondly, the hydrolysis and denaturation of dietary proteins during normal digestion may lead to the appearance of previously sequestered antigen [75]. However, it is still unclear whether chronic aspiration in the context of GERD causes and/or exacerbates pulmonary disease, or vice versa; the beginning and end of this vicious circle remain a mystery (Fig. 12.2).

In an acute aspiration model in rats previously sensitized with ovoalbumin, after 6 h the combined injury caused an additive, not synergistic, increase in airway hyperresponsiveness and neutrophil recruitment to the airways [73]. In chronic aspiration, the investigation of GERD-induced airway inflammation offers results that are

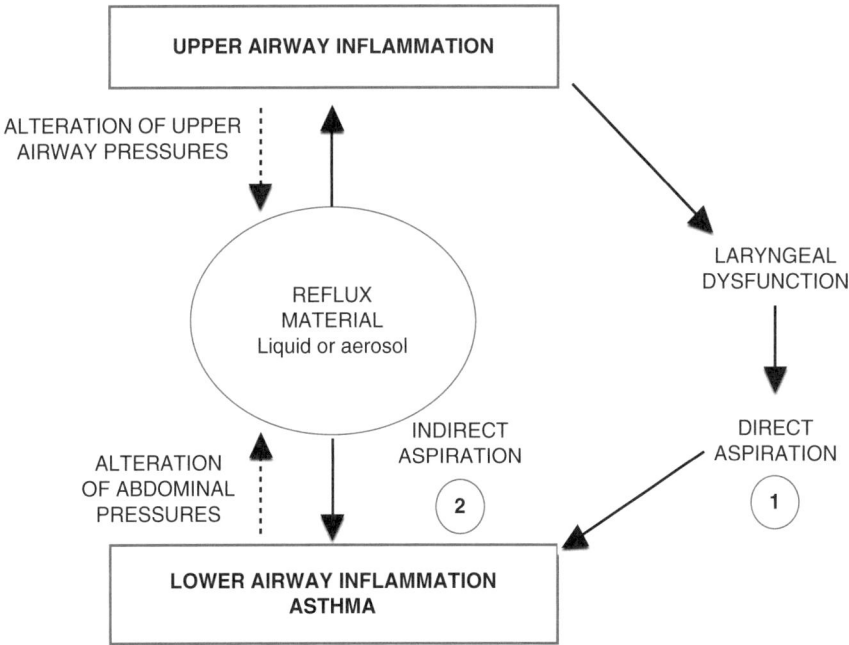

**Fig. 12.2** Relationships mechanisms leading to aspiration and asthma

particularly controversial, given the diversity of the findings. Studies in another rat model have shown that the particulate matter in gastric fluid is pivotal in the development of a macrophage-laden pathology [76]. Today, in view of the results obtained with numerous animal models, it is acknowledged that while aspiration profoundly decreases certain aspects of the T-cell-associated immune response, in others the effect is less pronounced and more variable. Lung histology from these rats indicates that chronic aspiration of whole gastric contents results in a granulomatous pneumonitis with prominent chronic inflammatory infiltrates and giant cell formation [77]. Those authors report that the interstitial pneumonitis and granuloma formation seen with whole gastric fluid aspiration were reproduced in rats receiving instillations of food particles and neutralized gastric fluid, but not with instillations of hydrochloric acid. This suggests that the particulate matter found in gastric contents is a major contributor to the histopathologic changes observed with repetitive aspiration. If we accept that it is the non-acidic components of the gastric fluid that mediate in the bronchial response, the failure of PPI to control asthma with concomitant GERD cannot be taken to indicate that GERD does not affect the evolution of asthma through the aspirated material [78]. Recently, using thorascopic biopsy (a procedure performed only very rarely in asthmatics) it has been demonstrated that a subset of severe asthma manifests a granulomatous pathology termed "asthmatic granulomatosis" [79].

In a recent comparative study of chronic aspiration, 60 rats were randomly divided into six equal groups: a GERD group, GERD-associated-asthma group, allergic asthma group, and their control groups. Cytokine levels and concentration of inflammatory cells in BAL were determined. The results demonstrated that assaying the concentrations of IL-5 and inflammatory cells in BAL may be an effective method of distinguishing GERD-associated asthma from allergic asthma [80]. Another group, however, found that GERD worsened IL13 (a Th2 cytokine) and eosinophil levels in BAL fluid of rats in the reflux esophagitis and asthma group compared with the asthma group; they also found that acid plays a major role in the deterioration of OVA-induced airway inflammation in rats with reflux esophagitis and asthma. These enhancements of OVA-induced airway inflammation were prevented by treatment with rabeprazole [81]. These inconsistent findings may be due to the species of rats used, since Brown–Norway rats are known to be Th2-predisposed [82, 83]. The extrapolation of these findings to humans might suppose that the response of the bronchial epithelium to the gastric aspirate may depend on the previous underlying asthmatic inflammation: type Th1 or Th2. In any case, it is possible that GERD does exacerbate asthma, possibly through vagally-mediated reflex bronchospasm [84]. Likewise reflux is reportedly more common among patients with 'difficult-to-control' asthma than in their well-controlled peers, suggesting that reflux may contribute to poor control [85].

## Aspiration Markers in Asthma

The effects of various components of gastric fluid (e.g., acid, bacteria, food, and enzymes) upon airway inflammation, hyper-responsiveness and hypersensitivity may have important implications for the clinical treatment of asthma and may provide insights into the underlying mechanisms associated with asthma pathogenesis. The current situation of aspiration markers such as pepsin, bile acids and intraalveolar macrophages in the lung and their possible connection with eosinophilic or non-eosinophilic asthmatic inflammation merits some comment.

## Pepsin

Salivary pepsin measurement has been used in the detection of GERD, especially in reflux-related laryngitis. A novel pepsin rapid test (Peptest-Biomed) is a convenient, non-invasive, quick and inexpensive technique in LPR diagnosis. As regards pepsin in the lower airway, Rosen et al. [86] found that 44% of patients with chronic cough or asthma had pepsin in the bronchoscopy fluid; however, the presence of pepsin did not correlate with any reflux parameters with the exception of non-acid reflux (0.04). Its sensitivity and specificity in predicting pathologic reflux by pH-MII or EGD were 57% and 65% respectively, with a positive predictive value of 50% and a negative predictive value of 71%. The authors propose that this association with non-acid reflux and pepsin positivity occurs because the non-acid reflux may not be sensed until it reaches the proximal esophagus or oropharynx, by which point the refluxate is already exposed to the airway.

## Bile Acids

D'Ovidio et al. showed that the presence of bile salts in BAL fluid 3 months after lung transplant was associated with the development of obliterative bronchiolitis in a time- and dose-dependent manner. This important study was the first to prospectively evaluate post-transplant patients and to show that aspiration markers are a risk factor for obliterative bronchiolitis [87]. However, the main limitation of using molecular aspiration markers such as pepsin and bile salts in BAL samples is the impossibility of standardizing the concentration.

## Alveolar Macrophages

A new analysis of the presence of alveolar macrophages (AMs) as markers of chronic aspiration has recently been proposed. Chlorophyllin-stained macrophages show the presence of green cytoplasmic pigments and appear to be highly specific for aspiration—much more so than the traditional approach of searching for lipid-laden macrophages which may in fact be a product of the endogenous metabolism [88]. This is an interesting finding but needs future validations.

AMs are among the main immune system cells found in the airways and have been implicated in the development and progression of asthma. AMs constitute a unique subset of pulmonary macrophages, which serve as a first line of defense against foreign invaders of the lung tissue. In addition, in human and animal studies, they have also been found to regulate pro- and anti-inflammatory responses in the airways, suggesting that they have a critical role in asthma [89]. The literature has established a substantial link between lung macrophages and airway remodeling and eosinophilic inflammation in asthma [90]. These findings show that CD11b(+) CD11c(int) macrophages expressing CCR3 as key pro-inflammatory cells are both necessary and sufficient for allergen-specific T cell stimulation during ongoing eosinophilic airway inflammation. Various parameters associated with asthmatic responses, including airway remodeling, the cellular immune response and the humoral immune response, are dependent upon the strain of mouse used, although a profound down-regulation of a broad array of T cell-associated cytokines and chemokines and up-regulation of macrophage-associated markers was observed as a result of aspiration [77]. These results suggest an interesting postulate that may impact human disease/asthma: chronic aspiration of gastric fluid has the potential to drive the immune response in the airways from adaptive to more innate. Another recent study indicated that the macrophages activated in the lung might become a source of IL-13 and thus increase mucous production and bronchial hyper-responsiveness [91].

Neutrophils in the broncho-alveolar area also have the capability to cause AHR. Coyle et al. demonstrated that neutrophil cathepsin G causes marked increases in AHR [92]. However, the triggers and mechanisms of neutrophilic forms of asthma remain unknown; growing evidence supports a role for the innate immune response with altered gene expression of toll-like receptors and increased expression of genes from the IL-1β pathway observed in patients with increased sputum neutrophils. This suggests that pathogen recognition and destruction processes may be altered and that in non-eosinophilic asthma, macrophage phagocytosis is impaired in patients with normal sputum eosinophil proportions [93].

## Influence of Other Entities on the Course of Asthma and Their Possible Interactions with GERD: Obesity, Obstructive Sleep Apnea and Chronic Cough

### OSA, GERD and Asthma

GERD has been associated with upper airway disorders such as rhinitis, sinusitis, and obstructive sleep apnea (OSA) [94, 95]. With regard to the association of OSA and GERD, treatment of nasal obstruction with continuous positive airway pressure (CPAP) has been shown to improve GERD symptoms [96]. It is doubtful that relieving upper airway obstruction would improve GERD unless the obstruction actually contributed to its pathophysiology. The association between GERD and OSA was assessed in a recent case-control study in Brisbane, Australia, of 237 patients with histologically confirmed Barrett's esophagus and 247 population controls. The study concluded that symptoms of OSA may be associated with an increased risk of Barrett's esophagus, an association that appears to be mediated entirely by GERD [97]. Interestingly, children with sleep-disordered breathing have also been shown to have a higher incidence of GERD [98]. Most children with OSA are not obese, but have large tonsils or adenoids that can cause upper airway obstruction.

Currently, sleep-related GERD is underappreciated from a clinical standpoint [99]. The only prospective study to have investigated whether nocturnal GERD (nGERD) induces respiratory disorders, including asthma and OSA, is the 9-year population-based study by Emilsson et al. [100]. Subjects with persistent nGERD had an independent increased risk of new asthma at follow-up (OR 2.3, 95% CI 1.1–4.9). The risk of developing symptoms of OSA was increased in subjects with new and persistent nGERD (OR 2.2, 95% CI 1.3–1.6, and OR 2.0, 95% CI 1.0–3.7 respectively). Therefore, this study suggests that nGERD is a risk factor for developing asthma.

As regards the mechanism connecting OSA and asthma, the recent literature has suggested a central role for tLESRs. Contrary to former belief, nocturnal reflux is not caused by negative intrathoracic pressure during apnea; recent studies have reported that the lower esophageal sphincter contracts during apneic episodes and thus inhibits gastric acid reflux. Therefore, nGERD is more likely caused by transient tLESRs [101]. However several factors may drive the unusual physiopathology of OSA. It appears to be more common in patients with obstructive lung diseases, perhaps as a result of shared risk factors—for example, obesity, smoking, increased airway resistance, local and systemic inflammation. Recently a new syndrome has attracted attention: OLDOSA (obstructive lung disease and obstructive sleep apnea syndrome) [102]. OSA has also been shown to be an independent risk factor for asthma exacerbations [103]. A recent study found OSA in 88% of patients with severe asthma, a significantly higher rate than in both moderate asthmatics and non-asthmatic controls matched for age and body mass index [104]. While the exact pathophysiological mechanism for this association remains to be determined, one possible explanation would be that OSA leads to GERD which exacerbates asthma in a kind of vicious circle [105] (Fig. 12.3).

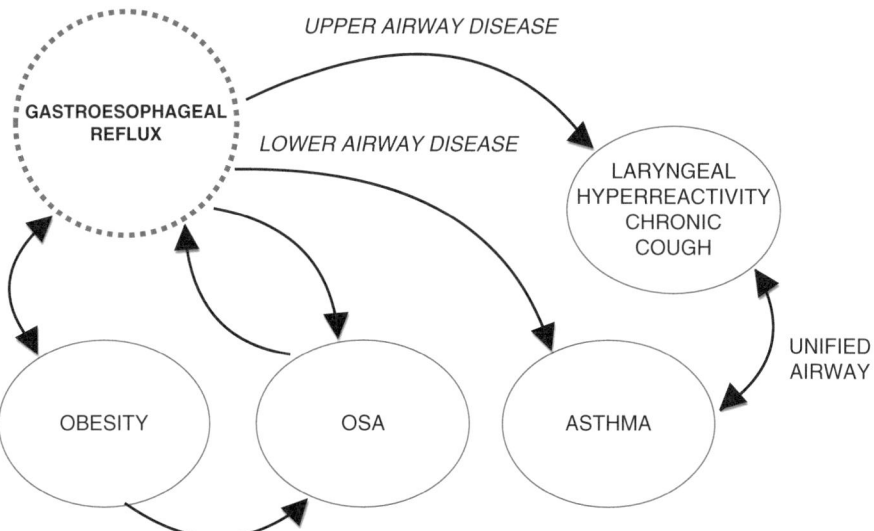

**Fig. 12.3** The complex integration of various entities through the reflux material

## Obesity, GERD and Asthma

The risk of asthma increases by 50% in the overweight or obese [106]. A recent meta-analysis found obesity to be a significant risk factor for incident asthma (OR, 1.51; 95% CI, 1.27–1.80) [107]. In the Obstructive Lung disease In Northern Sweden study, a variety of risk factors for new-onset asthma were studied in people living in three countries [108]. In addition to the known asthma risk factors such as family history of asthma, prior smoking, and allergic rhinitis, the study found that obesity was associated with twofold to threefold increases in the odds of developing asthma in the future. The effect was seen in both allergic and non-allergic individuals, suggesting that the mechanisms of obese asthma are different from the Th2 lymphocyte processes associated with allergic asthma.

In obese asthma there is an increased prevalence of comorbidities related to obesity, such as obstructive sleep apnea and gastro-esophageal reflux. Although these comorbidities should be treated in their own right, their role in worsening asthma and in symptom generation is unclear. More research is required to investigate these associations. One more variable that should be considered is how the upper airway obstruction, frequently present in obese patients during sleep, may act on the esophagus to exacerbate asthma. Another possible explanation of how obesity might lead to asthma is that adipokines, inflammatory cytokines derived from adipose tissue, contribute to increasing airway hyper-responsiveness [109]. Other authors believe that asthma may simply be over-diagnosed in obese patients. Clearly, multiple factors contribute to the asthma-obesity link, and no single factor is likely to explain it.

## Chronic Cough, GERD and Asthma

An interesting association which has not been analysed in depth so far is the coexistence of asthma and chronic cough. In a fair number of medical histories of asthmatics of varying degrees of severity, patients are unable to state which symptom is predominant. In humans, esophageal acid perfusion causes cough only in subjects with prior states of airway irritation such as asthma, not in healthy subjects [110]. The current body of evidence broadly supports the concept that neuronal interference between the esophagus and the airway drives the relationships between gastroesophageal reflux and cough. Chronic cough presents the diagnostic triad of eosinophilic airway inflammation, GERD and upper airway cough syndrome, although it has been hypothesized that the last two of these conditions may be connected through the reflux that reaches the upper airway, since patients with chronic cough, and asthmatics as well, very frequently report laryngeal symptoms such as inspiratory dyspnea, stridor, throat tightness and laryngeal itching, tickling, plugging and mucus dysphagia. Many asthma patients report developing "sensitivity" to various non-specific triggers such as cigarette smoking, cold air, exercise, perfume, clearing agents, odors and emotional stress, and these triggers should be routinely investigated in all asthmatics. Chronic cough often leads to misdiagnosis of asthma or multiple chemical sensitivity. The disorder may be long-lasting, as patients may be unsuccessfully treated for asthma and other comorbidities before correct diagnosis is made. Some patients present asthma but chronic cough is usually associated with other extra-esophageal symptoms, episodic choking or shortness of breath, and often the breathing problems begin at the same time. In these cases the reflux reaching the upper airway seems to be the cause of, or at least a decisive factor in, the breathing problems, especially in refractory neutrophilic asthma.

## The Role of Anti-GERD Treatment in the Course of Asthma: Antacid (PPI) Therapy, Life-Style Modifications and Surgery

### Antacid PPI Therapy

In general physicians treating asthma must address the following important considerations when standard therapy is ineffective: (1) Is the diagnosis correct? (2) Have environmental exposures been minimized? (3) Is medication adherence optimal? (4) Is inhaler technique correct? (5) Have factors that can exacerbate asthma been controlled—such as drugs (e.g., non-steroidal anti-inflammatory drugs, beta-blockers), rhinosinusitis, and GERD? In the last case, the treatment options include empiric acid suppression therapy, lifestyle modification, and surgery. The 2007 National Asthma Education and Prevention Program Guidelines for the diagnosis and management of asthma recommend that clinicians consider treatment of reflux to improve asthma control in patients with poorly controlled disease [111]. The American College of Gastroenterology guidelines suggest treatment with PPI for patients with extra-esophageal symptoms who also have typical symptoms of GERD [112]. Pharmacological therapies for acid suppression have been shown to greatly reduce esophageal exposure to low pH. In a study of the treatment of 82 patients with pH-confirmed diagnosis of extra-esophageal reflux who underwent an 8-week trial of 20 mg omeprazole twice daily, Patterson et al. reported failure to respond in over half of subjects [113]. Another controlled trial suggested a therapeutic benefit for PPIs in the subgroup of patients with both nocturnal respiratory and GERD symptoms but was largely negative [114]. Nonetheless, in a later randomized, placebo-controlled study the same authors found that only esomeprazole 40 mg twice daily led to a significant improvement when FEV 1 was calculated over the entire 26-week period (+0.07 L; $p = 0.0042$) [115]. Not all studies have shown improvement in asthma symptoms with PPIs. Littner et al. followed 207 patients with moderate-to-severe asthma and symptomatic reflux, who were treated with either placebo or a PPI b.i.d. for 24 weeks; these authors found that medical treatment did not reduce daily asthma symptoms, but did reduce asthma exacerbation and improved asthma-related quality of life [116].

PPI therapies reduce the total volume of the gastric juice [117] but may also increase the concentration of pepsin, bile acids and other putatively damaging digestive factors due to the lower volume of gastric secretion. However, the modest effects of PPI treatment of GERD in asthmatics may rather be attributed to a relative irreversibility of GERD-induced airway damage. Indeed, as many authors have pointed out, PPIs do not stop reflux but just make it less acidic; they limit, but do not eliminate, the potential damage to the airways caused by other components of the reflux and in addition they may compromise the competence of the stomach–esophagus barrier. However, PPI treatment may require considerable time, and this is an issue that has not been assessed in depth in studies of the relation between asthma and GERD. Bucknall et al. showed that the impact of the normalization of abnormal esophageal acid exposure on asthma symptoms is progressive and is greater at 3 months than at 2 months; a third of the patients in their series had persistent abnormal esophageal acid exposure despite daily PPI doses up to 80 mg. Therefore, tailoring GERD therapy with repeated pH studies may be beneficial, given the diversity in the presence of esophageal acid. Nonetheless, additional randomized controlled studies of this issue are needed [118]. In studies of the effectiveness of anti-GERD treatment in asthma, the vast majority only analyse medical treatment (essentially PPI) and not other anti-reflux measures.

Nevertheless, effective treatment strategies for supraesophageal reflux disease remain inadequately defined. It has been demonstrated that the mucosa of the upper airway is more sensitive to an acidic environment than the esophagus, and so small amounts of mildly acidic refluxate may be enough to result in inflammation [119]. In a randomized placebo-controlled trial of PPI for suspected extra-esophageal reflux, Vaezi et al. found no significant improvement with PPI treatment [120]. A possible confusion is the limit established for the pH of the reflux in extra-esophageal areas, as demonstrated in a recent study in which a nasopharyngeal pH cutoff of 6 correlated with symptoms of supra-esophageal reflux disease [121].

The treatment of the combination of asthma and GERD presents several methodological problems. Due to the poor sensitivity of endoscopy and pH monitoring, empiric therapy with PPIs is now considered the initial diagnostic step in patients suspected of having GERD-related symptoms. If unresponsive, diagnostic testing with pH monitoring off therapy may be reasonable in order to assess the baseline presence of reflux, and/or impedance/pH monitoring on therapy to exclude continued acid or weakly acid reflux. PPI-unresponsive asthmatics, without overt regurgitation, usually have either no reflux or causes other than GERD. In this group, PPI therapy should be discontinued [37]. However to complicate the situation of research into GERD treatment even further, there are patients with respiratory disease who have a normal reflux burden but respond to anti-reflux surgery. This suggests that even with pH-MII, catheter-based reflux monitoring is suboptimal for establishing causality between gastro-esophageal reflux and lung disease, and other tools to measure reflux related lung disease are needed [122]. Furthermore, when pepsin in the airway was assessed as an aspiration marker and potential aggravating factor in asthma, the relationship with lung pepsin and reflux monitoring was inconsistent [123].

In general, the criticism levelled at studies that compare the influence of anti acid treatment on asthma, and even though antisecretory treatment in difficult-to-control asthmatics with presence of acid reflux demonstrated by pHmetry has not been effective in the asthma [124] is that their results only support the idea that acid reflux is not important in asthma and that their design did not bear in mind other factors: the effect of pepsin on the laryngeal epithelium on non-acid reflux [125], esophageal distension and the stimulation of neurogen inflammation that is not mitigated by PPI [126], or the ineffective esophageal motility as a part of treatment-refractory esophageal reflux due to the presence of nocturnal gastric acid [27]. Thus, further studies are needed to determine the exact mechanism of this bilateral process, to better stratify patient populations (via pulmonary function testing, symptom scores or age) and to determine dose and duration of therapy.

## Life-Style Modifications

As regards the other measures for combating the effect of reflux in the airway, an interesting recent double blind randomized trial of patients with endoscopic signs and symptoms of LPR compared 2 months of rabeprazole with placebo control. The study found that lifestyle modifications significantly improved chronic and symptoms (hoarseness, throat clearing, non-productive cough, globus sensation and sore throat) compared to baseline but that the improvement in reflux symptoms, health status or laryngeal appearance was not significantly greater in the PPI group with additional lifestyle modifications. The modifications were: avoidance of fatty meals, caffeine, alcohol, smoking, and oral intake within 2 h of lying down or bedtime, as well as addition of extra pillows to raise the head of the bed by 6 in. [127]. Another recent study supported the role of lifestyle modifications in patients who had undergone overnight nasopharyngeal pH monitoring with a commercially available nasopharyngeal pH monitoring device (Dx-pH Measurement System, Restech). The study provided new evidence that supra-esophageal symptoms frequently occur in the supine position; 55% of patients with positive studies had supine-only reflux and 6 in. of head-of-bed elevation was effective in reducing symptoms such as throat clearing, cough, asthma, postnasal drainage, sinusitis, laryngo-pharyngitis, and sleep disturbance [128]. When effective, treatment with head-of-bed elevation has the additional advantage of eliminating both acidic and nonacidic reflux, which potentially makes it superior to treatment with PPI. This is in contrast to the treatment of GERD, for which nonacidic reflux is less of a concern due to the more robust defense mechanisms of the esophageal mucosa. Nonacidic reflux contains several potentially harmful constituents, including bile, pancreatic enzymes, and pepsin [129].

## Surgery in GERD

However, the true gold standard method for demonstrating reflux-related lung disease is the performance of fundoplication in patients, with resulting symptomatic improvement. Francis et al. performed a retrospective cohort study to establish which patients would benefit the most from Nissen fundoplication, [130]. They found that patients with both heartburn with or without regurgitation and esophageal pH <4 more than 12% of a 24-h period were more likely to present post-fundoplication resolution of the extra-esophageal reflux symptoms. Hence, surgical fundoplication may be useful in selected patients who continue to have regurgitation despite PPI therapy, have moderate-to-severe reflux measured by pH monitoring off therapy, and who may have a mechanical defect such as a moderate-sized hiatal hernia (>4 cm). Surgical fundoplication is not recommended for patients who are unresponsive to aggressive medical treatment. In another prospective review of the effects of anti-reflux surgery, data from a prospective, randomized, open-label trial comparing the efficacy and safety of laparoscopic anti-reflux surgery (LARS) vs esomeprazole (20 mg or 40 mg daily) over 5 years in patients with chronic GERD were analysed. The authors found esophageal acid reflux to be greatly reduced by LARS or esomeprazole therapy. However, patients receiving LARS had significantly greater reductions in 24-h esophageal acid exposure after 6 months and after 5 years. Esophageal and gastric pH, off and on therapy, did not predict long-term outcomes of patients and the authors concluded that abnormal supine acid exposure predicted esomeprazole dose escalation [131].

In summary, it is generally accepted that patients with poorly controlled asthma despite corticosteroid therapy without symptoms of reflux, as well as children, do not respond to aggressive PPI therapy. This is likely due to the fact that acid reflux does not contribute to their symptoms, although this concept, proposed by gastroenterologists, refers only to antacid treatment and to typical reflux symptoms, and not to atypical symptoms more related to extra-esophageal involvement. However there is a clear need for a clinical trial with inclusion criteria of objective evidence of acidic and nonacidic esophageal reflux and with randomized assignment of patients to medication and life style modifications or surgical repair of gastro-esophageal reflux. Until a trial of this nature is undertaken, empirical treatment with proton-pump inhibitors does not make sense [132].

## Summary and Conclusions

The trajectory of the reflux material from the stomach-duodenum to the airways causes esophageal and extra-esophageal symptoms, due to the direct action of the reflux material on the respiratory epithelial tissue or via reflex mechanisms involved in neuronal inflammation.

As an obstructive airway disorder, asthma also induces mechanistic changes which can also lead to GERD.

The relationship between asthma and GERD and the associated comorbidities such as obesity or OSA create numerous vicious circles. As it is not known whether the role of GERD is primary or secondary, the relationship is particularly problematic.

The suboptimal sensitivity and specificity of current diagnostic methods such as upper endoscopy, pH monitoring and impedance monitoring makes the diagnosis of the asthma—GERD relationship particularly difficult.

The current paradigm includes empiric therapy for GERD with high dose PPI twice a day. But attention should also be paid to other features of GERD such as gaseous material and nonacid material, and to aspects of its physiopathology of such as esophageal dysmotility, excessive gastric filling and the physical mechanism of the invalidation of the gastro-esophageal barrier which is common to all obstructive airway processes including COPD, laryngeal hyper-responsiveness and OSA.

There is no predictive model available to determine which patients will benefit from complete anti-reflux therapy. The results regarding treatment dose, duration and utility have varied widely from study to study.

Asthma and GERD are both multifactorial. In the two-way relationship between the two entities, close cooperation is required between pulmonologists, ENT specialists and gastroenterologists to achieve a fuller understanding of the problem and thus improve its management.

## References

1. Osler W. Bronchial asthma. In: The principles and practice of medicine. New York: Appleton; 1892. p. 497–501.
2. Lipan MJ, Reidenberg JS, Laitman JT. Anatomy of reflux: a growing health problem affecting structures of the head and neck. Anat Rec B New Anat. 2006;289((6):261–70.
3. Vakil N, van Zanten SV, Kahrilas P, et al. The Montreal definition and classification of gastro-esophageal reflux disease (GERD)—a global evidence-based consensus. Am J Gastroenterol. 2006;101:1900–20.
4. Gislason T, Janson C, Vermeire P, et al. Respiratory symptoms and nocturnal gastro-esophageal reflux: a population-based study of young adults in three European countries. Chest. 2002;121:158–63.
5. Stein MR. Possible mechanisms of influence of esophageal acid on airway hyper-responsiveness. Am J Med. 2003;115(3A):55S–9S.
6. Zerbib F, Guisset O, Lamouliatte H, et al. Effects of bronchial obstruction on lower esophageal sphincter motility and gastro-esophageal reflux in patients with asthma. Am J Respir Crit Care Med. 2002;166:1206–11.
7. Bateman ED, Boushey HA, Bousquet J, GOAL Investigators Group, et al. Can guideline-defined asthma control be achieved? The Gaining Optimal Asthma ControL Study. Am J Respir Crit Care Med. 2004;170(8):836–44.
8. Sin DD, Anthonisen NR, Soriano JB, et al. Mortality in COPD: role of comorbidities. Eur Respir J. 2006;28:1245–57.
9. Cazzola M, Calzetta L, Bettoncelli G, et al. Asthma and comorbid medical illness. Eur Respir J. 2011;38:42–9.
10. Pavord ID, Birring SS, Berry M, et al. Multiple inflammatory hits and the pathogenesis of severe airway disease. Eur Respir J. 2006;27:884–8.
11. Chan-Yeung M, Malo J-L. Occupational asthma. N Engl J Med. 1995;333:107–12.
12. Saritas Yuksel E, Vaezi MF. Extra-esophageal manifestations of gastro-esophageal reflux disease: cough, asthma, laryngitis, chest pain. Swiss Med Wkly. 2012;142:w13544.
13. Cheng YM, Wang HW, Cao AL, et al. Airway hyper-responsiveness induced by repeated esophageal infusion of HCl in Guinea pigs. Am J Respir Cell Mol Biol. 2014;51(5): 701–8.
14. Moayyedi P, Talley NJ. Gastro-esophageal reflux disease. Lancet. 2006;367:2086–100.
15. Akinbami LJ, Moorman JE, Bailey C, et al. Trends in asthma prevalence, health care use, and mortality in the United States, 2001–2010. NCHS Data Brief. 2012;94:1–8.
16. Havemann BD, Henderson CA, El-Serag HB. The association between gastro-esophageal reflux disease and asthma: a systematic review. Gut. 2007;56:1654–64.

17. Field SK, Underwood M, Brant R, et al. Prevalence of gastro-esophageal reflux symptoms in asthma. Chest. 1996;109:316–22.
18. Nordenstedt H, Nilsson M, Johansson S, et al. The relation between gastro-esophageal reflux and respiratory symptoms in a population-based study: the Nord-Trøndelag health survey. Chest. 2006;129:1051–6.
19. Mulrennan S, Knuiman M, Divitini M, et al. Gastro-esophageal reflux and respiratory symptoms in Busselton adults: the affects of body weight and sleep apnoea. Intern Med J. 2012;42(7):722–9.
20. Jordan HT, Stellman SD, Reibman J, et al. Factors associated with poor control of 9/11-related asthma 10-11 years after the 2001 World Trade Center terrorist attacks. J Asthma. 2015;21:1–8.
21. Ruigomez A, Rodriguez LA, Wallander MA, et al. Gastro-esophageal reflux disease and asthma: a longitudinal study in UK general practice. Chest. 2005;128(1):85–93.
22. Jack CI, Calverley PM, Donnelly RJ, et al. Simultaneous tracheal and esophageal pH measurements in asthma patients with gastro-esophageal reflux. Thorax. 1995;50(2):201–4.
23. Patterson RN, Johnston BT, Ardill JE, et al. Increased tachykinin levels in induced sputum from asthmatic and cough patients with acid reflux. Thorax. 2007;62:491–5.
24. Schneider JH, Kuper MA, Konigsrainer A, et al. Transient lower esophageal sphincter relaxation and esophageal motor response. J Surg Res. 2010;159:714–9.
25. Trudgill NJ, Riley SA. Transient lower esophageal sphincter relaxations are no more frequent in patients with gastro-esophageal reflux disease than in asymptomatic volunteers. Am J Gastroenterol. 2001;96:2569–74.
26. Beaumont H, Bennink RJ, De Jong J, et al. The position of the acid pocket as a major risk factor for acidic reflux in healthy subjects and patients with GORD. Gut. 2010;59:441–51.
27. Fouad YM, Katz PO, Hatlebakk JG, et al. Ineffective esophageal motility: the most common motility abnormality in patients with GERD-associated respiratory symptoms. Am J Gastroenterol. 1999;94(6):1464.
28. Sanger GJ, Lee K. Hormones of the gut-brain axis as targets for the treatment of upper gastrointestinal disorders. Nat Rev Drug Discov. 2008;7:241–54.
29. McGrath KW, Icitovic N, Boushey HA, et al. A large subgroup of mild-to-moderate asthma is persistently noneosinophilic. Am J Respir Crit Care Med. 2012;185:612–9.
30. Simpson JL, Scott R, Boyle MJ, et al. Inflammatory subtypes in asthma: assessment and identification using induced sputum. Respirology. 2006;11:54–61.
31. Simpson JL, Baines KJ, Ryan N, et al. Neutrophilic asthma is characterised by increased rhinosinusitis with sleep disturbance and GERD. Asian Pac J Allergy Immunol. 2014;32(1):66–74.
32. Thakkar K, Boatright RO, Gilger MA, et al. Gastro-esophageal reflux and asthma in children: a systematic review. Pediatrics. 2010;125(4):e925–30.
33. Harding SM. Gastro-esophageal reflux: a potential asthma trigger. Immunol Allergy Clin N Am. 2005;25:131–48.
34. Kastelik JA, Jackson W, Davies TW, et al. Measurement of gastric emptying in gastroesophageal reflux-related chronic cough. Chest. 2002;122:2038–437.
35. De Vita C, Berni Canani F, et al. "Silent" gastro-esophageal reflux and upper airway pathologies in childhood. Acta Otorhinolaryngol Ital. 1996;16:407–11.
36. Herregods TV, Bredenoord AJ, Smout AJ. Pathophysiology of gastro-esophageal reflux disease: new understanding in a new era. Neurogastroenterol Motil. 2015;27(9):1202–13.
37. Naik RD, Vaezi MF. Extra-esophageal reflux disease and asthma: understanding this interplay. Expert Rev Gastroenterol Hepatol. 2015;9(7):969–82.
38. Poelmans J, Tack J. Extra-esophageal manifestations of gastro-esophageal reflux. Gut. 2005;54(10):1492–9.
39. Bor S, Kitapcioglu G, Solak ZA, et al. Prevalence of gastro-esophageal reflux disease in patients with asthma and chronic obstructive pulmonary disease. J Gastroenterol Hepatol. 2010;25(2):309–13.
40. Kiljander TO, Salomaa ER, Hietanen EK, et al. Gastro-esophageal reflux in asthmatics: a double-blind, placebo-controlled crossover study with omeprazole. Chest. 1999;116(5):1257–64.

41. Morice AH, Faruqi S, Wright CE, et al. Cough hypersensitivity syndrome: a distinct clinical entity. Lung. 2011;189(1):73–9.
42. de Bortoli N, Nacci A, Savarhino E, et al. How many cases of laryngo-pharyngeal reflux suspected by laryngoscopy are gastro-esophageal reflux disease-related? World J Gastroenterol. 2012;18:4363–70.
43. Wilshire CL, Salvador R, Sepesi B, et al. Reflux-associated oxygen desaturations: usefulness in diagnosing reflux-related respiratory symptoms. J Gastrointest Surg. 2013;17:30–8.
44. Mise K, Capkun V, Jurcev-Savicevic A, et al. The influence of gastro-esophageal reflux in the lung: a case-control study. Respirology. 2010;15(5):837–42.
45. Turbyville JC. Applying principles of physics to the airway to help explain the relationship between asthma and gastro-esophageal reflux. Med Hypotheses. 2010;74:1075–80.
46. Garcia Rodriguez LA, Ruigomez A, Martin-Merhino E, et al. Relationship between gastro-esophageal reflux disease and COPD in UK primary care. Chest. 2008;134:1223–30.
47. Moote DW, Lloyd DA, McCourtie DR, et al. Increase in gastro-esophageal reflux during methacholine induced bronchospasm. J Allergy Clin Immunol. 1986;78:619–23.
48. Harding SM, Guzzo MR, Richter JE. The prevalence of gastro-esophageal reflux in asthma patients without reflux symptoms. Am J Respir Crit Care Med. 2000;162:34–9.
49. Kiljander TO, Laitinen JO. The prevalence of gastro-esophageal reflux disease in adult asthmatics. Chest. 2004;126:1490–4.
50. Leggett JJ, Johnston BT, Mills M, et al. Prevalence of gastro-esophageal reflux in difficult asthma: relationship to asthma outcome. Chest. 2005;127:1227–31.
51. Ronkainen J, Aro P, Storskrubb T, et al. High prevalence of gastro-esophageal reflux symptoms and esophagitis with or without symptoms in the general adult Swedish population: a Kalixanda study report. Scand J Gastroenterol. 2005;40:275–85.
52. Kavitt RT, Higginbotham T, Slaughter JC, et al. Symptom reports are not reliable during ambulatory reflux monitoring. Am J Gastroenterol. 2012;107(12):1826–32.
53. Woodcock A, Young EC, Smith JA. New insights in cough. Br Med Bull. 2010;96:61–73.
54. DiMango E, Holbrook JT, Simpson E, et al. Effects of asymptomatic proximal and distal gastro-esophageal reflux on asthma severity. Am J Respir Crit Care Med. 2009;180(9):809–16.
55. Roberts JR, Aravapalli A, Pohl D, et al. Extra-esophageal gastro-esophageal reflux disease (GERD) symptoms are not more frequently associated with proximal esophageal reflux than typical GERD symptoms. Dis Esophagus. 2012;25(8):678–81.
56. Wiener GJ, Tsukashima R, Kelly C, et al. Oropharyngeal pH monitoring for the detection of liquid and aerosolized supraesophageal gastric reflux. J Voice. 2009;23:498–504.
57. Montuschi P. Analysis of exhaled breath condensate in respiratory medicine: methodological aspects and potential clinical applications. Ther Adv Respir Dis. 2007;1:5–23.
58. Golub JS, Johns MM, Lim JH, et al. Comparison of an oropharyngeal pH probe and a standard dual pH probe for diagnosis of laryngo-pharyngeal reflux. Ann Otol Rhinol Laryngol. 2009;118(1):1–5.
59. Murry T, Bransky RC, Yu K, et al. Laryngeal sensory deficits in patients with chronic cough and paradoxical vocal fold movement disorder. Laryngoscope. 2010;120:1576–81.
60. Pacheco A, Cobeta R. Refractory chronic cough, or the need to focus on the relationship between the larynx and the esophagus. Cough. 2013;9(1):10.
61. Phua SY, McGarvey LPA, Ngu MC, et al. Patients with gastro-esophageal reflux disease and cough have impaired laryngo-pharyngeal mechanosensitivity. Thorax. 2005;60:488–91.
62. Nishino T. The role of the larynx in defensive airway reflexes in humans. Eur Respir Rev. 2002;12:231–5.
63. Phua SY, McGarvey L, Ngu M, et al. The differential effect of gastro-esophageal reflux disease on mechanostimulation and chemostimulation of the laryngo-pharynx. Chest. 2010;138:1180–5.
64. Blondeau K, Dupont LJ, Mertens V, et al. Improved diagnosis of gastro-esophageal reflux in patients with unexplained chronic cough. Aliment Pharmacol Ther. 2007;25:723–32.
65. Komatsu Y, Hoppo T, Jobe BA. Abnormal proximal reflux as a cause of adult-onset asthma: the case for hypopharyngeal impedance testing to improve the sensitivity of diagnosis. JAMA Surg. 2013;148(1):50–8.

66. Ryan NM, Vertigan AE, Gibson PG. Chronic cough and laryngeal dysfunction improve with specific treatment of cough and paradoxical vocal fold movement. Cough. 2009;5:4.
67. Smith J, Woodcock A, Houghton L. New developments in reflux-associated cough. Lung. 2010;188(Suppl 1):S81–6.
68. Good JT Jr, Kolakowski CA, Groshong SD, et al. Refractory asthma: importance of bronchoscopy to identify phenotypes and direct therapy. Chest. 2012;141(3):599–606.
69. Kotby MN, Hassan O, El-Makhzangy M, et al. Gastro-esophageal reflux / laryngopharyngeal reflux disease: a critical analysis of the literature. Eur Arch Otorhinolaryngol. 2010;267:171–9.
70. Johnston N, Dettmar PW, Bishwokarma B, et al. Activity/stability of human pepsin: implications for reflux attributed laryngeal disease. Laryngoscope. 2007;117:1036–9.
71. Low K, Lau KK, Holmes P, et al. Abnormal vocal cord function in difficult-to-treat asthma. Am J Respir Crit Care Med. 2011;184:50–6.
72. Terada K, Muro S, Ohara T, et al. Abnormal swallowing reflex and COPD exacerbations. Chest. 2010;137(2):326–32.
73. Nemzek JA, Kim J. Pulmonary inflammation and airway hyper-responsiveness in a mouse model of asthma complicated by acid aspiration. Comp Med. 2009;59:321–30.
74. Smith JA, Houghton LA. The esophagus and cough: laryngo-pharyngeal reflux, microaspiration and vagal reflexes. Cough. 2013;9(1):12.
75. Brownlee IA, Aseeri A, Ward C, et al. From gastric aspiration to airway inflammation. Monaldi Arch Chest Dis. 2010;73:54–63.
76. Appel JZ 3rd, Lee SM, Hartwig MG, et al. Characterization of the innate immune response to chronic aspiration in a novel rodent model. Respir Res. 2007;8:87.
77. Su KY, Thomas AD, Chang JC, et al. Chronic aspiration shifts the immune response from adaptive immunity to innate immunity in a murine model of asthma. Inflamm Res. 2012;61:863–73.
78. Downing TE, Sporn TA, Bollinger RR, et al. Pulmonary histopathology in an experimental model of chronic aspiration is independent of acidity. Exp Biol Med (Maywood). 2008;233:1202–129.
79. Wenzel SE, Vitari CA, Shende M, et al. Asthmatic granulomatosis: a novel disease with asthmatic and granulomatous features. Am J Respir Crit Care Med. 2012;186(6):501–7.
80. Zhu GC, Gao X, Wang ZG, et al. Experimental study for the mechanism of gastro-esophageal-reflux-associated asthma. Dis Esophagus. 2014;27(4):318–24.
81. Sugawa T, Fujiwara Y, Yamagami H, et al. A novel rat model to determine interaction between reflux esophagitis and bronchial asthma. Gut. 2008;57:575–81.
82. Brewer JP, Kisselgof AB, Martin TR. Genetic variability in pulmonary physiological, cellular, and antibody responses to antigen in mice. Am J Respir Crit Care Med. 1999;160:1150–6.
83. Hylkema M, Hoekstra M, Luinge M, et al. The strength of the OVA-induced airway inflammation in rats is strain dependent. Clin Exp Immunol. 2002;129:390–6.
84. Wright RA, Miller SA, Corsello BF. Acid-induced esophagobronchial- cardiac reflexes in humans. Gastroenterology. 1990;99:71–3.
85. Chopra K, Matta SK, Madan N, et al. Association of gastro-esophageal reflux with bronchial asthma. Indian Pediatr. 1995;32:1083–6.
86. Rosen R, Johnston N, Hart K, et al. The presence of pepsin in the lung and its relationship to pathologic gastro-esophageal reflux. Neurogastroenterol Motil. 2012;24(2):129–33.
87. D'Ovidio F, Mura M, Ridsdale R, et al. The effect of reflux and bile acid aspiration on the lung allograft and its surfactant and innate immunity molecules SP-A and SP-D. Am J Transplant. 2006;6(8):1930.
88. Alves LR, Soares EG, Aprile LR, et al. Chlorophyllin-stained macrophages as markers of pulmonary aspiration. Am J Respir Crit Care Med. 2013;188(12):1470–2.
89. Balhara J, Gounni AS. The alveolar macrophages in asthma: a double-edged sword. Mucosal Immunol. 2012;5(6):605–9.
90. Moon KA, Kim SY, Kim TB, et al. Allergen-induced CD11b+ CD11c(int) CCR3+ macrophages in the lung promote eosinophilic airway inflammation in a mouse asthma model. Int Immunol. 2007;19:1371–81.

91. Byers DE, Holtzman MJ. Alternatively activated macrophages and airway disease. Chest. 2011;140(3):768–74.
92. Coyle AJ, Ackerman SJ, Irvin CG. Cationic proteins induce airway hyper-responsiveness dependent on charge interactions. Am Rev Respir Dis. 1993;147:896–900.
93. Simpson JL, Gibson PG, Yang IA, et al. Impaired macrophage phagocytosis in non-eosinophilic asthma. Clin Exp Allergy. 2013;43:29–35.
94. Theodoropoulus DS, Ledford DK, Lockey RF, et al. Prevalence of upper respiratory symptoms in patients with symptomatic gastro-esophageal reflux. Am J Respir Crit Care Med. 2001;164:72–6.
95. Demeter P, Pap A. The relationship between gastro-esophageal reflux disease and obstructive sleep apnea. J Gastroenterol. 2004;39:815–20.
96. Kerr P, Shoenut JP, Millar T, et al. Nasal CPAP reduces gastro-esophageal reflux in obstructive sleep apnea syndrome. Chest. 1992;101:1539–44.
97. Lindam A, Kendall BJ, Thrift AP, et al. Symptoms of obstructive sleep apnea, gastro-esophageal reflux and the risk of Barrett's esophagus in a population-based case-control study. PLoS One. 2015;10(6):e0129836.
98. Bandla H, Splaingard M. Sleep problems in children with common medical disorders. Pediatr Clin N Am. 2004;51:203–27.
99. Shaker R, Castell DO, Schoenfeld PS, et al. Nighttime heartburn is an under-appreciated clinical problem that impacts sleep and daytime function: the results of a Gallup survey conducted on behalf of the American Gastroenterological Association. Am J Gastroenterol. 2003;98:1487–93.
100. Emilsson ÖI, Bengtsson A, Franklin KA, et al. Nocturnal gastro-esophageal reflux, asthma and symptoms of OSA: a longitudinal, general population study. Eur Respir J. 2013;41(6):1347–54.
101. Kuribayashi S, Kusano M, Kawamura O, et al. Mechanism of gastro-esophageal reflux in patients with obstructive sleep apnea syndrome. Neurogastroenterol Motil. 2010;22: e611–172.
102. Ioachimescu OC, Teodorescu M. Integrating the overlap of obstructive lung disease and obstructive sleep apnoea: OLDOSA syndrome. Respirology. 2013;18(3):421–31.
103. Ten Brinke A, Sterk PJ, Masclee AA, et al. Risk factors of frequent exacerbations in difficult-to treat-asthma. Eur Respir J. 2005;26:812–8.
104. Julien JY, Martin JG, Ernst P, et al. Prevalence of obstructive sleep apneahypopnea in severe versus moderate asthma. J Allergy Clin Immunol. 2009;124:371–6.
105. Puthalapattu S, Ioachimescu OC. Asthma and obstructive sleep apnea: clinical and pathogenic interactions. J Investig Med. 2014;62(4):665–75.
106. Beuther DA, Sutherland ER. Overweight, obesity, and incident asthma: a meta-analysis of prospective epidemiologic studies. Am J Respir Crit Care Med. 2007;175:661–6.
107. Buether DA, Sutherland ER. Overweight, obesity, and incident asthma. Am J Respir Crit Care Med. 2007;175:661–6.
108. Rönmark E, Andersson C, Nyström L, et al. Obesity increases the risk of incident asthma among adults. Eur Respir J. 2005;25:282–8.
109. Dixon AE. Adipokines and asthma. Chest. 2009;135:255–6.
110. Wu DN, Yamauchi K, Kobayashi H, et al. Effects of esophageal acid perfusion on cough responsiveness in patients with bronchial asthma. Chest. 2002;122:505–9.
111. National Heart Lung and Blood Institute National Asthma Education and Prevention Program Expert Panel Report 3: Guidelines for the Diagnosis and Management of Asthma. Full report; 2007. http://www.nhlbi.nih.gov/guidelines/ asthma/asthgdln.htm.
112. Katz PO, Gerson LB, Vela MF. Guidelines for the diagnosis and management of gastro-esophageal reflux disease. Am J Gastroenterol. 2013;108(3):308–28.
113. Patterson RN, Johnston BT, MacMahon J, et al. Esophageal pH monitoring is of limited value in the diagnosis of "reflux-cough". Eur Respir J. 2004;24:724–7.
114. Kiljander TO, Harding SM, Field SK, et al. Effects of esomeprazole 40 mg twice daily on asthma: a randomized placebo-controlled trial. Am J Respir Crit Care Med. 2006;173: 1091–7.

115. Kiljander TO, Junghard O, Beckman O, et al. Effect of esomeprazole 40 mg once or twice daily on asthma: a randomized, placebo-controlled study. Am J Respir Crit Care Med. 2010;181(10):1042–8.
116. Littner MR, Leung FW, Ballard ED 2nd, Lansoprazole Asthma Study Group. Effects of 24 weeks of lansoprazole therapy on asthma symptoms, exacerbations, quality of life, and pulmonary function in adult asthma patients with acid reflux symptoms. Chest. 2005;128(3):1128–35.
117. Gursoy O, Memis D, Sut N. Effect of proton pump inhibitors on gastric juice volume, gastric pH and gastric intramucosal pH in critically ill patients: a randomized, double-blind, placebo-controlled study. Clin Drug Invest. 2008;28:777–82.
118. Bucknall C, Stanton A, Miller G, et al. The impact of normalization of esophageal acid profile by incremental protein pump inhibitors dosing in difficult asthma patients with proven gastro-esophageal acid reflux. J Asthma. 2009;46:506–11.
119. Bulmer DM, Ali MS, Brownlee IA, et al. Laryngeal mucosa: its susceptibility to damage by acid and pepsin. Laryngoscope. 2010;120:777–82.
120. Vaezi MF, Richter JE, Stasney CR, et al. Treatment of chronic posterior laryngitis with esomeprazole. Laryngoscope. 2006;116:254–60.
121. Yuksel ES, Slaughter JC, Mukhtar N, et al. An oropharyngeal pH monitoring device to evaluate patients with chronic laryngitis. Neurogastroenterol Motil. 2013;25:315–23.
122. Mainie I, Tutuian R, Agrawal A, et al. Combined multichannel intraluminal impedance-pH monitoring to select patients with persistent gastro-esophageal reflux for laparoscopic Nissen fundoplication. Br J Surg. 2006;93:1483–7.
123. Potluri S, Friedenberg F, Parkman HP, et al. Comparison of a salivary/sputum pepsin assay with 24-hour esophageal pH monitoring for detection of gastric reflux into the proximal esophagus, oropharynx, and lung. Dig Dis Sci. 2003;48:1813–7.
124. Mastronade JG, Anthonisen NR, Castro M, et al. Efficacy of esomeprazole for treatment of poorly controlled asthma. N Engl J Med. 2009;360:1487–99.
125. Johnston N, Samuels TL, Blumin JH. Pepsin in nonacidic refluxate can damage hypopharyngeal epithelial cells. Ann Otol Rhinol Laryngol. 2009;118:677–85.
126. Canning BJ, Mazzone SB. Reflex mechanisms in gastro-esophageal reflux disease and asthma. Am J Med. 2003;115(Suppl 3A):S45–8.
127. Steward DL, Wilson KM, Kelly DH, et al. Proton pump inhibitor therapy for chronic laryngo-pharyngitis: a randomized placebo-control trial. Otolaryngol Head Neck Surg. 2004;131:342–50.
128. Scott DR, Simon RA. Supraesophageal reflux: correlation of position and occurrence of acid reflux-effect of head-of-bed elevation on supine reflux. J Allergy Clin Immunol Pract. 2015;3(3):356–61.
129. Ali MS, Parikh S, Chater P, et al. Bile acids in laryngo-pharyngeal refluxate: will they enhance or attenuate the action of pepsin? Laryngoscope. 2013;123:434–9.
130. Francis DO, Goutte M, Slaughter JC, et al. Traditional reflux parameters and not impedance monitoring predict outcome after fundoplication in extra-esophageal reflux. Laryngoscope. 2011;121(9):1902–9.
131. Hatlebakk JG, Zerbib F, Bruley des Varannes S, et al. LOTUS study group gastro-esophageal acid reflux control 5 years after anti-reflux surgery, compared with long-term esomeprazole therapy. Clin Gastroenterol Hepatol. 2016;14(5):678–85.
132. Asano K, Suzuki HN. Silent acid reflux and asthma control. N Engl J Med. 2009;360(15):1551–3.

# Gastroesophageal Reflux Disease (GERD) and COPD

## 13

Nabid Zaer and John R. Hurst

## Introduction

In this chapter we will consider the relevance of gastroesophageal reflux (GER) to Chronic Obstructive Pulmonary Disease (COPD), particularly with regard to COPD exacerbations. COPD is a long-term condition, progressive in its clinical course, characterised by persistent airflow limitation and chronic airway inflammation. Exacerbations contribute to the clinical severity in individual patients and are defined as episodic deteriorations in respiratory health. GERD, being common in the general population, is also highly prevalent in COPD. However, GERD has emerged as a potential risk factor for exacerbations of COPD in many studies employing diverse methodology.

## Definition of COPD, Exacerbation and GERD in COPD

COPD is a chronic, progressive condition, characterized by an increased inflammatory response within the airway and airflow limitation that is not fully reversible [1]. It is part of a spectrum of lung disease that develops when a genetically susceptible individual meets a sufficient environmental stimulus. In the developed world this stimulus is usually tobacco smoke but exposure to biomass fuel is important globally. The clinical course is progressive and often punctuated by exacerbations, with exacerbations having detrimental effects on patient quality of life, survival, accelerating lung function decline and therefore also being responsible for much of the heath-care costs associated with COPD [2]. The Global Initiative for Chronic Obstructive Lung Disease (GOLD) defines a COPD exacerbation as *"an acute event characterized by a worsening of the patient's respiratory symptoms that is beyond normal day-to-day variations and*

N. Zaer · J. R. Hurst (✉)
UCL Respiratory Medicine, University College London, London, UK
e-mail: j.hurst@ucl.ac.uk

*leads to a change in medication"*. Our understanding of the pathological mechanisms of COPD and COPD exacerbation is evolving. They appear often to be triggered by acquisition of respiratory viruses, or by alterations in the lung microbiome. Underlying mechanisms relevant in COPD and COPD exacerbations include unopposed action of proteases and oxidants leading to destruction of alveoli, and increased circulating inflammatory markers. The genetic susceptibility to COPD is best exemplified by alpha-1 antitrypsin deficiency.

For the purposes of this chapter we will defined GER as the retrograde movement of stomach contents through the lower esophageal sphincter (LOS) [3] into the esophagus or more proximally. According to the Montreal consensus definition GERD is *"a condition which develops when the reflux of stomach contents causes troublesome symptoms and/or complications"* [4]. The mechanisms of GER have been explored elsewhere in this text.

## Epidemiology and Prevalence of GERD in COPD Patients

A range of methodologies have been used in studies examining the prevalence of GER in COPD, and associations between the two conditions, including symptom questionnaires and objective measurements. The area is complex because of the poor correlation between symptom-based and objective assessments and whether purely peptic/acid reflux is assessed or non-acid reflux also considered. Using peptic symptom-based approaches, the prevalence of GERD ranges from 17% to 54% [5–13]. However, whilst over 90% sensitive, the use of symptoms is poorly specific—perhaps less than 50%—which limits the diagnostic value [14]. Symptoms may be up to three times more prevalent than the general population [15] including smoking controls [16]. Symptoms are more common with increasing COPD severity, and COPD patients are more likely than controls to be prescribed therapy for GERD.

Taking an epidemiological approach, using a large UK primary care database, incident GERD was positively associated with a prior diagnosis of COPD [17]: the relative risk of an incident GERD diagnosis among COPD patients over 5 years of follow up was 1.46 (95% CI 1.19–1.78). However, the relative risk of an incident COPD diagnosis in patients with GERD was not significantly elevated [18].

Studies using esophageal pH monitoring report the prevalence in COPD at between 19% and 78% [9, 19–22], up to five times more prevalent than the non-COPD population for proximal and distal reflux [23, 24]. The first study reporting 24 h pH monitoring in COPD patients and controls was published in 2004 [25]. Sixty two percent of the COPD patients had distal acidic reflux compared to 19% of age-similar controls ($p = 0.003$). In 58% of the COPD patients GERD symptoms were absent suggesting a high prevalence of asymptomatic acid reflux. In some patients, acidic GERD episodes were associated with oxygen desaturation, particularly when supine. A subsequent distal and proximal probe study found similar results and also noted abnormal proximal reflux [26].

There are no sufficiently large, comprehensive studies exploring GERD in COPD and control populations to be able to definitely answer questions regarding comparative prevalence of GERD in COPD versus control populations.

## Potential Mechanisms of Interaction Between GERD and COPD

There are a number of potential mechanisms by which GER and GERD may be more common in subjects with COPD than controls and these are summarised and illustrated in Fig. 13.1.

First, hyperinflation which flattens the diaphragm necessitates increased respiratory muscle effort may amplify the pressure gradient between the thorax and abdomen, impacting lower esophageal sphincter (LES) tone and predisposing to reflux [27, 28]. In support of this, indices of hyperinflation correlate negatively

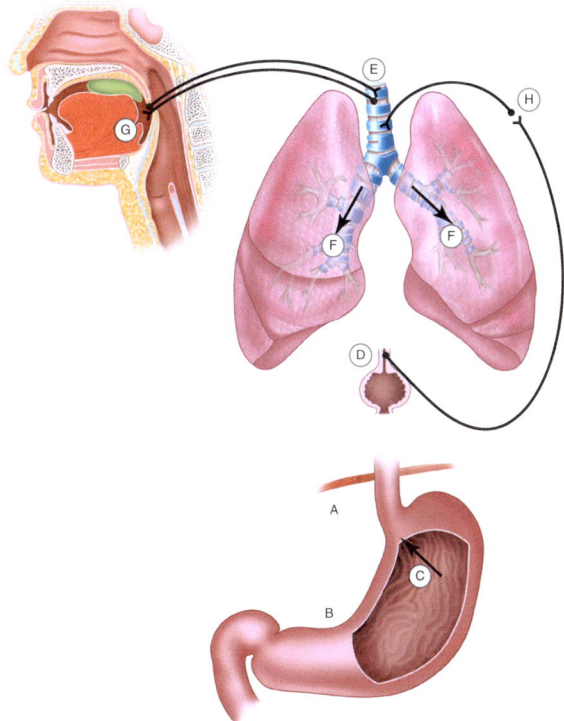

**Fig. 13.1** Potential mechanisms of association between GER and exacerbations of COPD. Displacement of the diaphragm (A) from hyper inflated lung results in additional extrinsic pressure on the stomach. Increased used of abdominal muscles from dyspnea and cough results in additional pressure on the stomach (B). This facilitates passage of stomach contents retrograde through the lower oesophageal sphincter (C), the competency of which may be affected by alterations in vagal tone either directly or with COPD therapy. Increased intrathoracic pressure from hyperinflation may exert additional extrinsic pressure on the esophagus (D), facilitating retrograde movement of refluxate to the proximal esophagus. Small quantities of liquid refluxate therefore spill over into the airway (E) and constituents of aspirated refluxate (F) enhance inflammation and increase susceptibility to exacerbation. Alternative mechanisms include impairment in swallowing (G) and vagal neuronal reflex from esophageal stimulation (H)

with resting sphincter tone [22] however indices of hyperinflation are not necessarily correlated with the presence of GERD in COPD [29]. Such effects may be increased further at COPD exacerbations when there may be additional dynamic hyperinflation together with increased cough. Second, mechanisms may be active that reduce LES tone. This may be seen, for example, in association with smoking, and with cough, the former associated with nicotine-induced relaxation of the LES circular muscle [30]. Smoking may also affect saliva production, and therefore the ability to neutralize acidic reflux events [30]. Medications commonly used in COPD including beta-2 agonists, anti-cholinergics and theophylline may also affect LES tone [6, 31–36]. A more general autonomic dysfunction, which may include effects on LOS tone, has been described as a feature of COPD [37]. The limited number of studies examining esophageal peristalsis in COPD suggest that motility may be altered, at least in severe disease [22, 26, 38–41]. There are no data to suggest that hiatus hernia is more common in COPD patients than controls.

Third, pulmonary micro-aspiration may arise from proximal GER, or from swallowing dysfunction. A higher frequency of exacerbations has been reported in individuals with an abnormal swallowing reflex (OR 4.86 [95% CI 1.45–18.43]) [41] and the swallowing reflex may be abnormal in a proportion of patients with COPD compared to controls [42]. Increased breathing frequency, as seen at exacerbations for example, may also impact the ability to swallow normally [43]. Our understanding of the airway microbiome is evolving rapidly and it is yet to be established how micro-aspiration affects microbial diversity and dysbiosis within the airway.

Fourth, GER may heighten bronchial reactivity [44]—perhaps through a vago-vagal mechanism as in the induction of cough [45, 46]—although the concept of bronchial reactivity in COPD is less well understood than in asthma.

Lastly, it is important to remark that risk factors for GER in the general population may also be relevant in patients with COPD. Such factors include increasing age, female gender and elevated BMI. Elevated BMI is a predictor of GERD in severe COPD (OR 1.2 [95% CI 1.0–1.6]) [26].

## GERD and Exacerbations of COPD

The first report of a relationship between symptoms of GERD and COPD exacerbations was published in 2006 [9]. In a small, selected group of 86 patients self-reported exacerbation frequency was higher in patients with self-reported GERD (3.2 vs. 1.6/year, $p = 0.02$). Results were confirmed in a 2007 study that quantified GERD using the FSSG questionnaire [5], demonstrating a significant association between symptom score and exacerbation frequency ($r = 0.24$, $p = 0.03$). Multiple studies have since examined associations between the presence of GERD—usually by self-report—and exacerbations of COPD. Seven of these have been combined as a meta-analysis reporting that the risk of exacerbation is over seven times higher in people with GERD (Risk Ratio 7.57 [95% CI 3.84–14.94]) [47].

Subsequently, studies in COPD have been greatly facilitated by the collection of data in large collaborative cohorts of patients, including the Copenhagen City Heart Study, *COPDGene* and *ECLIPSE* datasets. More recent data have therefore emerged evaluating the prevalence and associations of GERD in patients with COPD from these cohorts.

It is now recognized that susceptibility to exacerbation in COPD may be considered a phenotype or endotype of the disease, and in comprehensive multi-variable assessments the presence of GERD independently predicted exacerbation in the ECLIPSE cohort [48]. The presence of self-reported GERD increased the risk of exacerbation in a multi-variate analysis: OR for $\geq 2$ vs. 0 exacerbations of 2.07 (1.58–2.72), $p < 0.001$. GERD was the only novel modifiable risk factor in the analysis. This is important since currently available interventions to prevent exacerbation are poorly effective and GERD provides an alternative therapeutic approach. Whether this underlies the effectiveness of macrolide exacerbation is discussed in Chap. 25.

Further and more detailed analysis of the *ECLIPSE* data [29], specifically looking at GERD, showed that self-reported GERD was more common in women (OR = 1.80, 95% CI 1.41–2.29), older people (OR = 1.20, 95% CI 1.02–1.41 per 10 year increase), and those who were overweight or obese (OR = 1.40 [1.08–1.80], and 1.48 [1.11–1.98], respectively, for 25–29.9 and 30+ kg/m$^2$, when compared to 18.5–24.9 kg/m$^2$). GERD was also seen more frequently in those with milder COPD as assessed by less severe impairment in FEV$_1$ (OR = 0.95, 95% CI 0.93–0.97), and was associated with poorer health status (OR = 1.06, 95% CI 1.04–1.09), and a history of wheeze (OR = 1.33, 95% CI 1.05–1.68) and asthma (OR = 1.65, 95% CI 1.29–2.12). Although GERD was more common in women, the variables associated with GERD did not vary by sex. In an analysis from the Copenhagen City Heart Study, subjects with COPD and GERD had a greater prevalence of chronic bronchitis (31 vs 21%, $p = 0.004$), more breathlessness (39% vs 22%, $p < 0.001$), and more experienced exacerbation (6.8% vs 1.4%, $p < 0.001$) than those with COPD and no GERD [49].

The *COPDGene* cohort analysis reported that the prevalence of GERD was 29% and more common in women, and in those with chronic bronchitis [6]. The presence of GERD was associated with increased breathlessness, poorer quality of life, cardiovascular events and frequent exacerbations both at baseline and during follow-up.

It must be acknowledged that the relationships between GERD and exacerbation is complex: exacerbations may also predispose to increased GER through additional cough and dynamic hyperinflation. However, it will be appreciated from the above that the signal between GERD and exacerbation events in COPD is present in many different studies, suggesting that the association is robust.

Exacerbations are not the only relevant outcome measure in COPD and associations between COPD and quality-of-life, and symptoms have been described above. It is also possible that reflux may be associated with disease progression (FEV$_1$ decline), as seen post lung-transplantation for example, but there are at present no data to support this in COPD.

## Implications for Practice

A thorough medical history provides the most important initial assessment to detect the presence of GER in COPD in clinical practice [50, 51]. Because of the overlap between GERD and COPD symptoms, relationships between symptoms and provoking factors such as body position and meals should be carefully examined. History may be supplemented by the use of GERD symptom-questionnaires [51, 52]. Several have been validated for use in the diagnosis of acidic GERD, and most respond to antacid therapy [53]. Non acid airway reflux may be better assessed in validated questionnaires (see Chap. 7).

The gold standard investigation in the eyes of many, as in a non-COPD population, is 24-h pH-manometry testing. However, this clearly does not detect non acid reflux. Many clinicians and patients prefer an empiric trial of antacid therapy but antacid therapy does not alter the number of reflux events. Thus the sensitivity and specificity of empiric approaches has been questioned [54].

Direct visualization of the oesophagus may be considered, and in patients with severe COPD where endoscopy may be hazardous the use of camera-pills could provide a safer alternative. As outlined above, the relationships between symptoms, esophageal mucosal appearances and findings on physiological studies are variable such that in a population survey of 1000 subjects, 2/3 of those with symptoms had no esophagitis and only 1/3 of those with visible esophagitis reported symptoms [55]. Perhaps a better investigation is high resolution oesophageal manometry where oesophageal dysmotility can also be assessed (see Chap. 10).

Finally, assessments of swallow such as contrast swallow and detection of aspiration using scintigraphy may be considered. Pepsin and bile-acids can be been detected in sputum as evidence of reflux, but such investigations are still largely a research tool [56].

## Does Treating GER Affect Outcomes in COPD?

This remains a key question, and there have been few studies of anti-reflux therapy specifically in patients with COPD. In the main, trials of antacid therapy have been undertaken in the mistaken belief that these treatments prevent reflux and aspiration.

A 12 month single-blind randomized trial of lansoprazole in 100 patients with COPD was associated with a reduction in exacerbation frequency (0.34 vs. 1.18/year $p < 0.001$), and the frequency of colds in patients randomized to the PPI [57]. This study was predicated on the anti-inflammatory actions, of acid-suppression of the drug and thus patients with symptomatic GERD were excluded [58].

Macrolide antibiotics reduce exacerbation frequency in COPD [59, 60] and whilst the potential mechanisms for this clearly include antibacterial and anti-inflammatory action, macrolides are also pro-kinetic and it is possible that this mechanism may also be relevant (see Chap. 25).

Epidemiologic studies provide conflicting data. The Copenhagen City Heart study reported that people with COPD and GERD who did not use acid suppression therapy had an increased risk of exacerbations Hazards Ratio (HR): HR = 2.7 (1.3–5.4, $p = 0.006$) which was not present in those who did use acid suppression [49]. In contrast, the *COPDGene Investigators* [6] reported that use of PPI did not influence the positive association they had also reported between GERD and exacerbations in COPD. This was also the finding of a further analysis in the large *ECLIPSE* dataset which noted that patients with GORD and taking acid suppression therapy actually had an increased risk of exacerbation (HR = 1.58, 95% CI 1.35–1.86) [29]. These conflicting data are no substitute for a properly powered and conducted clinical trial of anti-reflux intervention in COPD. No such trial yet exists.

## Conclusions

GER is a common comorbidity in those with COPD and patients may or may not be symptomatic. Multiple mechanisms are likely to be relevant. Self-reported GERD symptoms robustly increase the risk of exacerbations in COPD, across multiple studies. Key unanswered questions remain including whether acidic or neutral, proximal or distal, liquid or gaseous, and reflux, reflex or micro-aspiration mechanisms are most important, and therefore which anti-reflux strategies may be most beneficial in managing GER-related COPD events.

## References

1. Global initiative for chronic obstructive pulmonary disease [homepage on the Internet]. Global strategy for the diagnosis, management and prevention of chronic obstructive pulmonary disease. 2014.
2. Vos T, Flaxman A, Naghavi M. Years lived with disability (YLDs) for 1160 sequelae of 289 diseases and injuries 1990–2010: a systematic analysis for the Global Burden of Disease Study 2010. Lancet. 2012;380:2163–96.
3. Mittal RK, Balaban DH. The esophagogastric junction. N Engl J Med. 1997;336:924–32.
4. Vakil N, van Zanten SV, Kahrilas P, Dent J, Jones R. The Montreal definition and classification of gastroesophageal reflux disease: a global evidence-based consensus. Am J Gastroenterol. 2006;101:1900–20.
5. Terada K, Muro S, Sato S, et al. Impact of gastro-oesophageal reflux disease symptoms on chronic obstructive pulmonary disease exacerbation. Thorax. 2008;63:951–5.
6. Martinez CH, Okajima Y, Murray S, COPDGene Investigators, et al. Impact of self-reported gastroesophageal reflux disease in subjects from COPD Gene cohort. Respir Res. 2014;15:62.
7. Liang B-M, Feng Y-L. Association of gastroesophageal reflux disease symptoms with stable chronic obstructive pulmonary disease. Lung. 2012;190:277–82.
8. Rogha M, Behravesh B, Pourmoghaddas Z. Association of gastroesophageal reflux disease symptoms with exacerbations of chronic obstructive pulmonary disease. J Gastrointestin Liver Dis. 2010;19(3):253–6.
9. Rascon-Aguilar IE, Pamer M, Wludyka P, Cury J, Coultas D, Lambiase LR, et al. Role of gastroesophageal reflux symptoms in exacerbations of COPD. Chest. 2006;130:1096–101.

10. Bor S, Kitapcioglu G, Solak Z, Ertilav M, Erdinc M. Prevalence of gastroesophageal reflux disease in patients with asthma and chronic obstructive pulmonary disease. J Gastroenterol Hepatol. 2010;25:309–13.
11. Shimizu Y, Dobashi K, Kusano M, Mori M. Different gastroesophageal reflux symptoms of middle-aged to elderly asthma and chronic objective pulmonary disease patients. J Clin Biochem Nutr. 2011;50(2):169–75.
12. Takada K, Matsumoto S, Kojima E, et al. Prospective evaluation of the relationship between acute exacerbations of COPD and gastroesophageal reflux disease diagnosed by questionnaire. Respir Med. 2011;105:1531–6.
13. Phulpoto M, Ozyyum S, Rizvi N, Khuhaware S. Proportion of gastroesophageal symptoms in patients with chronic obstructive pulmonary disease. J Pak Med Assoc. 2005;55:276–9.
14. Sweet M, Patti M, Hoopes C, Hayes SR, Golden JA. Gastro-oesophageal reflux and aspiration in patients with advanced lung disease. Thorax. 2009;64:167–73.
15. Barr RG, Celli BR, Mannino DM, Petty T, Rennard SI, Sciurba FC, et al. Comorbidities, patient knowledge, and disease management in a national sample of patients with COPD. Am J Med. 2009;122:348–55.
16. Mokhlesi B, Morris AL, Huang CF, Curcio AJ, Barrett TA, Kamp DW. Increased prevalence of gastroesophageal reflux symptoms in patients with COPD. Chest. 2001;119:1043–8.
17. El-Serag H, Hill C, Jones R. Systematic review: the epidemiology of gastro-oesophageal reflux disease in primary care, using the UK general practice research database. Aliment Pharmacol Ther. 2009;29:470–80.
18. García-Rodríguez LA, Ruigómez A, Martín-Merino E, Johansson S, Wallander MA. Relationship between gastroesophageal reflux disease and COPD in UK primary care. Chest. 2008;134:1223–30.
19. Sweet MP, Herbella FA, Leard L, et al. The prevalence of distal and proximal gastroesophageal reflux in patients awaiting lung transplantation. Ann Surg. 2006;244(4):491–7.
20. Lee AL, Button B, Denehy L, et al. Proximal and distal gastro-oesophageal reflux in chronic obstructive pulmonary disease and bronchiectasis. Respirology. 2014;19(2):211–7.
21. Kamble N, Khan N, Kumar N, Nayak H, Daga M. Study of gastro-oesophageal reflux disease in patients with mild-to-moderate chronic obstructive pulmonary disease in India. Respirology. 2013;18:463–7.
22. Gadel AA, Mostafa M, Younis A, Haleem M. Esophageal motility pattern and gastroesophageal reflux in chronic obstructive pulmonary disease. Hepatogastroenterology. 2012;59(120):2498–502.
23. El-Serag H, Sweet S, Winchester C, Dent J. Update on the epidemiology of gastro-oesophageal disease: a systematic review. Gut. 2014;63(6):871–80.
24. Dent J, El-Serag H, Wallander M, Johansson S. Epidemiology of gastro-oesophageal reflux disease: a systematic review. Gut. 2005;54:710–7.
25. Casanova C, Baudet JS, del Valle Velasco M, Martin JM, Aguirre-Jaime A, de Torres JP, et al. Increased gastro-oesophageal reflux disease in patients with severe COPD. Eur Respir J. 2004;23:841–5.
26. Kempainen RR, Savik K, Whelan TP, Dunitz JM, Herrington CS, Billings JL. High prevalence of proximal and distal gastroesophageal reflux disease in advanced COPD. Chest. 2007;131:1666–71.
27. Pauwels A, Blondeau K, Dupont L, Sifrim D. Mechanisms of increased gastroesophageal reflux in patients with cystic fibrosis. Am J Gastroenterol. 2012;107(9):1346–53.
28. Turbyville J. Applying principles of physics to the airway to help explain the relationship between asthma and gastroesophageal reflux. Med Hypotheses. 2010;74:1075–80.
29. Benson VS, Müllerová H, Vestbo J, Wedzicha JA, Patel A, Hurst JR, Evaluation of COPD Longitudinally to Identify Predictive Surrogate Endpoints (ECLIPSE) Investigators. Associations between gastro-oesophageal reflux, its management and exacerbations of chronic obstructive pulmonary disease. Respir Med. 2015;109(9):1147–54.
30. Pandolfino JE, Kahrilas PJ. Smoking and gastro-esophageal reflux disease. Eur J Gastroenterol Hepatol. 2000;12:837–42.

31. Kim J, Lee JH, Kim Y, et al. Association between chronic obstructive pulmonary disease and gastroesophageal reflux disease: a national cross-sectional cohort study. BMC Pulm Med. 2013;13:51.
32. Stein M, Towner T, Weber R. The effect of theophylline on the lower esophageal sphincter pressure. Ann Allergy. 1980;45:238.
33. Crowell M, Zayat E, Lacy B. The effects of an inhaled B2-adrenergic agonist on lower esophageal function: a dose-response study. Chest. 2001;121:1024–7.
34. Ruzkowski C, Sanowski R, Austin J, Rohwedder JJ, Waring JP. The effects of inhaled albuterol and oral theophylline on gastroesophageal reflux in patients with gastroesophageal reflux disease and obstructive lung disease. Arch Intern Med. 1992;152(4):783–5.
35. Niklasson A, Strid H, Simren M, Engstrom C-P, Bjornsson E. Prevalence of gastrointestinal symptoms in patients with chronic obstructive pulmonary disease. Eur J Gastroenterol Hepatol. 2008;20(4):335–41.
36. Sontag S, O'Connell S, Khandelwal S, Miller T, Nemchausky B, Schnell T. Most asthmatics have gastroesophageal reflux with or without bronchodilator therapy. Gastroenterology. 1990;99:613–20.
37. Emerenziani S, Sifrim D. Gastroesophageal reflux and gastric emptying, revisited. Curr Gastroenterol Rep. 2005;7:190–5.
38. Sifrim D, Silny J, Holloway R, Janssens J. Patterns of gas and liquid reflux during transient lower esophageal sphincter relaxation. A study using intraluminal electrical impedance. Gut. 1999;44:47–54.
39. Orr W, Elsenbruch S, Harnish M, Johnson L. Proximal migration of esophageal acid perfusions during waking and sleep. Am J Gastroenterol. 2000;95:37–42.
40. Fortunato G, Machado M, Andrade C, Felicetti J, Camargo J, Cardoso P. Prevalence of gastroesophageal reflux in lung transplant candidates with advanced lung disease. J Bras Pneumol. 2008;34(10):772–8.
41. Terada K, Muro S, Ohara T, et al. Abnormal swallowing reflex and COPD exacerbations. Chest. 2010;137(2):326–32.
42. Teramoto S, Kume H, Ouchi Y. Altered swallowing physiology and aspiration in COPD. Chest. 2002;122(3):1104–5.
43. Mokhlesi B, Logemann JA, Rademaker AW, Stangl CA, Corbridge TC. Oropharyngeal deglutition in stable COPD. Chest. 2002;121(2):361–9.
44. Wu DN, Tanifuji Y, Kobayashi H, Yamauchi K, Kato C, Suzuki K, et al. Effects of esophageal acid perfusion on airway hyperresponsiveness in patients with bronchial asthma. Chest. 2000;118:1553–6.
45. Wu DN, Yamauchi K, Kobayashi H, Tanifuji Y, Kato C, Suzuki K, et al. Effects of esophageal acid perfusion on cough responsiveness in patients with bronchial asthma. Chest. 2002;122:505–9.
46. Javorkova N, Varechova S, Pecova R, Tatar M, Balaz D, Demeter M, et al. Acidification of the oesophagus acutely increases the cough sensitivity in patients with gastro-oesophageal reflux and chronic cough. Neurogastroenterol Motil. 2008;20:119–24.
47. Sakae T, Pizzichini M, Teixeira P, de Silva R, Trevisol D, Pizzichini E. Exacerbations of COPD and symptoms of gastroesophageal reflux: a systematic review and meta-analysis. J Bras Pneumol. 2013;39(3):259–71.
48. Hurst JR, Vestbo J, Anzueto A, Locantore N, Müllerova H, Tal-Singer R, et al. Susceptibility to exacerbation in chronic obstructive pulmonary disease. N Engl J Med. 2010;363: 1128–38.
49. Ingebrigtsen T, Marott J, Vestbo J, Nordestgaard B, Hallas J, Lange P. Gastroesophageal reflux disease and exacerbations in chronic obstructive pulmonary disease. Respirology. 2015;20:101–7.
50. Katz PO, Gerson LB, Vela MF. Corrigendum: guidelines for the diagnosis and management of gastroesophageal reflux disease. Am J Gastroenterol. 2013;108:308–28.
51. Stanghellini V, Armstrong D, Monnikes H, Bardhans K. Systematic review: do we need a new gastro-oesophageal reflux disease questionnaire? Aliment Pharmacol Ther. 2004;19:463–89.

52. Fraser A, Delaney B, Moayyedi P. Symptom-based outcome measures for dyspepsia and GERD trials: a systematic review. Am J Gastroenterol. 2005;100:442–52.
53. Modlin IM, Moss SF. Symptom evaluation in gastroesophageal reflux disease. J Clin Gastroenterol. 2008;42:558–63.
54. Bytzer P, Jones R, Vakil N, Junghard O, Lind T, Wernersson B, et al. Limited ability of the proton-pump inhibitor test to identify patients with Gastroesophageal reflux disease. Clin Gastroenterol Hepatol. 2012;10(12):1360–6.
55. Ronkainen J, Aro P, Storskrubb T, Johansson S-E, Lind T, Bolling-Sternevald E, et al. Prevalence of Barrett's esophagus in the general population: an endoscopic study. Gastroenterology. 2005;129:1825–31.
56. Pacheco-Galván A, Hart SP, Morice AH. Relationship between gastro-oesophageal reflux and airway diseases: the airway reflux paradigm. Arch Bronconeumol. 2011;47:195–203.
57. Sasaki T, Nakayama K, Yasuda H, et al. A randomised, single-blind study of lansoprazole for the prevention of exacerbations of chronic obstructive pulmonary disease in older patients. J Am Geriatr Soc. 2009;57(8):1453–7.
58. Kedika RR, Souza RF, Spechler SJ. Potential anti-inflammatory effects of proton pump inhibitors: a review and discussion of the clinical implications. Dig Dis Sci. 2009;54:2312–7.
59. Seemungal TAR, Wilkinson TMA, Hurst JR, Perera WR, Sapsford RJ, Wedzicha JA. Long-term erythromycin therapy is associated with decreased chronic obstructive pulmonary disease exacerbations. Am J Respir Crit Care Med. 2008;178:1139–47.
60. Albert RK, Connett J, Bailey WC, Casaburi R, JAD C Jr, Criner GJ, et al. Azithromycin for prevention of exacerbations of COPD. N Engl J Med. 2011;365:689–98.

# Gastro Oesophageal Reflux and Bronchiectasis

Kirsty L. Hett and Ben Hope-Gill

## Introduction

Bronchiectasis was first described in 1819 by the French physician Rene Laënnec [1]. William Osler offered a more detailed description in the late nineteenth century [2] and it is suspected that he died from complications of undiagnosed bronchiectasis [3]. Bronchiectasis is a disease characterised by abnormal, permanent dilatation of the small and medium sized airways, leading to symptoms of chronic cough, mucopurulent sputum production, haemoptysis, breathlessness and fatigue [4] (Fig. 14.1).

The pathophysiology of bronchiectasis has been described as a vicious cycle of events [5]; following an initial event to damage the airways, there is abnormal mucous clearance leading to bacterial colonisation, infection and on-going inflammation (Fig. 14.2).

## The Aetiology of Gastroesophageal Reflux and Bronchiectasis

The causes of bronchiectasis depend upon the population being studied. A case series of 25 patients, published in 1962, highlighted the association between proven cases of gastro oesophageal reflux (GOR), with or without hiatus hernia and bronchitis, bronchiectasis, pneumonitis and empyema [7].

A UK based study of 150 patients with bronchiectasis showed that chronic GOR disease led to the development of bronchiectasis in 4% of the study population [4]. A separate UK study of 165 patients with bronchiectasis suggested aspiration was the cause in 1% of the study population [8] (Table 14.1).

K. L. Hett · B. Hope-Gill (✉)
Department of Respiratory Medicine, Cardiff and Vale University Health Board, Cardiff, UK
e-mail: Ben.Hope-gill@wales.nhs.uk

© Springer International Publishing AG, part of Springer Nature 2018
A. H. Morice, P. W. Dettmar (eds.), *Reflux Aspiration and Lung Disease*,
https://doi.org/10.1007/978-3-319-90525-9_14

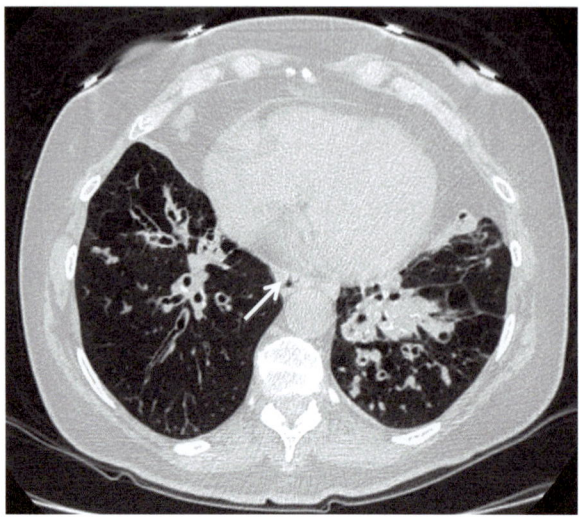

**Fig. 14.1** HRCT showing bronchial wall thickening, mucoid impaction and dilated airways and a hiatus hernia (arrow)

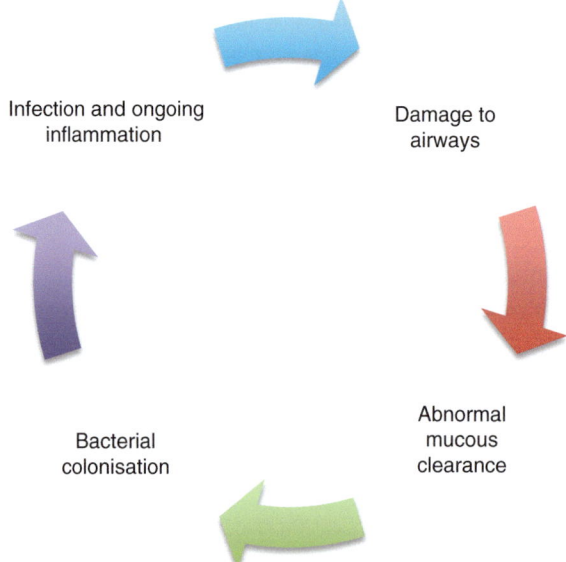

**Fig. 14.2** Adapted from Mc Shane [6]

However, the method of diagnosis of GOR was mainly based on clinical assessment. None of the studies used gastro-oesophageal impedance monitoring; which measures both acid and non-acid reflux or oesophageal manometry. Therefore it is likely that the true prevalence of reflux in patients with bronchiectasis is underestimated.

**Table 14.1** Aetiology of bronchiectasis of adults

| Author | Year published | Country | Method of diagnosis | Total number | % aspiration/GOR |
|---|---|---|---|---|---|
| Guan [9] | 2015 | South China | History simplified reflux questionnaire 24 h pH monitoring | 148 | 4 |
| McDonnell [10] | 2015 | UK | History | 81 | 7 |
| Anwar [11] | 2013 | UK | History | 189 | 1 |
| McShane [12] | 2012 | USA | History | 106 | 11 |
| Shoemark [8] | 2007 | UK | History video fluoroscopy | 165 | 1 |
| Pasteur [4] | 2000 | UK | History | 150 | 4 |

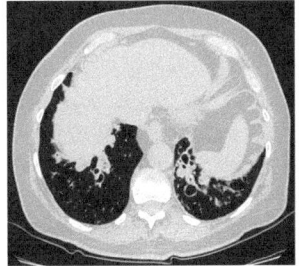 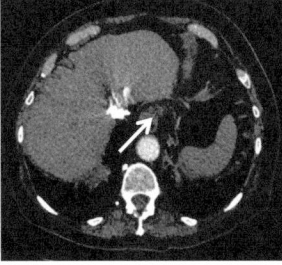 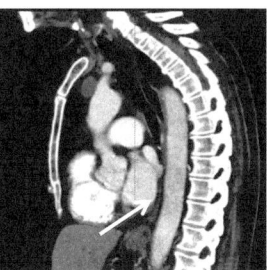

**Fig. 14.3** HRCT showing bronchiectasis, contrast enhanced images demonstrate a small hiatus hernia (arrows)

Oesophageal acid exposure and the severity of oesophagitis is greater in patients with a hiatus hernia, than in those without [13–15]. The role of hiatal hernias (HH) in the development of bronchiectasis has been suggested, although a causal link is unproven [10]. A retrospective, cross–sectional, observational study of 81 stable patients with a diagnosis of bronchiectasis, found that a HH was present in 36%. Patients with HH had a higher prevalence of GOR symptoms (62% vs 29%, $p < 0.01$). The newly developed bronchiectasis scoring systems were used (Bronchiectasis Severity Index [16] and FACED [17]) and showed a higher bronchiectasis severity score in patients with HH. It has previously been shown that symptomatic GOR in bronchiectasis is related to reduced lung function [18]. This study shows that patients with HH also had greater lung function impairment with increased extent and severity of bronchiectasis on high-resolution computed tomography (HRCT). Interestingly there was no predilection for any particular lobe being affected. An alternative explanation is that HH is caused by underlying bronchiectasis; as patients with severe disease have more hyperinflated lungs, potentially altering the diaphragm-oesophageal interface [12] (Fig. 14.3).

In 1992, a small study evaluated the effects of hiatal hernia and lower oesophageal sphincter (LOS) pressure on the competence of the gastroesophageal junction during abrupt increases in intra-abdominal pressure, such cough and Valsalva manoeuvre. They found that susceptibility to GOR induced by sudden increases in pressure were strongly associated with the size of hiatus hernia and LOS pressure [19].

It is unclear whether bronchiectasis and its associated cough, leads to incompetence of the diaphragm-oesophageal interface causing GOR or whether it is the GOR itself that leads to bronchiectasis. It is likely that both mechanisms contribute to worsening bronchiectasis and exacerbation of GOR disease.

## Gastroesophageal Reflux and the Bacteriology of Bronchiectasis

Different bacterial pathogens require different conditions to thrive; for example the airway microbiome may be altered by either refluxate or conditions created by anti-acid pharmacotherapy. A recent study using 24 h impedance monitoring has shown that high dose acid suppression therapy increases proximal non-acid reflux [20].

Humans secrete approximately 2.5 l of gastric juice per day, generating a fasting pH of 1.5, which increases to between pH 3.0 and 5.0 during feeding. There has been investigation into the bactericidal properties of gastric acid since the early 1920s. Interestingly, a pH of less than 2.0 has generally been accepted as the requirement for killing bacteria, which is not maintained during eating, when most bacteria enter the stomach [21]. Some conditions such as achlorydia or hypochlorydia lead to an increased risk of infection; with gastrectomy and chronic gastritis being identified as risk factors for the development of tuberculosis [22–24]. This raises the question whether iatrogenic increase in gastric pH leads to greater proliferation of bacteria and subsequently respiratory infection, from aspiration of gastric contents.

The presence of bacteria in the stomach has been associated with the development of hospital-acquired infection, particularly ventilation associated pneumonia [25, 26]. Patients undergoing intensive care are routinely given acid suppression therapy to prevent the development of stress ulcers but this appears to pre-dispose them to respiratory infections [27–31].

The most commonly cultured bacterial pathogens in bronchiectasis are nonenteric gram-negative bacteria; mainly Haemophilus influenza (55%) and Pseudomonas aeruginosa (26%) [32]. Other organisms include Moraxella catarrhalis, Streptococcus pneumonia and *Staphylococcus aureus* [33]. On longitudinal follow up, the microorganisms isolated do not change but there is a higher incidence of pseudomonas [33]. Patients colonised with pseudomonas aeruginosa have an accelerated decline in lung function [34].

Reflux can have an alkaline or neutral pH due to its complex composition; including gastric acid, gastric enzymes, bile acids and pancreatic enzymes from the duodenum. The gastric pH influences activity and toxicity of enzymes and subsequent damage to the epithelium [20]. However, whether it is the acidic or alkaline refluxate itself that cause bronchiectasis or associated bacteria aspirated with it, is not clear. Little is also known about the proliferation of bacteria in relation to pH or refluxate and further studies to identify which bacteria commonly isolated in bronchiectasis thrive in acid versus alkaline conditions would improve our understanding of disease mechanisms.

Overall, there is currently little data regarding the bacteriology of patients with bronchiectasis specifically due to GOR or aspiration to inform our understanding of the underlying mechanisms of disease. Further studies are needed to identify potential pathogenetic relationships. However, it is possible that microenvironmental factors, such as refluxate pH, contribute to the observation that enteric organisms are not usually cultured in sputum in bronchiectasis.

## Nontuberculous Mycobacterial Lung Disease

Nontuberculous mycobacteria (NTM) are opportunistic organisms commonly found in the human environment, particularly water and it's distribution systems, biofilms, soil and aerosols [35]. Mycobacterium avium complex (MAC) is a NTM that typically causes respiratory infection, in patients with chronic lung disease or those that are immunosuppressed. MAC is the most commonly isolated NTM in patients with non-cystic fibrosis bronchiectasis [36].

It is unclear whether MAC causes bronchiectasis or whether MAC occurs as a consequence of bronchiectatic disease [37, 38].

The radiographic features associated with MAC have been described as reticulonodular infiltrates [39], particularly within the right middle lobe and lingula [40, 41]. This was initially described as Lady Windermere syndrome; it was postulated that the voluntary suppression of cough, a behaviour that befitted ladies of good breeding in England, led to the development of non-specific inflammatory processes in these poorly draining regions of the lung [40].

Gastroesophageal reflux is common in patients with NTM disease [42]. Thomson and colleagues hypothesised that as MAC can be found in contaminated water, reflux aspiration may be a point of entry into the respiratory tract. As described above, MAC more commonly infects the right middle lobe and lingula [40, 41]. The bronchi to these areas are long and narrow and at particular risk from aspiration. Although this was not confirmed in a more recent study [43].

It is possible that acid suppression enhances survival of MAC within the stomach, leading to respiratory tract infection. Thompson et al. studied the prevalence of GOR, symptoms of reflux and acid-suppression therapy in patients with MAC compared with controls. They showed that GOR (44% vs 28% $p < 0.019$), medication to suppress acid production and clinically suspected aspiration are more common in patients with MAC, than in patients without. However, there were cofounding factors which need to be taken into account when considering this data (including use of steroids) and it is possible that use of acid suppressive therapy may reflect more severe GOR [43].

Koh et al. investigated the prevalence of GOR disease in patients with NTM disease using 24 h oesophageal pH monitoring. In patients with NTM disease, prevalence of GOR was 26%, although without symptoms of heartburn (27%). Patients with GOR were more likely to have a positive sputum smear for acid fast bacilli (80 vs 44%, $p = 0.008$) and the involvement of bronchiectasis on HRCT was more extensive [44]. However, it is not clear whether GOR is causative or secondary to more severe lung disease and increased cough frequency [45].

The above data raises the possibility that the presence of GOR influences which organisms infect the lung in bronchiectasis and that acid suppressive treatment may also play a role by altering the micro environment within the upper gastrointestinal tract and the lungs.

## Helicobacter Pylori

*Helicobacter pylori* (HP) was first identified in tracheobronchial aspirates in mechanically ventilated patients in 1993, suggesting a potential link with ventilator-associated pneumonia [46]. However, it was only identified in 2 of 20 patients (10%) so subsequent studies were designed to evaluate the seroprevalence of HP in bronchiectasis and to directly investigate the presence of HP within respiratory samples.

*Helicobacter Pylori* is a slow growing microaerophilic gram-negative spiral shaped bacterium that causes chronic inflammation of the gastric mucosa. It has been causally related to some digestive diseases such as gastritis, peptic ulcers [47], gastric mucosa-associated lymphoid tissue lymphoma and gastric carcinoma [48–51]. There is also increasing recognition of its role in extra-gastrointestinal diseases, including ischaemic heart disease [52], cerebrovascular disease [52], rosacea [53, 54], urticaria [55], idiopathic thrombocytopenia [56] and Henoch-Schonlein purpura [57]. *Helicobacter Pylori* is also associated with several chronic respiratory diseases; particularly asthma, chronic bronchitis, pulmonary fibrosis and bronchiectasis [58–61]. A meta-analysis of nine case control studies comprising 782 cases and 815 controls showed a significant association between HP infection and the presence of chronic respiratory disease (bronchitis OR 2.90 (95% CI: 2.04–4.13) [62]. There are also similarities between the pathogenesis of peptic ulcers within the upper gastrointestinal tract and bronchiectasis [63, 64]; including the recruitment of polymorphs and T lymphocytes into the sub-mucosa and the release of cytokines, particularly IL-8, TNF$\alpha$ and IL-1$\beta$ [65, 66].

In 1998, seropositivity for HP was found to be significantly higher in patients with bronchiectasis (76%), than in healthy volunteers (54.3%) and in those with active pulmonary tuberculosis (52.9%), when measuring HP specific IgG using an ELISA assay. Seropositivity for HP was also higher in patients with greater volumes of expectorated sputum. However, the investigators were unable to isolate HP directly from the sputum of bronchiectatic patients [67] so the significance of seropositivity remains unclear.

Tsang et al. [18] evaluated 100 patients with bronchiectasis and 94 controls, who tested positive for HP. They found that one third of bronchiectatic patients suffered from upper GI symptoms. There was an inverse relationship between the presence of upper gastrointestinal symptoms and lung function; patients who had acid regurgitation or upper abdominal distension had significantly lower FEV1 and FVC compared with those that didn't. The presence of upper abdominal pain and distension was also associated with the number of lobes affected by bronchiectasis. This further supports a link between upper abdominal pathology and the development of bronchiectasis [18].

In 2007, Gulhan et al. performed polymerase chain reaction assays on bronchoalveolar lavage fluid (BALF) and surgically resected preserved lung tissue from patients with bronchiectasis and controls. The study aimed to determine the prevalence of HP in addition to evaluating serum IgG against HP using an ELISA. Contradictory to previous studies, HP was not detected in either BALF or lung tissue samples and anti-HP IgG did not significantly differ from controls [68]. These conflicting results question a clear association between HP infection and the development of bronchiectasis.

An indirect role for other toxic products of HP has also been considered. These include urease, catalase, phospholipidase, alcohol dehydrogenase, haemolysin, platelet aggravating factor and mucolytic factor [69]. Some strains of HP express a virulence factor known as cytotoxin-associated gene A (CagA), which is an outer membrane protein that leads to the production of a vacuolating cytotoxin [70]. Detection of serum anti HP CagA is currently the most practical investigation for predicting bacterial virulence and disease development by HP [71]. Patients that are seropositive for anti-HP CagA are associated with increased incidence of peptic ulcer disease [72]. The role of serum anti-HP CagA has also been evaluated in patients with bronchiectasis compared with controls. Although anti-HP CagA was elevated in patients with bronchiectasis, there was no significant difference in clinical parameters such as sputum volume, lung function or the number of lobes affected by bronchiectasis between CagA positive and CagA negative patients. This suggests that if HP does play a significant pathogenic role in bronchiectasis, it probably does so via a non-CagA and non-vacuolating toxin-mediated mechanism [18].

## Gastroesophageal Reflux, Quality of Life and Bronchiectasis

Mandal et al. used the Hull Airway Reflux Questionnaire, a validated tool, to assess whether symptoms of reflux predicted exacerbation frequency and quality of life in patients with bronchiectasis [58]. Using this assessment tool reflux was reported in approximately one third of patients, although the presence of GOR was not confirmed by oesophageal physiology tests. In addition, symptoms of reflux were associated with more severe bronchiectasis; including poorer lung function and greater disease extent as assessed by HRCT scans. Patients with reflux also had higher levels of inflammatory mediators and pathogenic organisms in the sputum. In addition, there was an increased risk of exacerbation. Overall, symptoms of reflux were associated with reduced health-related quality of life [73].

## Investigation of GOR in Bronchiectasis

There is currently no gold standard test for the diagnosis of GOR in respiratory disease. In relation to COPD and bronchiectasis, Lee et al. developed the idea of measuring pepsin in exhaled breath condensate (EBC) [74]. Pepsin is a proteolytic enzyme produced in the stomach which has also been isolated from saliva, tracheal aspirates and bronchoalveolar lavage fluid. It causes mucosal injury to the exposed tissue and is more damaging than gastric acid alone [75]. The investigators undertook a small study of 30 patients undergoing synchronous 24 h oesophageal pH monitoring and EBC sampling to measure pH and pepsin concentration. In this study GOR was not associated with a higher concentration of EBC pepsin and also did not correlate with DeMeester score (a measure of lower oesophageal acidity and a surrogate indicator of the severity of GOR). However, pepsin concentrations in EBC and sputum were moderately correlated suggesting it may have a role as a non-invasive marker of pulmonary microaspiration [74]. A previous study by the same investigators in 2014 found pepsin to be present in 26% of patients with bronchiectasis but the presence of pepsin in sputum was not related to a diagnosis of GOR based on oesophageal monitoring [76].

## The Effect of Treatment on GOR and Bronchiectasis

As discussed, anatomical upper gastrointestinal disorders, such as hiatus hernia, are common in patients with bronchiectasis [10]. Pitney and Callahan published an interesting case report in 2001, describing resolution of bronchiectasis after treatment of the underling GOR. A child with Cri du Chat Syndrome, had bronchiectasis on HRCT secondary to recurrent aspiration. This was confirmed on barium swallow, nuclear scintiscan and bronchoalveolar lavage. The child underwent Nissen fundoplication with gastrostomy tube placement. Several months later a repeat HRCT showed near resolution of the bronchiectasis [77].

An earlier study evaluated the success, complication rates and comorbidities following a modified Thal fundoplication in children with reflux associated respiratory disease; of which 10% had bronchiectasis. The results were not analysed according to specific disease category but overall 88% of children "felt better" after the procedure [78]. A study was also performed to evaluate the effect of Nissen fundoplication in adult cystic fibrosis patients, who had failed conventional medical therapies. There was a significant improvement in cough symptoms; assessed using the Leicester Cough Questionnaire. Interestingly, spirometry also improved and the number of exacerbations was halved [79]. These findings highlight the potential benefits of anti-reflux procedures for the treatment of GOR in patients with bronchiectasis. However, further prospective studies are required.

The use of mechanical aids, including chest physiotherapy with postural drainage, active breathing cycles, oscillatory positive pressure devices and high frequency assisted airway clearance constitute potential adjunct therapies for patients with bronchiectasis. A small study of 6 patients showed that airway clearance techniques to facilitate sputum expectoration involving gravity-assisted drainage with head down tilt provoked GOR in patients with cystic fibrosis (CF). The use of adjuncts in CF is well established but their role is less well understood in non-CF bronchiectasis. However, it is not unreasonable to hypothesise that this is also a relevant factor in patients with non-CF bronchiectasis.

## Conclusions

There has been a recent surge in interest in the relationship between GOR and bronchiectasis. The evidence presented suggests that underlying bronchiectasis is exacerbated by the presence of coexistent GOR resulting in reduced health-related quality of life. Therefore, the identification and treatment of GOR should be a priority for treating clinicians. Although, such treatment should not necessarily mean lone acid-suppression therapy as the effect of non-acid reflux on the airways remains unknown. Well-conducted clinical trials are needed. Whilst evidence of GOR is common in patients with bronchiectasis there remains much work to be done before a clear understanding of the role of GOR in the pathogenesis of bronchiectasis is achieved. This includes the influence of both acid and non-acid refluxate on the airway microbiome and airway colonisation. The use of newer reflux assessment methods such as impedance manometry and EBC sampling in this patient group will help this.

## References

1. Laennec RTH. A treatise on the diseases of the chest and on mediate auscultation. London: Thomas & George Underwood; 1829. https://archive.org/stream/treatiseondiseas1829laen#page/n5/mode/2up.
2. Stafler P, Carr SB. Non-cystic fibrosis bronchiectasis: its diagnosis and management. Arch Dis Child Educ Pract Ed. 2010;95(3):73–82.
3. Wrong O. Osler and my father. J R Soc Med. 2003;96(9):462–4.
4. Pasteur MC, Helliwell SM, Houghton SJ, Webb SC, Foweraker JE, Coulden RA, et al. An investigation into causative factors in patients with bronchiectasis. Am J Respir Crit Care Med. 2000;162(4 Pt 1):1277–84.
5. Cole PJ. Inflammation: a two-edged sword--the model of bronchiectasis. Eur J Respir Dis Suppl. 1986;147:6–15.
6. McShane PJ, Naureckas ET, Tino G, Strek ME. Non-cystic fibrosis bronchiectasis. Am J Respir Crit Care Med. 2013;188(6):647–56.
7. Kennedy JH. "Silent" gastroesophageal reflux: an important but little known cause of pulmonary complications. Chest. 1962;42:42–5.
8. Shoemark A, Ozerovitch L, Wilson R. Aetiology in adult patients with bronchiectasis. Respir Med. 2007;101(6):1163–70.
9. Guan WJ, Gao YH, Xu G, Lin ZY, Tang Y, Li HM, et al. Aetiology of bronchiectasis in Guangzhou, southern China. Respirology. 2015;20(5):739–48.
10. McDonnell MJ, Ahmed M, Das J, Ward C, Mokoka M, Breen DP, et al. Hiatal hernias are correlated with increased severity of non-cystic fibrosis bronchiectasis. Respirology. 2015;20(5):749–57.
11. Anwar GA, McDonnell MJ, Worthy SA, Bourke SC, Afolabi G, Lordan J, et al. Phenotyping adults with non-cystic fibrosis bronchiectasis: a prospective observational cohort study. Respir Med. 2013;107(7):1001–7.
12. McShane PJ, Naureckas ET, Strek ME. Bronchiectasis in a diverse US population: effects of ethnicity on etiology and sputum culture. Chest. 2012;142(1):159–67.
13. Sontag SJ, Schnell TG, Miller TQ, Nemchausky B, Serlovsky R, O'Connell S, et al. The importance of hiatal hernia in reflux esophagitis compared with lower esophageal sphincter pressure or smoking. J Clin Gastroenterol. 1991;13(6):628–43.

14. Kasapidis P, Vassilakis JS, Tzovaras G, Chrysos E, Xynos E. Effect of hiatal hernia on esophageal manometry and pH-metry in gastroesophageal reflux disease. Dig Dis Sci. 1995;40(12):2724–30.
15. DeMeester TR, Lafontaine E, Joelsson BE, Skinner DB, Ryan JW, O'Sullivan GC, et al. Relationship of a hiatal hernia to the function of the body of the esophagus and the gastroesophageal junction. J Thorac Cardiovasc Surg. 1981;82(4):547–58.
16. Chalmers JD, Goeminne P, Aliberti S, McDonnell MJ, Lonni S, Davidson J, et al. The bronchiectasis severity index. An international derivation and validation study. Am J Respir Crit Care Med. 2014;189(5):576–85.
17. Martínez-García M, de Gracia J, Vendrell Relat M, Girón RM, Máiz Carro L, de la Rosa Carrillo D, et al. Multidimensional approach to non-cystic fibrosis bronchiectasis: the FACED score. Eur Respir J. 2014;43(5):1357–67.
18. Tsang KW, Lam WK, Kwok E, Chan KN, Hu WH, Ooi GC, et al. *Helicobacter pylori* and upper gastrointestinal symptoms in bronchiectasis. Eur Respir J. 1999;14(6):1345–50.
19. Sloan S, Rademaker AW, Kahrilas PJ. Determinants of gastroesophageal junction incompetence: hiatal hernia, lower esophageal sphincter, or both? Ann Intern Med. 1992;117(12):977–82.
20. Kilduff CE, Counter MJ, Thomas GA, Harrison NK, Hope-Gill BD. Effect of acid suppression therapy on gastroesophageal reflux and cough in idiopathic pulmonary fibrosis: an intervention study. Cough. 2014;10:4.
21. Zhu H, Hart CA, Sales D, Roberts NB. Bacterial killing in gastric juice–effect of pH and pepsin on *Escherichia coli* and *Helicobacter pylori*. J Med Microbiol. 2006;55(Pt 9):1265–70.
22. Thorn PA, Brookes VS, Waterhouse JA. Peptic ulcer, partial gastrectomy, and pulmonary tuberculosis. Br Med J. 1956;1(4967):603–8.
23. Steiger Z, Nickel WO, Shannon GJ, Nedwicki EG, Higgins RF. Pulmonary tuberculosis after gastric resection. Am J Surg. 1976;131(6):668–71.
24. Hsu WH, Kuo CH, Wang SS, Lu CY, Liu CJ, Chuah SK, et al. Acid suppressive agents and risk of Mycobacterium tuberculosis: case-control study. BMC Gastroenterol. 2014;14:91.
25. Simms HH, DeMaria E, McDonald L, Peterson D, Robinson A, Burchard KW. Role of gastric colonization in the development of pneumonia in critically ill trauma patients: results of a prospective randomized trial. J Trauma. 1991;31(4):531–6.
26. Inglis TJ, Sherratt MJ, Sproat LJ, Gibson JS, Hawkey PM. Gastroduodenal dysfunction and bacterial colonisation of the ventilated lung. Lancet. 1993;341(8850):911–3.
27. Driks MR, Craven DE, Celli BR, Manning M, Burke RA, Garvin GM, et al. Nosocomial pneumonia in intubated patients given sucralfate as compared with antacids or histamine type 2 blockers. The role of gastric colonization. N Engl J Med. 1987;317(22):1376–82.
28. Tryba M, Cook DJ. Gastric alkalinization, pneumonia, and systemic infections: the controversy. Scand J Gastroenterol Suppl. 1995;210:53–9.
29. Cook D, Guyatt G, Marshall J, Leasa D, Fuller H, Hall R, et al. A comparison of sucralfate and ranitidine for the prevention of upper gastrointestinal bleeding in patients requiring mechanical ventilation. Canadian critical care trials group. N Engl J Med. 1998;338(12):791–7.
30. Steinberg KP. Stress-related mucosal disease in the critically ill patient: risk factors and strategies to prevent stress-related bleeding in the intensive care unit. Crit Care Med. 2002;30(6 Suppl):S362–4.
31. Rousseau MC, Catala A, Blaya J. Association between pulmonary and digestive infections in patients receiving gastric acid-lowering medications for a long duration. Brain Inj. 2003;17(10):883–7.
32. Angrill J, Agustí C, de Celis R, Rañó A, Gonzalez J, Solé T, et al. Bacterial colonisation in patients with bronchiectasis: microbiological pattern and risk factors. Thorax. 2002;57(1):15–9.
33. King PT, Holdsworth SR, Freezer NJ, Villanueva E, Holmes PW. Microbiologic follow-up study in adult bronchiectasis. Respir Med. 2007;101(8):1633–8.
34. Martínez-García MA, Soler-Cataluña JJ, Perpiñá-Tordera M, Román-Sánchez P, Soriano J. Factors associated with lung function decline in adult patients with stable non-cystic fibrosis bronchiectasis. Chest. 2007;132(5):1565–72.

35. Falkinham JO. Nontuberculous mycobacteria in the environment. Clin Chest Med. 2002;23(3):529–51.
36. Mirsaeidi M, Hadid W, Ericsoussi B, Rodgers D, Sadikot RT. Non-tuberculous mycobacterial disease is common in patients with non-cystic fibrosis bronchiectasis. Int J Infect Dis. 2013;17(11):e1000–4.
37. Swensen SJ, Hartman TE, Williams DE. Computed tomographic diagnosis of Mycobacterium avium-intracellulare complex in patients with bronchiectasis. Chest. 1994;105(1):49–52.
38. Wallace RJ. Mycobacterium avium complex lung disease and women. Now an equal opportunity disease. Chest. 1994;105(1):6–7.
39. Prince DS, Peterson DD, Steiner RM, Gottlieb JE, Scott R, Israel HL, et al. Infection with Mycobacterium avium complex in patients without predisposing conditions. N Engl J Med. 1989;321(13):863–8.
40. Reich JM, Johnson RE. Mycobacterium avium complex pulmonary disease presenting as an isolated lingular or middle lobe pattern. The Lady Windermere syndrome. Chest. 1992;101(6):1605–9.
41. Dhillon SS, Watanakunakorn C. Lady Windermere syndrome: middle lobe bronchiectasis and Mycobacterium avium complex infection due to voluntary cough suppression. Clin Infect Dis. 2000;30(3):572–5.
42. Ilowite J, Spiegler P, Chawla S. Bronchiectasis: new findings in the pathogenesis and treatment of this disease. Curr Opin Infect Dis. 2008;21(2):163–7.
43. Thomson RM, Armstrong JG, Looke DF. Gastroesophageal reflux disease, acid suppression, and Mycobacterium avium complex pulmonary disease. Chest. 2007;131(4):1166–72.
44. Koh WJ, Lee JH, Kwon YS, Lee KS, Suh GY, Chung MP, et al. Prevalence of gastroesophageal reflux disease in patients with nontuberculous mycobacterial lung disease. Chest. 2007;131(6):1825–30.
45. Sexton P, Harrison AC. Susceptibility to nontuberculous mycobacterial lung disease. Eur Respir J. 2008;31(6):1322–33.
46. Mitz HS, Farber SS. Demonstration of *Helicobacter pylori* in tracheal secretions. J Am Osteopath Assoc. 1993;93(1):87–91.
47. Marshall BJ, Warren JR. Unidentified curved bacilli in the stomach of patients with gastritis and peptic ulceration. Lancet. 1984;1(8390):1311–5.
48. Parsonnet J, Friedman GD, Vandersteen DP, Chang Y, Vogelman JH, Orentreich N, et al. *Helicobacter pylori* infection and the risk of gastric carcinoma. N Engl J Med. 1991;325(16):1127–31.
49. Wotherspoon AC, Ortiz-Hidalgo C, Falzon MR, Isaacson PG. *Helicobacter pylori*-associated gastritis and primary B-cell gastric lymphoma. Lancet. 1991;338(8776):1175–6.
50. Isaacson PG, Spencer J. Is gastric lymphoma an infectious disease? Hum Pathol. 1993;24(6):569–70.
51. EUROGAST Study Group. An international association between *Helicobacter pylori* infection and gastric cancer. The EUROGAST Study Group. Lancet. 1993;341(8857):1359–62.
52. Whincup PH, Mendall MA, Perry IJ, Strachan DP, Walker M. Prospective relations between *Helicobacter pylori* infection, coronary heart disease, and stroke in middle aged men. Heart. 1996;75(6):568–72.
53. Rebora A, Drago F, Picciotto A. *Helicobacter pylori* in patients with rosacea. Am J Gastroenterol. 1994;89(9):1603–4.
54. Utaş S, Ozbakir O, Turasan A, Utaş C. *Helicobacter pylori* eradication treatment reduces the severity of rosacea. J Am Acad Dermatol. 1999;40(3):433–5.
55. Wedi B, Wagner S, Werfel T, Manns MP, Kapp A. Prevalence of *Helicobacter pylori*-associated gastritis in chronic urticaria. Int Arch Allergy Immunol. 1998;116(4):288–94.
56. Gasbarrini A, Franceschi F, Tartaglione R, Landolfi R, Pola P, Gasbarrini G. Regression of autoimmune thrombocytopenia after eradication of *Helicobacter pylori*. Lancet. 1998;352(9131):878.
57. Reinauer S, Megahed M, Goerz G, Ruzicka T, Borchard F, Susanto F, et al. Schönlein-Henoch purpura associated with gastric *Helicobacter pylori* infection. J Am Acad Dermatol. 1995;33(5 Pt 2):876–9.

58. Ayres JG, Miles JF. Oesophageal reflux and asthma. Eur Respir J. 1996;9(5):1073–8.
59. Shi G, Bruley des Varannes S, Scarpignato C, Le Rhun M, Galmiche JP. Reflux related symptoms in patients with normal oesophageal exposure to acid. Gut. 1995;37(4):457–64.
60. DeMeester TR, Wang CI, Wernly JA, Pellegrini CA, Little AG, Klementschitsch P, et al. Technique, indications, and clinical use of 24 hour esophageal pH monitoring. J Thorac Cardiovasc Surg. 1980;79(5):656–70.
61. Barish CF, Wu WC, Castell DO. Respiratory complications of gastroesophageal reflux. Arch Intern Med. 1985;145(10):1882–8.
62. Wang L, Guan Y, Li Y, Liu X, Zhang Y, Wang F, et al. Association between chronic respiratory diseases and *Helicobacter pylori*: a meta-analysis. Arch Bronconeumol. 2015;51(6):273–8.
63. Silva JR, Jones JA, Cole PJ, Poulter LW. The immunological component of the cellular inflammatory infiltrate in bronchiectasis. Thorax. 1989;44(8):668–73.
64. Rauws EA, Langenberg W, Houthoff HJ, Zanen HC, Tytgat GN. Campylobacter pyloridis-associated chronic active antral gastritis. A prospective study of its prevalence and the effects of antibacterial and antiulcer treatment. Gastroenterology. 1988;94(1):33–40.
65. Eller J, Lapa e Silva JR, Poulter LW, Lode H, Cole PJ. Cells and cytokines in chronic bronchial infection. Ann N Y Acad Sci. 1994;725:331–45.
66. Noach LA, Bosma NB, Jansen J, Hoek FJ, van Deventer SJ, Tytgat GN. Mucosal tumor necrosis factor-alpha, interleukin-1 beta, and interleukin-8 production in patients with *Helicobacter pylori* infection. Scand J Gastroenterol. 1994;29(5):425–9.
67. Tsang KW, Lam SK, Lam WK, Karlberg J, Wong BC, Hu WH, et al. High seroprevalence of *Helicobacter pylori* in active bronchiectasis. Am J Respir Crit Care Med. 1998;158(4):1047–51.
68. Gülhan M, Ozyilmaz E, Tarhan G, Demirağ F, Capan N, Ertürk A, et al. *Helicobacter pylori* in bronchiectasis: a polymerase chain reaction assay in bronchoalveolar lavage fluid and bronchiectatic lung tissue. Arch Med Res. 2007;38(3):317–21.
69. Mégraud F. Toxic factors of *Helicobacter pylori*. Eur J Gastroenterol Hepatol. 1994;6(Suppl 1):S5–10.
70. Cover TL, Cao P, Lind CD, Tham KT, Blaser MJ. Correlation between vacuolating cytotoxin production by *Helicobacter pylori* isolates in vitro and in vivo. Infect Immun. 1993;61(12):5008–12.
71. Peura DA. *Helicobacter pylori* and ulcerogenesis. Am J Med. 1996;100(5A):19S–25S.
72. Tee W, Lambert JR, Dwyer B. Cytotoxin production by *Helicobacter pylori* from patients with upper gastrointestinal tract diseases. J Clin Microbiol. 1995;33(5):1203–5.
73. Mandal P, Morice AH, Chalmers JD, Hill AT. Symptoms of airway reflux predict exacerbations and quality of life in bronchiectasis. Respir Med. 2013;107(7):1008–13.
74. Lee AL, Button BM, Denehy L, Roberts S, Bamford T, Mu FT, et al. Exhaled breath condensate pepsin: potential noninvasive test for gastroesophageal reflux in COPD and bronchiectasis. Respir Care. 2015;60(2):244–50.
75. Tobey NA, Hosseini SS, Caymaz-Bor C, Wyatt HR, Orlando GS, Orlando RC. The role of pepsin in acid injury to esophageal epithelium. Am J Gastroenterol. 2001;96(11):3062–70.
76. Lee AL, Button BM, Denehy L, Roberts SJ, Bamford TL, Ellis SJ, et al. Proximal and distal gastro-oesophageal reflux in chronic obstructive pulmonary disease and bronchiectasis. Respirology. 2014;19(2):211–7.
77. Pitney AC, Callahan CW, Ruess L. Reversal of bronchiectasis caused by chronic aspiration in cri du chat syndrome. Arch Dis Child. 2001;85(5):413–4.
78. Ahrens P, Heller K, Beyer P, Zielen S, Kühn C, Hofmann D, et al. Antireflux surgery in children suffering from reflux-associated respiratory diseases. Pediatr Pulmonol. 1999;28(2):89–93.
79. Fathi H, Moon T, Donaldson J, Jackson W, Sedman P, Morice AH. Cough in adult cystic fibrosis: diagnosis and response to fundoplication. Cough. 2009;5:1.

# Reflux Aspiration and Cystic Fibrosis

## 15

Ans Pauwels

### Abstract

Chronic airway infections are the hallmark of cystic fibrosis (CF), an autosomal recessive disease, however it is defined as a multi-organ disease, with characteristic abnormalities in the lung, pancreas and the gastro-intestinal tract. Gastro-oesophageal reflux (GOR) is the retrograde bolus movement into the oesophagus and beyond and can be accompanied by typical symptoms such as heartburn and regurgitation.

## Introduction

Increased GOR has been demonstrated in a large proportion of CF patients, both in children as well as in adults, with a prevalence ranging from 15 up to 90%. A substantial subgroup of CF patients have so called silent reflux, i.e. increased reflux without having typical peptic reflux symptoms. Aspiration of (duodeno)-gastric contents into the airways has been suggested in CF patients: bile acids have been found in saliva and sputum of CF patients. More important, aspiration of bile acids in the lungs of CF patients was associated with more airway inflammation, by means of higher interleukin-8 levels, and the degree of aspiration appears to be related to the extent of the airway inflammation. Treatment with proton pump inhibitors (PPI) is common practice in CF patients, however, this will not prevent reflux and consequently aspiration from occurring. PPIs decrease the acidity in the stomach, hence leading to more bacteria or bacterial products in the stomach. When this is aspirated into the lungs, it will lead to higher grades of inflammation, ultimately questioning the efficacy of PPI use in patients with CF.

---

A. Pauwels
Translational Research Center for Gastrointestinal Disorders (TARGID),
University of Leuven, Leuven, Belgium
e-mail: ans.pauwels@med.kuleuven.be

© Springer International Publishing AG, part of Springer Nature 2018
A. H. Morice, P. W. Dettmar (eds.), *Reflux Aspiration and Lung Disease*,
https://doi.org/10.1007/978-3-319-90525-9_15

## Cystic Fibrosis (CF)

Cystic fibrosis (CF) is an autosomal recessive disease occurring in approximately 1/2000–1/4000 live births in the Western world. The characteristics of this disease were first described in 1938, but it was only in 1989 that the CF-gene was discovered [1]. It is now widely known that recessive mutations of the CF transmembrane conductance regulator gene (CFTR-gene) mapped on chromosome 7 entail CF. This gene encodes a chloride channel expressed in epithelial cells of multiple organs. Mutations in the CFTR-gene will lead to the production of an abnormal CFTR-protein. Although CF remains a life-threatening disease survival of CF patients has substantially improved in the last 20 years, with a median survival of 37 years in 2005 [2].

## Airway Inflammation

Airway inflammation is the main characteristic of CF lung disease. The traditional concept in CF is the defect in the CFTR-gene leading to hyperviscous secretions in the airways, which impairs mucociliary clearance, leading to chronic bacterial infection and eventually causing inflammation [3]. In respect to healthy individuals, airway fluids, such as broncho-alveolar lavage fluid (BALF) of patients with CF show an increased number of neutrophils and increased levels of pro-inflammatory cytokines, such as interleukin-8 (IL-8) [4]. Since the lungs of CF patients are inflamed and infected at a young age, it is debated whether infection is the cause or consequence of the pulmonary inflammation in CF [5–8].

Patients with CF can have a variety of gastro-intestinal tract symptoms. Two entities are common: gastro-oesophageal reflux (GOR) and an obstruction of the small bowel. It has been suggested that CF is primarily a GI disorder which effects the lungs. Small bowel obstruction presents problems in approximately 10% of the CF patients over the age of 5 and distal intestinal obstruction syndrome (DIOS) is the most common cause of obstruction in CF adults [9]. CF patients with DIOS typically present with pain in the lower abdomen and a decreased frequency of defecation.

## Gastro-oesophageal Reflux (GOR)

The occurrence of GOR, the retrograde bolus flow in the esophagus, in CF was first described by Feigelson in 1975 [10]. There is a high variation of prevalence of GOR in CF in literature, which is probably due to the different age groups studied and different techniques used to study reflux in CF. The prevalence of increased acid exposure varies from 15 to 76% in infants with CF, from 20 to 55% in CF children and up to 90% in adults [11–19]. The 'gold standard' to detect reflux in the 1980s and 1990s was 24 h oesophageal pH-monitoring. Since the development of a newer technique, impedance-pH monitoring, it is possible to determine not only acid reflux, but also non-acidic reflux episodes [20, 21]. Using this technique, increased reflux was found in 20/23 (87%) CF patients. Acid reflux was most common, however, there appeared to be a subgroup of CF patients (21%) having increased weakly acidic reflux [22]. In a group of 24 CF children, increased reflux was found in 67%, with the majority of reflux events being acidic [23]. It is important to notice that a substantial subgroup of CF patients have increased reflux without having typical GOR symptoms, i.e. so called silent reflux. Button et al. described silent GOR in 60% of CF adults and Blondeau et al. previously reported silent GOR in 57% of adult CF patients [13, 22].

The mechanisms of increased reflux have been extensively studied in GORD, but much less is known about the pathophysiology of GORD in CF. Low LES pressure is an important factor in the pathogenesis of reflux in CF, however the predominant mechanism of reflux in CF is the increased occurrence of transient lower oesophageal sphincter relaxations (TLOSRs) [14, 16, 24]. During TLOSRs, gastro-oesophageal pressure gradients were higher in 12 CF patients compared to healthy subjects. This was suggested to be due to a more negative intra-thoracic pressure [24]. This increased inspiratory effort in CF can favour reflux, suggesting that in adult CF reflux can be a secondary phenomenon to respiratory dysfunction.

The highest concern about increased reflux in CF is the alleged occurrence of aspiration of (duodeno)-gastric contents into the lungs. The gastro-oesophageal refluxate contains mostly acid, aerosolised chyme and food particles; however, other components might also be present, such as pepsin, bile and other duodeno-gastric enzymes. Several methods have been used to detect gastric aspiration into the lungs, like pulmonary scintigraphy, ambulatory 24 h laryngeal or pharyngeal pH-measurements, lipid-laden macrophages and the presence of (duodeno)-gastric components in BALF [25–30].

## Detection of Aspiration

Pulmonary scintigraphy has been used to detect aspiration by measuring radiolabelled gastric material in the lungs, however, it has a low sensitivity [30].

Laryngeal or pharyngeal pH-measurements have the limitation of being able to only detect proximal reflux of acidic components. Therefore, Ledson et al. performed simultaneous ambulatory 24 h tracheal and oesophageal pH-measurements in a group of 11 adult CF patients and described tracheal acidification in 36%, suggesting that acidic components are frequently aspirated into the trachea [29].

The presence of lipid-laden macrophages in BALF has been used to determine aspiration, but it has a low sensitivity and specificity, varying from 57 to 69% and from 75 to 79% [31, 32].

Aspiration can also be determined by detection of (duodeno)-gastric components, such as pepsin and bile acids, in saliva, sputum or BALF. The golden standard in detecting aspiration, measuring (duodeno)-gastric contents in BALF collected during bronchoscopy is invasive and not routinely performed in CF. Blondeau et al. showed the presence of bile acids in saliva of almost half of the CF adults and in 35% of CF children [22, 23]. Although measuring the presence of (duodeno)-gastric markers in saliva is simple, if positive, it indicates regurgitation of gastric contents

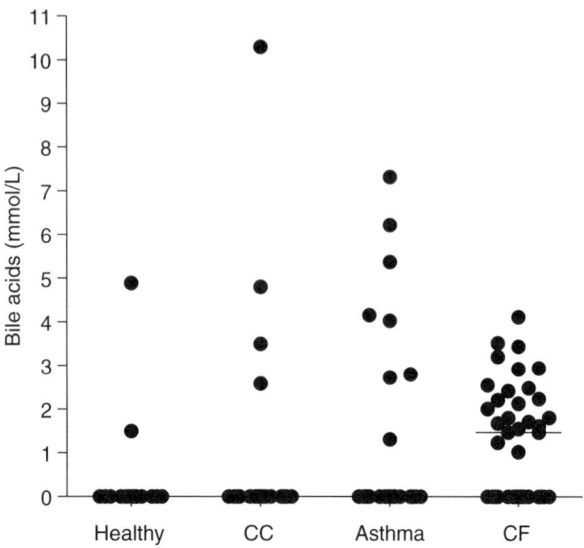

**Fig. 15.1** Concentration of bile acids in sputum of healthy controls (n = 15), patients with chronic cough (CC), asthma patients and patients with CF (n = 41) [33]

and only suggests a higher risk for aspiration. In contrast, detection of (duodeno)-gastric components in sputum is non-invasive and can confirm aspiration in the airways. In a recent study, bile acids were found in sputum of 23/41 (56%) CF patients, in 2/15 (13%) healthy controls, in 4/28 (14%) patients with chronic cough and in 8/29 (28%) asthma patients (Fig. 15.1). The concentration of bile acids in sputum of patients with CF was significantly higher compared to healthy controls and patients with chronic cough [33].

Presence and concentration of (duodeno)-gastric markers in the airway theoretically depends on volume and proximal extent of the refluxate, failure of the anti-aspiration protective mechanisms and bronchial mucociliary clearance. Aspiration does not occur with every reflux event. Normal protective mechanisms against aspiration are reflex contraction of the UES and closure of the glottis and vocal cords and cough [34].

## Lung Function

Since impairment of lung function in CF is determined by a variety of parameters (i.e. recurrent infection with *Pseudomonas aeruginosa*, poor weight for height values, development of CF related diabetes mellitus), it is challenging to assess the impact of an isolated factor, e.g. GOR of aspiration, on the pathophysiology of lung disease in CF.

An early study by Stringer et al. performed in a group of 57 CF children, reported lower lung function values in those with proven reflux compared to those without reflux [35]. These results were confirmed in 2001 in a study using data from the European Epidemiologic Registry of CF, where Navarro et al. conducted a survey in 7010 CF patients older than 6 years and found that patients with peptic GOR have a slightly lower lung function compared to patients without GOR [36].

A more recent study however was unable to confirm a significant correlation between quantitative severity of reflux and impairment of lung function in a group of 42 CF patients [33].

In the latter study, median concentrations of neutrophil elastase, a marker of inflammation, and neutrophilia were significantly higher in sputum from a group of 41 CF patients compared to healthy controls. Moreover, CF patients with proven aspiration (the presence of bile acids in sputum) had significantly higher levels of neutrophil elastase compared to those without aspiration. Although lung function at the time of the sputum sampling was not significantly different between patients with and without aspiration, a significant negative correlation was found between lung function values and bile acid concentrations. Furthermore, in these patients, there was a significant correlation between bile acid concentrations in sputum and the number of days of IV antibiotic therapy in 2 years preceding sputum collections [33]. Such studies are confounded by sampling error because of the episodic nature of reflux events.

## Aspiration

Aspiration of bile acids in CF is associated with more airway inflammation and the degree of aspiration appears to be related to the extent of the airway inflammation. It seems logical to assume that increased reflux will increase the likelihood of aspiration. However, even CF patients with a physiological amount of reflux might have aspiration with deleterious consequences for their lung function.

It has been hypothesized that aspiration can lead to chemical injury, which can provoke airway constriction and edema followed by an inflammatory response. Not only acid particulates and bile acids, but also pepsin has been linked to increased airway inflammation. It was shown by McNally et al. that high levels of pepsin in BALF of a group CF children was associated with high levels of IL-8, a potent activator for neutrophils [37].

## Treatment

Treatment with proton pump inhibitors (PPI) to reduce acid reflux is common practice in CF, but also to compensate for decreased bicarbonate secretion and to facilitate pancreatic enzymes supplementation. PPI treatment reduces both acidity as well as volume of the gastric contents, however, it does not eliminate reflux [38]. Consequently acid suppression will not prevent aspiration of non-acidic gastric components, like food particles, bile acids, trypsin and other duodeno-gastric components.

As mentioned above, there appears to be a link between reflux/aspiration and neutrophilic inflammation in the lungs, probably mediated via IL-8. A recent in vitro study showed that exposure of primary bronchial epithelial cells to gastric juice from patients treated with PPIs provoked a significantly higher grade of inflammation, by means of IL-8, compared to exposure to gastric juice from patients not treated with PPIs. Levels of endotoxins were significantly higher in gastric juice from patients on PPI compared to patients off PPI, suggesting that bacterial subproducts might be very important for the inflammatory reaction [39].

## Conclusions

Several studies proposed the hypothesis that CF lungs are more susceptible for inflammation compared to healthy lungs. Khan et al. and Rosenfeld et al. have revealed elevated levels of different cytokines and neutrophils in the lungs of CF patients, even in those who have only mild lung disease or in the absence of infection [4, 6]. Muhlebach et al. found higher levels of inflammatory cytokines in response to similar levels of pulmonary infection in CF children compared to non-CF controls and after stimulation of both CF and healthy airway epithelial cells with *Pseudomonas aeruginosa*, levels of IL-8 were found to be significantly higher in the CF cells compared to the healthy cells [7, 40]. A recent study could confirm these findings: CF primary bronchial epithelial cells secreted significantly higher levels of IL-8 compared to healthy primary bronchial epithelial cells, both after stimulation with gastric juice from patients on and off PPI [39].

Based on literature findings, we can hypothesize that CF patients, when treated with PPIs, have a gastric juice with a high pH and bacterial contamination. CF patients are known to have increased reflux and bronchial aspiration. The aspirated material has a significantly enhanced inflammatory effect on CF bronchial epithelial cells in culture. Chronic treatment with PPI does not prevent aspiration and may result in a paradoxically increased inflammatory effect in the airways. Alternative therapies, such as anti-reflux surgery, can be the treatment choice in CF patients. In a group of 25 CF children who underwent a Nissen fundoplication, those who had a forced expiratory volume in 1 s (FEV1) of less than 60% predicted at the time of the fundoplication showed an improvement in FEV1 slope as compared to those with a FEV1 of 60% and more [41]. A recent uncontrolled study by Fathi et al. showed beneficial effects of a Nissen fundoplication in a group of CF patients reducing both cough and exacerbation rate [42]. Based on these results, a non-invasive screening test for aspiration might be used to select CF patients that could benefit from anti-reflux surgery.

## References

1. Riordan JR, Rommens JM, Kerem B, et al. Identification of the cystic fibrosis gene: cloning and characterization of complementary DNA. Science. 1989;245(4922):1066–73.
2. Vender RL. Cystic fibrosis lung disease in adult patients. Postgrad Med. 2008;120(1):64–74.
3. De Rose V. Mechanisms and markers of airway inflammation in cystic fibrosis. Eur Respir J. 2002;19(2):333–40.

4. Rosenfeld M, Gibson RL, McNamara S, et al. Early pulmonary infection, inflammation, and clinical outcomes in infants with cystic fibrosis. Pediatr Pulmonol. 2001;32(5):356–66.
5. Balough K, McCubbin M, Weinberger M, et al. The relationship between infection and inflammation in the early stages of lung disease from cystic fibrosis. Pediatr Pulmonol. 1995;20(2):63–70.
6. Khan TZ, Wagener JS, Bost T, et al. Early pulmonary inflammation in infants with cystic fibrosis. Am J Respir Crit Care Med. 1995;151(4):1075–82.
7. Muhlebach MS, Stewart PW, Leigh MW, et al. Quantitation of inflammatory responses to bacteria in young cystic fibrosis and control patients. Am J Respir Crit Care Med. 1999;160(1):186–91.
8. Nixon GM, Armstrong DS, Carzino R, et al. Early airway infection, inflammation, and lung function in cystic fibrosis. Arch Dis Child. 2002;87(4):306–11.
9. Rubinstein S, Moss R, Lewiston N. Constipation and meconium ileus equivalent in patients with cystic fibrosis. Pediatrics. 1986;78(3):473–9.
10. Feigelson J, Sauvegrain J. Letter: Gastro-esophageal reflux in mucoviscidosis. Nouv Press Med. 1975;4(38):2729–30.
11. Bosheva M, Ivancheva D, Genkova N, et al. Gastroesophageal reflux in children with cystic fibrosis. Folia Med. 1998;40(3B Suppl 3):124–6.
12. Brodzicki J, Trawinska-Bartnicka M, Korzon M. Frequency, consequences and pharmacological treatment of gastroesophageal reflux in children with cystic fibrosis. Med Sci Monit. 2002;8(7):CR529–37.
13. Button BM, Roberts S, Kotsimbos TC, et al. Gastroesophageal reflux (symptomatic and silent): a potentially significant problem in patients with cystic fibrosis before and after lung transplantation. J Heart Lung Transplant. 2005;24(10):1522–9.
14. Cucchiara S, Santamaria F, Andreotti MR, et al. Mechanisms of gastro-oesophageal reflux in cystic fibrosis. Arch Dis Child. 1991;66(5):617–22.
15. Heine RG, Button BM, Olinsky A, et al. Gastro-oesophageal reflux in infants under 6 months with cystic fibrosis. Arch Dis Child. 1998;78(1):44–8.
16. Ledson MJ, Tran J, Walshaw MJ. Prevalence and mechanisms of gastro-oesophageal reflux in adult cystic fibrosis patients. J R Soc Med. 1998;91(1):7–9.
17. Scott RB, O'Loughlin EV, Gall DG. Gastroesophageal reflux in patients with cystic fibrosis. J Pediatr. 1985;106(2):223–7.
18. Vic P, Tassin E, Turck D, et al. Frequency of gastroesophageal reflux in infants and in young children with cystic fibrosis. Arch Pediatr. 1995;2(8):742–6.
19. Vinocur CD, Marmon L, Schidlow DV, et al. Gastroesophageal reflux in the infant with cystic fibrosis. Am J Surg. 1985;149(1):182–6.
20. Sifrim D, Castell D, Dent J, et al. Gastro-oesophageal reflux monitoring: review and consensus report on detection and definitions of acid, non-acid, and gas reflux. Gut. 2004;53(7):1024–31.
21. Silny J. Intraluminal multiple electric impedance procedure for measurement of gastrointestinal motility. Neurogastroenterol Motil. 1991;3:151–62.
22. Blondeau K, Dupont LJ, Mertens V, et al. Gastro-oesophageal reflux and aspiration of gastric contents in adult patients with cystic fibrosis. Gut. 2008;57(8):1049–55.
23. Blondeau K, Pauwels A, Dupont L, et al. Characteristics of gastroesophageal reflux and potential risk of gastric content aspiration in children with cystic fibrosis. J Pediatr Gastroenterol Nutr. 2010;50(2):161–6.
24. Pauwels A, Blondeau K, Dupont LJ, et al. Mechanisms of increased gastroesophageal reflux in patients with cystic fibrosis. Am J Gastroenterol. 2012;107(9):1346–53.
25. Blondeau K, Mertens V, Vanaudenaerde BA, et al. Gastro-oesophageal reflux and gastric aspiration in lung transplant patients with or without chronic rejection. Eur Respir J. 2008;31(4):707–13.
26. Farrell S, McMaster C, Gibson D, et al. Pepsin in bronchoalveolar lavage fluid: a specific and sensitive method of diagnosing gastro-oesophageal reflux-related pulmonary aspiration. J Pediatr Surg. 2006;41(2):289–93.
27. Koksal D, Ozkan B, Simsek C, et al. Lipid-laden alveolar macrophage index in sputum is not useful in the differential diagnosis of pulmonary symptoms secondary to gastroesophageal reflux. Arch Med Res. 2005;36(5):485–9.

28. Krishnan U, Mitchell JD, Tobias V, et al. Fat laden macrophages in tracheal aspirates as a marker of reflux aspiration: a negative report. J Pediatr Gastroenterol Nutr. 2002;35(3):309–13.
29. Ledson MJ, Wilson GE, Tran J, et al. Tracheal microaspiration in adult cystic fibrosis. J R Soc Med. 1998;91(1):10–2.
30. Ravelli AM, Panarotto MB, Verdoni L, et al. Pulmonary aspiration shown by scintigraphy in gastroesophageal reflux-related respiratory disease. Chest. 2006;130(5):1520–6.
31. Bauer ML, Lyrene RK. Chronic aspiration in children: evaluation of the lipid-laden macrophage index. Pediatr Pulmonol. 1999;28(2):94–100.
32. Ding Y, Simpson PM, Schellhase DE, et al. Limited reliability of lipid-laden macrophage index restricts its use as a test for pulmonary aspiration: comparison with a simple semiquantitative assay. Pediatr Dev Pathol. 2002;5(6):551–8.
33. Pauwels A, Decraene A, Blondeau K, et al. Bile acids in sputum and increased airway inflammation in patients with cystic fibrosis. Chest. 2012;141(6):1568–74.
34. Shaker R, Dodds WJ, Ren J, et al. Esophagoglottal closure reflex: a mechanism of airway protection. Gastroenterology. 1992;102(3):857–61.
35. Stringer DA, Sprigg A, Juodis E, et al. The association of cystic fibrosis, gastroesophageal reflux, and reduced pulmonary function. Can Assoc Radiol J. 1988;39(2):100–2.
36. Navarro J, Rainisio M, Harms HK, et al. Factors associated with poor pulmonary function: cross-sectional analysis of data from the ERCF. Eur Respir J. 2001;18(2):298–305.
37. McNally P, Ervine E, Shields MD, et al. High concentrations of pepsin in bronchoalveolar lavage fluid from children with cystic fibrosis are associated with high interleukin-8 concentrations. Thorax. 2011;66(2):140–3.
38. Vela MF, Camacho-Lobato L, Srinivasan R, et al. Simultaneous intraesophageal impedance and pH measurement of acid and nonacid gastroesophageal reflux: effect of omeprazole. Gastroenterology. 2001;120(7):1599–606.
39. Pauwels A, Verleden S, Farre R, et al. The effect of gastric juice on interleukin-8 production by cystic fibrosis primary bronchial epithelial cells. J Cyst Fibros. 2013;12(6):700–5.
40. Joseph T, Look D, Ferkol T. NF-kappaB activation and sustained IL-8 gene expression in primary cultures of cystic fibrosis airway epithelial cells stimulated with Pseudomonas aeruginosa. Am J Physiol Lung Cell Mol Physiol. 2005;288(3):L471–9.
41. Boesch RP, Acton JD. Outcomes of fundoplication in children with cystic fibrosis. J Pediatr Surg. 2007;42(8):1341–4.
42. Fathi H, Moon T, Donaldson J, et al. Cough in adult cystic fibrosis: diagnosis and response to fundoplication. Cough. 2009;5:1.

# Gastroesophageal Reflux and Idiopathic Pulmonary Fibrosis

## 16

Lawrence A. Ho and Ganesh Raghu

**Abstract**

Idiopathic pulmonary fibrosis (IPF) is a specific form of chronic and progressive fibrosing interstitial pneumonia of unknown cause. IPF is the most common form of idiopathic interstitial pneumonia (IIP) and accounts for 50–60% of these diseases. Even though the cause of IPF is unknown, various exposures such cigarette smoking, metal/wood dust, certain drugs and importantly gastroesophageal reflux (GER) have been associated with IPF. There is an increasing body of literature regarding the relationship between GER and IPF, particularly over the last decade. This has culminated in anti-acid medications receiving a conditional recommendation for use in patients with IPF in the most recent American Thoracic Society/European Respiratory Society/Japanese Respiratory Society and Latin American Thoracic Associate guidelines for the treatment of IPF. This chapter will explore the proposed pathologic relationship between IPF and GER as well as treatments, outcomes and future directions.

## Idiopathic Pulmonary Fibrosis

Idiopathic pulmonary fibrosis (IPF) is a chronic and progressive fibrosing interstitial pneumonia of unknown cause that is associated with the histopathologic and radiographic pattern of an usual interstitial pneumonia (UIP) pattern [1]. A median survival of 3–5 years from the time of diagnosis has been widely described [2]. Clinical features of IPF include progressive dyspnea, cough and a restrictive pulmonary physiology. The incidence and prevalence of IPF worldwide is increasing with

L. A. Ho · G. Raghu (✉)
Center for Interstitial Lung Disease, Division of Pulmonary, Critical Care and Sleep Medicine, University of Washington, Seattle, WA, USA
e-mail: laho@uw.edu; graghu@uw.edu

recent estimates of prevalence in the US being 18.2 cases per 100,000 persons [3]. IPF occurs in adults over 50 years old with the onset typically in the sixth and seventh decade of life [1]. There is a male predominance; males with IPF outnumber females with IPF by nearly 1.5:1 [1]. Although studies in the western hemisphere have a higher prevalence in Caucasians of European origin, there does not appear to be any known racial, ethnic, geographic, or cultural predilection for IPF. In the appropriate clinical setting, a confident diagnosis of IPF can be made based on clinical features—an UIP pattern on high-resolution computed tomography (HRCT) combined with clinical criteria including the absence alternative causes [1]. Based on current guidelines for the diagnosis of IPF, histopathologic features of an UIP pattern on surgical lung biopsy is required for definitive diagnosis of IPF in patients who do not have the definitive UIP pattern on HRCT images [1].

Until recently, treatment options for IPF have been limited [1]. In 2014, the results of two randomized controlled clinical trials were published demonstrating that both the medications studied, pirfenidone and nintedanib, attenuated the rate of decline in the forced vital capacity (FVC) over 52 weeks [4, 5]. These two medications have been given a conditional recommendation for use in the 2015 updated American Thoracic Society guidelines for the treatment of IPF [6]. In addition to these two medications, anti-acid medications were the only other type of medication to receive a conditional recommendation in these updated guidelines. This highlights the growing link between IPF and abnormal gastroesophageal reflux (GER).

## GER and Idiopathic Pulmonary Fibrosis

Although the understanding of the pathogenesis of IPF is incomplete, the theory of inflammation playing a significant role in IPF has fallen out of favor. Instead, most investigators agree on a theory involving a lung injurious event with resultant continuous abnormal repair [7]. By definition, IPF is a disease of unknown etiology, but various factors have been associated with IPF as potential causes of lung injury. These factors include cigarette smoking, viral infections, environmental exposures and importantly GER and microaspiration [8–10] (Fig. 16.1).

## Studies Evaluating GER in Patients with IPF

The connection between GER and IPF is longstanding. Case series dating back to 1971 have described pulmonary fibrosis associated with hiatal hernia [11]. Since then, there have been numerous studies that have documented a strong relationship between GER and IPF. More recently, a study using multidetector computed tomography scans to identify hiatal hernias found hiatal hernias to be more prevalent in IPF patients compared to patients with asthma and chronic obstructive pulmonary disease (39% vs. 17% vs. 13%, p-value = 0.01 to <0.001) [12]. Perhaps most notably, a case-control study of over 100,000 patients in the Veterans Administration Hospitals reported that erosive esophagitis and esophageal stricture significantly

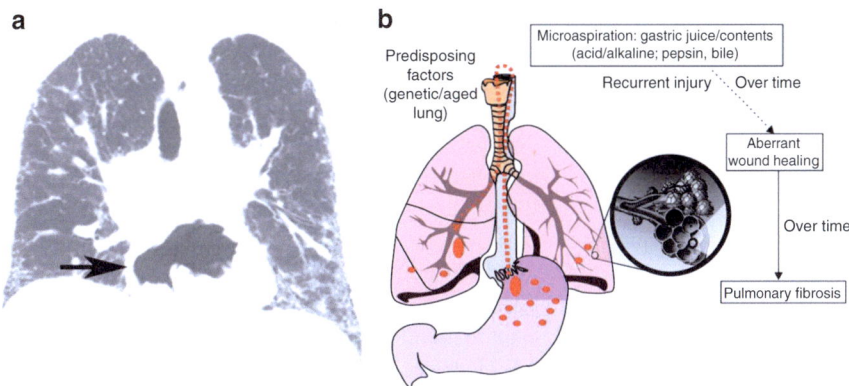

**Fig. 16.1** (**a**) High-resolution computed tomography (HRCT) image of the chest in a patient with idiopathic pulmonary fibrosis (IPF; diagnosis ascertained per criteria described) demonstrating the co-presence of hiatal hernia (arrow). (**b**) Concepts of gastro-oesophageal reflux (GER) and microaspiration in the pathogenesis of IPF and acute exacerbation of IPF. Note the schematic representation of the presence of a hiatal hernia (small) and the contents of gastric juice refluxate gaining access to the distal pulmonary parenchyma via GER and microaspiration (shown by the dots from the distal oesophagus into the proximal oesophagus and aspirating into the lung (arrowhead)), which can cause lung injury. Recurrent injury caused by intermittent microaspirations leads to aberrant wound healing and subsequent pulmonary fibrosis (which manifests as a usual interstitial pneumonia pattern on lung histopathology and a clinical diagnosis of IPF), especially in a genetically predisposed person and in elderly individuals, who are more susceptible to manifest IPF

increased the risk of pulmonary fibrosis [13]. Also, a series of 32 asymmetric IPF cases demonstrated increased reporting of overt GERD symptoms in those patients with asymmetric IPF compared to symmetric IPF (63% vs. 31%, p = 0.009) [14]. The patients with asymmetric IPF reported sleeping on the more affected side.

In an early study, Mays et al. indicated the incidence of both hiatal hernia and GER was higher in patients with radiographic evidence of pulmonary fibrosis when compared to age-matched control subjects [15]. In this study, GER was determined based on upper gastrointestinal series. Subsequently, more precise techniques of evaluating GER, including ambulatory esophageal pH monitoring, have been used to evaluate GER in studies with IPF patients. In a prospective study, Tobin et al. demonstrated increased distal and proximal acid exposure in 16 of 17 patients with well-defined IPF using ambulatory esophageal pH monitoring [16]. Additional studies utilizing similar techniques have demonstrated the prevalence of GER in IPF between 67 and 88% in the distal esophagus and 30–71% in the proximal esophagus [17–19].

## Cause and Effect Relationship of GER and IPF

While there is an ever-growing body of literature regarding IPF and GER, the exact relationship remains is unclear [20]. There are several theories regarding this relationship. The first theory involves GER as a sequlae of IPF. Decreased lung compliance in patients with IPF lead to increased swings in pleural pressure thus causing dysfunction of the lower esophageal sphincter and GER [21]. Alternatively, another theory revolves around chronic microaspiration of small droplets of gastric juice either triggering an acute exacerbation or leading to progressive injury and fibrosis. This hypothesis has been confirmed in animal models as pulmonary fibrosis has been induced by direct instillation of acid into the airways [22–24]. Specifically, gastric juice instillation in pig lungs has been shown to cause alveolar damage and subsequent intra-alveolar and interstitial fibrosis with gastric hydrochloric acid and pepsin speculated to be the causative agents [24]. Other components of refluxate may be implicated (see Chap. 3). Additionally, in rodent models, aspiration of gastric fluid can result in increased concentrations of inflammatory and profibrotic cytokines including IL-1, IL-2, TNF-alpha and TGF-beta [25]. Human studies, mainly in the post-lung transplant patient population, have demonstrated harmful effects such as airway inflammation, increased cell membrane permeability, lung remodeling and stimulation of immune response when the lungs are exposed to gastric juice [26–28].

## Asymptomatic GER and Non-acid Reflux

Despite the high prevalence of GER in IPF, IPF patients often demonstrate clinically occult disease. GER symptoms such as regurgitation, dysphagia and heartburn are poor predictors of GER in patients with IPF as several studies have documented only 25–47% of patients with IPF report symptoms of GER [16, 17, 29]. Additionally, using these symptoms to screen for the pathologic presence of GER on 24 h pH monitoring has a relatively low sensitivity (65%) and specificity (71%) [19]. Recently, Allaix et al. demonstrated that the prevalence of heartburn was significantly lower in patients with IPF than in patients with gastroesophageal reflux disease (GERD), but extra-esophageal manifestations of GERD including cough, chest pain and hoarseness were significantly more common among IPF patients [30].

Nonacid reflux could also play a role in lung injury as studies using multichannel intraluminal impedance and pH monitoring in IPF patients confirm the presence of non-acid refluxate [31, 32]. In a study comparing patients with IPF to control patients, a higher number of non-acid reflux events occurred in patients with IPF compared to controls [31]. Other studies have shown that laryngeal epithelial cells uptake pepsin. Once internalized, pepsin can induce an inflammatory response as well as cytotoxicity and airway remodeling [33, 34].

## GER and Acute Exacerbation of IPF

The natural history of IPF is classically described as a gradual decline and loss of function over years [1]. However, the course of IPF can be unpredictable and it is also recognized that patients can demonstrate periods of rapid deterioration. These periods of rapid deterioration are considered acute exacerbations if the following criteria is met: (1) acute worsening—typically symptoms persisting for less than 1 month (2) new bilateral ground glass opacities and/or consolidation on computed tomography and (3) deterioration not fully explained by cardiac failure or fluid overload [35]. Aspiration or occult aspiration of gastric contents has been proposed a mechanism of acute exacerbation of IPF. A study evaluating pepsin levels in BAL fluid of acute exacerbation of IPF patients versus stable IPF patients found that BAL pepsin levels were significantly increased in the group with acute exacerbations of IPF [36]. The BAL pepsin concentration was one standard deviation higher in the acute exacerbation group compared to the stable group with an odds ratio 1.46 (95% CI 1.03–2.09, $p = 0.04$). However, BAL pepsin levels were not predictive of survival and the increased pepsin levels were driven by a subgroup (33% of cases) with markedly elevated pepsin levels in BAL. See Chap. 8 for a discussion of pepsin as a marker of reflux.

## GER Control and IPF Progression

Although there is ample evidence to suggest that GER plays a role in the pathogenesis and progression of IPF, a causative relationship between GER and IPF has yet to be firmly established. Also, the severity of GER may not always correlate with the severity of lung disease in IPF. A study by Raghu et al. evaluated 65 patients with well-defined IPF and did not find any correlation between GER severity and impairment of lung function [17]. Regardless, several studies have addressed reflux control and disease progression. In 2006, Raghu et al. reported a small cases series of four patients. In this retrospective review, adequate treatment for acid GER by either proton pump inhibitor (PPI) or fundoplication (ascertained by 24-h esophageal pH monitoring) lead to stable or improved pulmonary function tests values including forced vital capacity (FVC) and diffusing capacity of the lung for carbon monoxide over a 2–6 year period [37]. A larger study published in the same year evaluated 14 pre-lung transplant IPF patients and demonstrated stabilization in oxygen requirements in patients who had undergone a pre-transplant Nissen Fundoplication [38]. More recently, Lee et al. preformed a retrospective study of 204 patients with IPF enrolled prospectively in longitudinal cohort studies [29]. GER suppression with medical therapy was found to be an independent predictor of longer survival time (HR 0.47, 95% CI 0.24–0.93, p-value = 0.03). Additionally medical therapy was associated with lower radiographic fibrosis scores on HRCT.

## Methods of GER Control

GER can be controlled by several measures; the main categories of GER suppression include lifestyle modifications, pharmacologic therapy (Chaps. 23, 24, 25, 26, and 27) and surgical interventions (Chap. 28). Lifestyle modifications are important in controlling reflux and strategies include sleeping in a bed that has been raised at the head, dietary modifications, and appropriate timing of meals (such as not eating 3–4 h from bedtime). From a pharmacologic standpoint, PPI and histamine2-receptor antagonists (H2RA) have long been used to suppress acid production and are indicated to suppress symptoms associated with abnormal acid GER. It should, however, be emphasized that the PPIs and/or H2RA are not "anti reflux medications" as they merely suppress the acidity of the refluxate of the GER. Emerging data, though, suggests that PPIs, and not H2RAs, have effects that extend beyond the gastrointestinal system [39, 40].

In addition to the known mechanism of blocking the hydrogen/potassium adenosine triphosphatase enzyme in the gastric parietal cells, PPIs also act as scavengers of reactive oxygen species and induce the production of antioxidants [41]. Additionally, PPIs are reported to suppress pro-inflammatory cytokines and inhibit the interaction of inflammatory cells with vascular endothelial cells [40, 42]. A recent in vitro study demonstrated that esomeprazole suppressed transcriptional expression of pro-fibrotic molecules including fibronectin and matrix metalloproteinase enzymes [43]. Also, esomeprazole strongly up-regulated cytoprotective enzymes such as heme oxygenase 1 [44] (Fig. 16.2).

As described in the previous section, anti-acid medications have been associated with improved outcomes in IPF patients in several studies. The majority of the patients in these studies have been maintained on PPIs as opposed to H2RA. A recent study evaluated PPI medications exclusively and also demonstrated a prolonged lung transplant-free survival compared to control patients [43]. Although several studies have reported positive outcomes with anti-acid medications, several other recent publications have cast some uncertainty on these benefits. Kreuter et al. preformed a post hoc analysis of 624 patients with IPF that were enrolled in three clinical trials [45]. This study showed no significant differences in disease progression, all-cause mortality, IPF-related mortality, all-cause hospitalization rate or mean change in percent FVC at 52 weeks in patients receiving antacid therapy versus those who did not receive antacid therapy. While the report indicated that severe gastrointestinal adverse events and pulmonary infections were apparently more frequent with anti-acid therapy, there were several limitations with the study and caution must be taken in interpretation such reports from post hoc analyses [46, 47].

PPI medications may also not sufficiently reduce acid refluxate. Raghu et al. demonstrated that 63% of patients with IPF treated with a standard dose of PPI continued to have abnormal acid based on repeat 24 h pH monitoring while on therapy [17]. Therefore, surgical interventions including fundoplication and hiatal hernia repair can also be considered for GER control. The benefit of fundoplication is that theoretically, this procedure effectively suppresses both acid and non-acid refluxate [48]. Fundoplication has a relatively long standing history of aiding symptoms.

Pellegrini et al. published a study of 100 patients with reflux in 1979 [49]. 5 patients with a primary respiratory disorder reported complete resolution of their respiratory symptoms after fundoplication. Subsequent studies have demonstrated improvement in several respiratory symptoms including cough as well as quality of life scores [50, 51]. Fundoplication also appears to be a relatively safe procedure

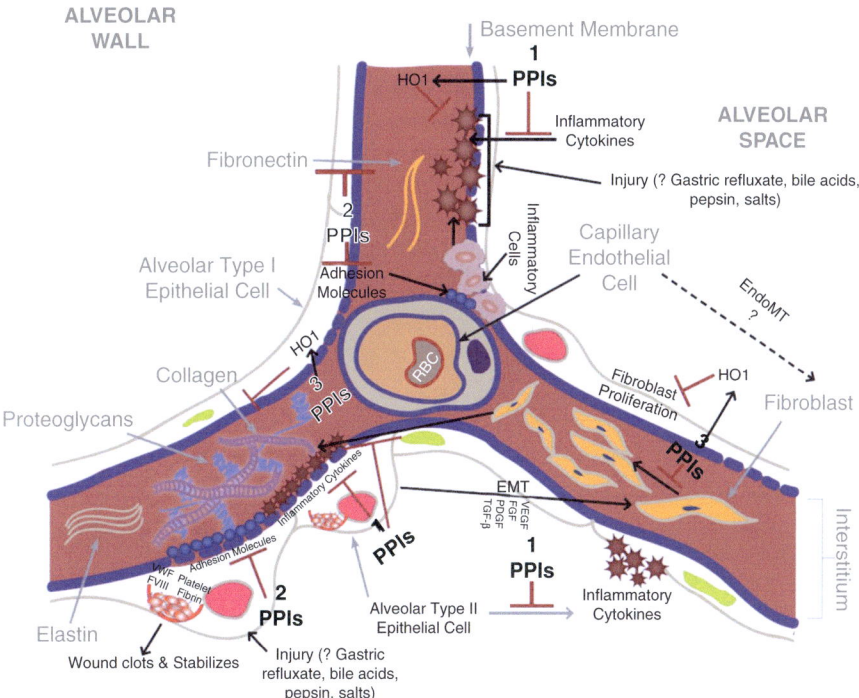

**Fig. 16.2** Schematic illustration of the key cellular and molecular events associated with an injured alveolar wall in genetically predisposed person manifesting pulmonary fibrosis. Note that proton pump inhibitors (PPIs) suppress key events in the lung inflammation and fibrosis including (1) release of proinflammatory molecules from injured epithelial cells; (2) expression of adhesion molecules and adherence of inflammatory cells into the vascular wall; (3) proliferation of fibroblasts including extracellular matrix deposition. The? indicates "unclear." *EMT* epithelial-to-mesenchymal transition, *EndoMT* endothelial-to-mesenchymal transition, *FGF* fibroblast growth factor, *FVIII* factor VIII, *HO1* heme oxyngease 1, *PDGF* platelet-derived growth factor, *RBC* red blood cell, *TGF-β* transforming growth factor-β, *VEGF* vascular endothelial growth factor, *VWF* Von Willenbrand factor

even in the IPF population who tend to have more advanced lung disease. Linden et al. retrospectively reviewed patients on the lung transplant wait list who underwent fundoplication. There were no perioperative complications in the 14 patients with IPF who underwent fundoplication. Most recently, Raghu et al. reported a retrospective review of 27 patients with progressive IPF despite antacid treatment for abnormal acid GER. These patients underwent fundoplication and there were no deaths at 90 day follow-up and 2 year survival was 81.5% [52]. Currently, an ongoing prospective multicenter randomized phase II trial—Weighing Risks and Benefits of Laparoscopic Anti-reflux Surgery in Patients with Idiopathic Pulmonary Fibrosis (WRAP-IPF) has completed enrollment. The results of this study will hopefully provide some clarity regarding the safety and efficacy of laparoscopic fundoplication in IPF patients with GER.

## Conclusion

There is a growing amount of literature linking GER and miroaspiration to IPF. Literature to date suggests that GER is highly associated with IPF. Given this prevalence, it is appropriate to consider formal esophagus and reflux studies in IPF patients even in patients with no GER symptoms as many patients with IPF have clinically occult GER. While several studies suggest stabilization or improvement in lung function with adequate control of acid reflux, there are significant unknowns regarding the GER and IPF as well treatment with antiacid medications for IPF [53]. It is hoped that ongoing clinical studies and future studies that are warranted will settle the issue of the need for treatment of GER in patients with IPF.

## References

1. Raghu G, Collard HR, Egan JJ, Martinez FJ, Behr J, Brown KK, et al. An official ATS/ERS/JRS/ALAT statement: idiopathic pulmonary fibrosis: evidence-based guidelines for diagnosis and management. Am J Respir Crit Care Med. 2011;183(6):788–824.
2. American Thoracic Society. Idiopathic pulmonary fibrosis: diagnosis and treatment. International consensus statement. American Thoracic Society (ATS), and the European Respiratory Society (ERS). Am J Respir Crit Care Med. 2000;161(2 Pt 1):646–64.
3. Raghu G, Chen S-Y, Hou Q, Yeh W-S, Collard HR. Incidence and prevalence of idiopathic pulmonary fibrosis in US adults 18–64 years old. Eur Respir J. 2016;48(1):179–86.
4. King TEJ, Bradford WZ, Castro-Bernardini S, Fagan EA, Glaspole I, Glassberg MK, et al. A phase 3 trial of pirfenidone in patients with idiopathic pulmonary fibrosis. N Engl J Med. 2014;370(22):2083–92.
5. Richeldi L, du Bois RM, Raghu G, Azuma A, Brown KK, Costabel U, et al. Efficacy and safety of nintedanib in idiopathic pulmonary fibrosis. N Engl J Med. 2014;370(22):2071–82.
6. Raghu G, Rochwerg B, Zhang Y, Garcia CAC, Azuma A, Behr J, et al. An official ATS/ERS/JRS/ALAT clinical practice guideline: treatment of idiopathic pulmonary fibrosis. An update of the 2011 clinical practice guideline. Am J Respir Crit Care Med. 2015;192(2):e3–19.
7. Hunninghake GW, Schwarz MI. Does current knowledge explain the pathogenesis of idiopathic pulmonary fibrosis?: a perspective. Proc Am Thorac Soc. 2007;4(5):449–52.
8. Baumgartner KB, Samet JM, Stidley CA, Colby TV, Waldron JA. Cigarette smoking: a risk factor for idiopathic pulmonary fibrosis. Am J Respir Crit Care Med. 1997;155(1):242–8.
9. Stewart JP, Egan JJ, Ross AJ, Kelly BG, Lok SS, Hasleton PS, et al. The detection of Epstein-Barr virus DNA in lung tissue from patients with idiopathic pulmonary fibrosis. Am J Respir Crit Care Med. 1999;159(4 Pt 1):1336–41.
10. Noth I, Zhang Y, Ma S-F, Flores C, Barber M, Huang Y, et al. Genetic variants associated with idiopathic pulmonary fibrosis susceptibility and mortality: a genome-wide association study. Lancet Respir Med. 2013;1(4):309–17.
11. Pearson JE, Wilson RS. Diffuse pulmonary fibrosis and hiatus hernia. Thorax. 1971;26(3):300–5.
12. Noth I, Zangan SM, Soares RV, Forsythe A, Demchuk C, Takahashi SM, et al. Prevalence of hiatal hernia by blinded multidetector CT in patients with idiopathic pulmonary fibrosis. Eur Respir J. 2012;39(2):344–51.
13. el-Serag HB, Sonnenberg A. Comorbid occurrence of laryngeal or pulmonary disease with esophagitis in United States military veterans. Gastroenterology. 1997;113(3):755–60.
14. Tcherakian C, Cottin V, Brillet P-Y, Freynet O, Naggara N, Carton Z, et al. Progression of idiopathic pulmonary fibrosis: lessons from asymmetrical disease. Thorax. 2011;66(3):226–31.
15. Mays EE, Dubois JJ, Hamilton GB. Pulmonary fibrosis associated with tracheobronchial aspiration. A study of the frequency of hiatal hernia and gastroesophageal reflux in interstitial pulmonary fibrosis of obscure etiology. Chest. 1976;69(4):512–5.

16. Tobin RW, Pope CE, Pellegrini CA, Emond MJ, Sillery J, Raghu G. Increased prevalence of gastroesophageal reflux in patients with idiopathic pulmonary fibrosis. Am J Respir Crit Care Med. 1998;158(6):1804–8.
17. Raghu G, Freudenberger TD, Yang S, Curtis JR, Spada C, Hayes J, et al. High prevalence of abnormal acid gastro-oesophageal reflux in idiopathic pulmonary fibrosis. Eur Respir J. 2006;27(1):136–42.
18. Salvioli B, Belmonte G, Stanghellini V, Baldi E, Fasano L, Pacilli AMG, et al. Gastro-oesophageal reflux and interstitial lung disease. Dig Liver Dis. 2006;38(12):879–84.
19. Sweet MP, Patti MG, Leard LE, Golden JA, Hays SR, Hoopes C, et al. Gastroesophageal reflux in patients with idiopathic pulmonary fibrosis referred for lung transplantation. J Thorac Cardiovasc Surg. 2007;133(4):1078–84.
20. Raghu G, Meyer KC. Silent gastro-oesophageal reflux and microaspiration in IPF: mounting evidence for anti-reflux therapy? Eur Respir J. 2012;39(2):242.
21. Lee JS, Collard HR, Raghu G, Sweet MP, Hays SR, Campos GM, et al. Does chronic microaspiration cause idiopathic pulmonary fibrosis? Am J Med. 2010;123(4):304–11.
22. Mitsuhashi T, Shimazaki M, Chanoki Y, Kuwahara H, Sakai T, Masuda H. Experimental pulmonary fibrosis induced by trisodium citrate and acid-citrate-dextrose. Exp Mol Pathol. 1985;42(2):261–70.
23. Schwartz DJ, Wynne JW, Gibbs CP, Hood CI, Kuck EJ. The pulmonary consequences of aspiration of gastric contents at pH values greater than 2.5. Am Rev Respir Dis. 1980;121(1):119–26.
24. Popper H, Juettner F, Pinter J. The gastric juice aspiration syndrome (Mendelson syndrome). Aspects of pathogenesis and treatment in the pig. Virchows Arch A Pathol Anat Histopathol. 1986;409(1):105–17.
25. Appel JZ, Lee SM, Hartwig MG, Li B, Hsieh C-C, Cantu E, et al. Characterization of the innate immune response to chronic aspiration in a novel rodent model. Respir Res. 2007;8(1):87.
26. Perng D-W, Chang K-T, Su K-C, Wu Y-C, Wu M-T, Hsu W-H, et al. Exposure of airway epithelium to bile acids associated with gastroesophageal reflux symptoms: a relation to transforming growth factor-β1 production and fibroblast proliferation. Chest. 2007;132(5):1548–56.
27. Blondeau K, Mertens V, Vanaudenaerde BA, Verleden GM, Van Raemdonck DE, Sifrim D, et al. Gastro-oesophageal reflux and gastric aspiration in lung transplant patients with or without chronic rejection. Eur Respir J. 2008;31(4):707.
28. D'Ovidio F, Mura M, Tsang M, Waddell TK, Hutcheon MA, Singer LG, et al. Bile acid aspiration and the development of bronchiolitis obliterans after lung transplantation. J Thorac Cardiovasc Surg. 2005;129(5):1144–52.
29. Lee JS, Ryu JH, Elicker BM, Lydell CP, Jones KD, Wolters PJ, et al. Gastroesophageal reflux therapy is associated with longer survival in patients with idiopathic pulmonary fibrosis. Am J Respir Crit Care Med. 2011;184(12):1390–4.
30. Allaix ME, Fisichella PM, Noth I, Herbella FA, Borraez Segura B, Patti MG. Idiopathic pulmonary fibrosis and gastroesophageal reflux. Implications for treatment. J Gastrointest Surg. 2014;18(1):100–4. Discussion 104-5.
31. Savarino E, Carbone R, Marabotto E, Furnari M, Sconfienza L, Ghio M, et al. Gastro-oesophageal reflux and gastric aspiration in idiopathic pulmonary fibrosis patients. Eur Respir J. 2013;42(5):1322–31.
32. Gavini S, Borges LF, Finn RT, Lo W-K, Goldberg HJ, Burakoff R, et al. Lung disease severity in idiopathic pulmonary fibrosis is more strongly associated with impedance measures of bolus reflux than pH parameters of acid reflux alone. Neurogastroenterol Motil. 2017;29(5):e13001.
33. Johnston N, Wells CW, Blumin JH, Toohill RJ, Merati AL. Receptor-mediated uptake of pepsin by laryngeal epithelial cells. Ann Otol Rhinol Laryngol. 2007;116(12):934–8.
34. Bathoorn E, Daly P, Gaiser B, Sternad K, Poland C, MacNee W, et al. Cytotoxicity and induction of inflammation by pepsin in acid in bronchial epithelial cells. Int J Inflamm. 2011;2011:5.
35. Collard HR, Ryerson CJ, Corte TJ, Jenkins G, Kondoh Y, Lederer DJ, et al. Acute exacerbation of idiopathic pulmonary fibrosis. An international working group report. Am J Respir Crit Care Med. 2016;194(3):265–75.
36. Lee JS, Song JW, Wolters PJ, Elicker BM, King TE, Kim DS, et al. Bronchoalveolar lavage pepsin in acute exacerbation of idiopathic pulmonary fibrosis. Eur Respir J. 2012;39(2):352–8.

37. Raghu G, Yang ST-Y, Spada C, Hayes J, Pellegrini CA. Sole treatment of acid gastroesophageal reflux in idiopathic pulmonary fibrosis: a case series. Chest. 2006;129(3):794–800.
38. Linden PA, Gilbert RJ, Yeap BY, Boyle K, Deykin A, Jaklitsch MT, et al. Laparoscopic fundoplication in patients with end-stage lung disease awaiting transplantation. J Thorac Cardiovasc Surg. 2006;131(2):438–46.
39. Kedika RR, Souza RF, Spechler SJ. Potential anti-inflammatory effects of proton pump inhibitors: a review and discussion of the clinical implications. Dig Dis Sci. 2009;54(11):2312–7.
40. Yoshida N, Yoshikawa T, Tanaka Y, Fujita N, Kassai K, Naito Y, et al. A new mechanism for anti-inflammatory actions of proton pump inhibitors – inhibitory effects on neutrophil-endothelial cell interactions. Aliment Pharmacol Ther. 2000;14(Suppl 1):74–81.
41. Takagi T, Naito Y, Okada H, Ishii T, Mizushima K, Akagiri S, et al. Lansoprazole, a proton pump inhibitor, mediates anti-inflammatory effect in gastric mucosal cells through the induction of heme oxygenase-1 via activation of NF-E2-related factor 2 and oxidation of kelch-like ECH-associating protein 1. J Pharmacol Exp Ther. 2009;331(1):255–64.
42. Sasaki T, Yamaya M, Yasuda H, Inoue D, Yamada M, Kubo H, et al. The proton pump inhibitor lansoprazole inhibits rhinovirus infection in cultured human tracheal epithelial cells. Eur J Pharmacol. 2005;509(2–3):201–10.
43. Ghebremariam YT, Cooke JP, Gerhart W, Griego C, Brower JB, Doyle-Eisele M, et al. Pleiotropic effect of the proton pump inhibitor esomeprazole leading to suppression of lung inflammation and fibrosis. J Transl Med. 2015;13:249.
44. Ghebre YT, Raghu G. Idiopathic pulmonary fibrosis: novel concepts of proton pump inhibitors as antifibrotic drugs. Am J Respir Crit Care Med. 2016;193(12):1345–52.
45. Kreuter M, Spagnolo P, Wuyts W, Renzoni E, Koschel D, Bonella F, et al. Antacid therapy and disease progression in patients with idiopathic pulmonary fibrosis who received pirfenidone. Respiration. 2017;93:415.
46. Raghu G. Anti-acid treatment in patients with IPF: interpret results from post-hoc, subgroup, and exploratory analyses with great caution. Lancet Respir Med. 2016;4(9):e46–7.
47. Johnson WC, Raghu G. Clinical trials in idiopathic pulmonary fibrosis: a word of caution concerning choice of outcome measures. Eur Respir J. 2005;26(5):755–8.
48. Dallemagne B, Weerts J, Markiewicz S, Dewandre J-M, Wahlen C, Monami B, et al. Clinical results of laparoscopic fundoplication at ten years after surgery. Surg Endosc. 2006;20(1):159–65.
49. Pellegrini CA, DeMeester TR, Johnson LF, Skinner DB. Gastroesophageal reflux and pulmonary aspiration: incidence, functional abnormality, and results of surgical therapy. Surgery. 1979;86(1):110–9.
50. Patti MG, Arcerito M, Tamburini A, Diener U, Feo CV, Safadi B, et al. Effect of laparoscopic fundoplication on gastroesophageal reflux disease-induced respiratory symptoms. J Gastrointest Surg. 2000;4(2):143–9.
51. Ciovica R, Gadenstatter M, Klingler A, Neumayer C, Schwab GP. Laparoscopic antireflux surgery provides excellent results and quality of life in gastroesophageal reflux disease patients with respiratory symptoms. J Gastrointest Surg. 2005;9(5):633–7.
52. Raghu G, Morrow E, Collins BF, Ho LAT, Hinojosa MW, Hayes JM, et al. Laparoscopic anti-reflux surgery for idiopathic pulmonary fibrosis at a single centre. Eur Respir J. 2016;48(3):826–32.
53. Johannson KA, Strambu I, Ravaglia C. Antacid therapy in idiopathic pulmonary fibrosis: more questions than answers. Lancet Respir Med. 2017;5:591.

# Gastro-Oesophageal Reflux Disease (GORD) and Chronic Cough

## 17

Lorcan McGarvey and Kian Fan Chung

## Introduction

Gastro-oesophageal reflux disease (GORD) as a syndrome arose from the attempt to understand peptic symptoms and pathology in the upper GI tract. Extra-oesophageal manifestations, such as LPR and airway reflux (discussed in other chapters in this volume) were initially unrecognised. In this chapter 'classic' GORD and its relationship or otherwise to the airways is discussed.

A recent consensus based statement defined GORD as the effortless movement of stomach contents into the oesophagus or mouth causing troublesome symptoms or complications [1]. Although most healthy people experience some degree of reflux from time to time such episodes are not usually bothersome and rarely lead to complications. In terms of bothersome symptoms, heartburn, and acid regurgitation are most typical but extra-oesophageal manifestations including cough, hoarseness, and frequent throat clearing have been belatedly recognised [2]. Complications arise from tissue damage due to the direct injurious effects of gastric refluxate and include oesophagitis and the development of strictures, Barrett's oesophagus and in some instances oesophageal carcinoma. These peptic complications have led to the paradigm that GORD = acid.

GORD is prevalent, occurring in 20% of the general population [3] and chronic cough is one of the commonest clinical problems encountered by

L. McGarvey (✉)
Centre for Experimental Medicine, Wellcome-Wolfson Institute for Experimental Medicine, School of Medicine, Dentistry and Biomedical Sciences, Queen's University, Belfast, UK
e-mail: l.mcgarvey@qub.ac.uk

K. F. Chung
Airway Disease Section, National Heart and Lung Institute, Imperial College London, London, UK

Royal Brompton Hospital, London, UK
e-mail: f.chung@imperial.ac.uk

© Springer International Publishing AG, part of Springer Nature 2018
A. H. Morice, P. W. Dettmar (eds.), *Reflux Aspiration and Lung Disease*,
https://doi.org/10.1007/978-3-319-90525-9_17

doctors [4]. Although GORD and chronic cough are both common and frequently co-exist, the precise clinical association between the two is often unclear. Current guidelines on the management of cough recommend that clinicians consider reflux as a possible aggravating factor and suggest empirical trials of anti-reflux treatment [5–7]. However, without exception each has highlighted the limited evidence base on which to recommend treatment and the need to clarify the pathophysiological mechanisms linking GORD and cough. Here we provide an overview of the existing literature on definition, epidemiology and clinical presentation of GORD and cough, highlighting the association between gut and lung and its relevance to GORD associated cough.

## Epidemiology

The lack of agreed standards for the diagnosis of GORD makes it difficult to provide precise data on its prevalence in the general population. In a population-based study, Locke et al., used a validated GORD questionnaire and found a prevalence rate of 18% for frequent heartburn, defined as occurring at least weekly [8]. Other studies have generated data much in line with this suggesting that between 10 and 20% of the general population report at least weekly heartburn [3, 9] that explains the considerable spend on antacid medical therapy (mainly proton pump inhibitors) which has been estimated to be $14 billion annually in the US alone [10]. GORD is considered as the most frequent reason for gastrointestinal outpatient clinic visits in the United States, with nearly 9 million visits reported in 2009 [11]. Risk factors include increasing age, male sex, abdominal obesity and tobacco use [2].

## Clinical Presentation

Heartburn and acid regurgitation typically occurring after meals are the most common presenting symptoms of GORD although respiratory symptoms in particular cough occur in between 15 and 18% of patients with abnormal pH manometry [12]. Among patients referred for specialist investigation of chronic cough, defined as one persisting for more than 8 weeks, GORD is thought to account for approximately a third of cases [13, 14]. However, up to 75% of patients with GORD associated cough don't have typical reflux symptoms and therefore clinicians might not consider this condition as the underlying cause [14, 15]. Certain clinical features including cough on talking (e.g. on the telephone), coughing on getting up out of bed and cough when eating are believed to characteristic of GORD associated cough [16] although this is not true if GORD related cough is limited to patients with abnormal oesophageal pH measurements [13].

## Pathophysiology of GORD

Reflux occurs due to a failure of the lower oesophageal sphincter (LES) to control the retrograde flow of gastric contents. An increased number of Transient Lower Esophageal Sphincter Relaxations (TLESRs) are considered the key factor responsible for GORD [17]. As the LES is sensitive to changes in intra-thoracic and intra-abdominal pressure, it is unsurprising that obesity is commonly associated with GORD. Elevated body mass index (BMI) is associated with the development of reflux oesophagitis and hiatus hernia [18]. Other factors such as smoking have been implicated and likely exert their effect by increasing TLESRs and the number of reflux events [19]. In addition, factors associated with oesophageal dysmotility and impaired gastric emptying contributes further to the likelihood of pathological reflux. The majority of acid reflux events detectable by pH studies are confined to the body of the oesophagus. Episodes traversing beyond the upper oesophageal sphincter (UES) and extending into the laryngopharynx are termed laryngopharyngeal reflux (LPR). LPR is associated with a range of clinical symptoms including hoarseness and frequent throat clearing which are frequently reported by patients with chronic cough.

## Mechanisms of GORD-Associated Cough

Two mechanisms have been proposed to explain how reflux may trigger cough. The first (reflux theory) involves the retrograde movement of gastric contents and subsequent 'direct' activation of neural receptors responsible for cough either in the larynx or lower airway. The inhalation of noxious substances into the larynx and into the lungs is prevented through the activation of protective upper airway neural reflexes which evoke upper oesophageal sphincter (UOS) contraction and closure of the glottis and vocal cords. Aspiration occurs when these protective mechanisms fail and recent evidence suggest that patients with GORD may be at increased risk of aspiration due to impairment of these protective reflexes [20]. However, support for the occurrence of pathological aspiration of gut contents as evidenced by increased levels of pepsin and bile salts in the airways of patients with cough compared to healthy controls is lacking [21, 22]. The numerous technical problems associated with such studies are discussed in Chap. 8.

An alternative hypothesis (reflex theory) considers that indirect stimulation through activation of neural pathways linking the oesophagus to the airway (the oesophageal-bronchial reflex). Experimental studies by Ing et al. compared distal acid oesophageal perfusion with saline perfusion and reported significantly more cough events when acid was perfused into the distal oesophagus. There was no evidence of proximal reflux of acid and coughing was prevented with pre-treatment of the oesophagus with topical lignocaine. Inhaled ipratropium bromide (anticholinergic) also inhibited cough suggesting acid activation of distal oesophageal receptors alone was responsible for vagally mediated cough [23]. Several additional lines of evidence support a neutrally-mediated mechanism for the association between acid reflux and cough in particular the evidence that oesophageal sensory stimulation can release tachykinins into the airways [24, 25]. Direct acidification of the lower oesophagus is also associated with other neurally-mediated responses such as bronchospasm, providing further support for the reflex theory [26, 27].

The temporal association of gastro-oesophageal reflux events with coughing episodes has been investigated and this temporal link occurs irrespective of the acid content of the refluxate or the presence of other conditions contributing to cough [28]. However, in those patients where the reflux event is followed on by a coughing episode, there is more erosive disease or evidence of oesophageal exposure to reflux, and also these patients have a greater tussive response to citric acid [29]. These observations also provide indirect support that the development of cough hypersensitivity may link acid reflux events to cough.

## Management of GORD-Associated Cough

Central to the clinical management of the GORD-associated cough is identifying the subgroups of patients most likely to respond to various medical or surgical treatments available for GORD. However, there are no readily identifiable clinical features that help and, although a number of investigational techniques have been developed, each has its limitations, often lacking in specificity and sensitivity. Recently, a more targeted approach to physiological testing in adult patients with suspected GORD associated cough has been recommended [30]. A brief summary of the utility of the most common investigations undertaken is provided below.

## Investigations

### Barium Swallow

While the reflux of gastric contents during barium swallow has been detected in 30% of normal subjects, it can be absent in up to 60% of patients with GORD [6]. However, in selected cases, in particular patients with chronic cough and symptomatic reflux despite intensive acid suppression, documenting structural abnormalities such as a hiatus hernia and determining the presence and extent of volume reflux using a barium swallow can be clinically useful. Such patients may benefit from pro-kinetic therapy.

### Oesophageal Manometry

Abnormal manometry has been reported in up to two-thirds of patients undergoing investigation for possible reflux associated cough [31]. Oesophageal manometry findings are not useful in identifying cough patients likely to respond to prokinetic agents but evidence of a major motility disorder such as absent peristalsis or achalasia would exclude such a patient from anti-reflux surgery. Nonacid oesophagopharyngeal reflux may be detected by combined manometry/impedance techniques discussed in detail in Chap. 10.

## 24-Hour Oesophageal pH Monitoring

Twenty-four hour oesophageal pH monitoring does not help to nor will it detect potential causative factors such as weakly acidic or alkaline reflux events nor responds to acid suppression [32]. Furthermore, while a number of symptom association parameters (SAP) have been developed, there is no consensus on how the temporal relationship between an acid reflux event and a cough episode should be categorised. In our opinion these limitations negate the utility of this investigation in the evaluation of patients with chronic cough. Consequently it is almost never requested in our practice.

## Multichannel Intraluminal Impedance

The capacity of multichannel intraluminal impedance (MII-pH) monitoring to detect non-acid (or weakly acidic) as well as acid liquid moving in both an antegrade and retrograde direction represents a more complete means of characterising reflux events within the oesophagus. Since the technique relies on contact of liquid with the proble electrodes it does not reliably detect gaseous reflux. Sifrim et al. were the first to use this technique to identify a subgroup of patients with chronic cough clearly associated with weakly acidic liquid gastro-oesophageal reflux [33]. In another study of MII-pH monitoring in asthmatics and chronic cough patients, those with a positive SAP for cough had evidence of greater number and a higher proportion of proximal reflux episodes in the pharynx compared to those with a negative SAP [34]. While MII-pH has not been not been widely adopted clinically, it continues to provide mechanistic insights into the factors responsible for the reflux-cough syndrome. Recently, in an attempt to identify the characteristics of refluxate most important in triggering cough, Herregods et al. reported that the presence of a larger volume of refluxate and oesophageal exposure to reflux for a longer period of time were important whereas the acidity of the refluxed material seemed less relevant. They interpreted their findings as an explanation for why most patients with chronic cough tend not to benefit from acid suppression therapy [35].

## Treatment of GORD-Associated Cough

The absence of clinical features or of a reflux test that reliably identifies the most effective treatment for a patient with suspected reflux associated cough has hampered any clear consensus. The existing literature on treatment has been focused on

**Table 17.1** Summary of recommendations for chronic cough due to gastroesophageal reflux in adults[a]

| |
|---|
| 1. In adult patients with chronic cough, we suggest that the cough be managed according to a published management guideline that initially considers the most common potential aetiologies as well as symptomatic gastroesophageal reflux (ungraded, consensus based) |
| 2. In adult patients with chronic cough suspected to be due to reflux-cough syndrome, we recommend that treatment include (1) diet modification to promote weight loss in overweight or obese patients; (2) head of bed elevation and avoiding meals within 3 h of bedtime; and (3) in patients who report heartburn and regurgitation, proton pump inhibitors (PPIs), H2-receptor antagonists, alginate, or antacid therapy sufficient to control these symptoms (grade 1C) |
| 3. In adult patients with suspected chronic cough due to reflux-cough syndrome, but without heartburn or regurgitation, we recommend against using PPI therapy alone because it is unlikely to be effective in resolving the cough (grade 1C) |
| 4. In adult patients with chronic cough potentially due to reflux-cough syndrome who are refractory to a 3-month trial of medical antireflux therapy and are being evaluated for surgical management (antireflux or bariatric), or in whom there is strong clinical suspicion warranting diagnostic testing for gastroesophageal reflux, we suggest that they undergo oesophageal manometry and pH-metry with conventional methodology (grade 2C) |
| 5. In adult patients with chronic cough and a major motility disorder (e.g., absent peristalsis, achalasia, distal oesophageal spasm, hypercontractility) and/or normal acid exposure time in the distal oesophagus, we suggest not advising antireflux surgery (grade 2C) |
| 6. In adult patients with chronic cough, adequate peristalsis, and abnormal oesophageal acid exposure determined by pH-metry in whom medical therapy has failed we suggest antireflux (or bariatric when appropriate) surgery for presumed reflux-cough syndrome (grade 2C) |

[a]From Reference [28], with permission

acid suppression and such studies where PPI therapy has been assessed have generally been of low quality (often open label, small, using ineffective doses for insufficient periods of time) [36–40]. Although the empirical use of antacid treatment has been advocated [5–7], there is a need to refine these recommendations. An example of such refinement would be targeting PPI therapy only for those with positive pH-metry where therapeutic benefit is considered more likely [41] (Table 17.1).

Two well conducted randomised controlled studies have demonstrated that PPIs have no effect greater than placebo in patients thought to have reflux cough [39, 42].

### Conclusion

GORD is associated with chronic cough. However, this association does not appear to be causative. Antacid treatment should only be given to carefully selected patients. If reflux is an important cause of chronic cough then it is a form of reflux outside the classic GORD paradigm.

## References

1. Vakil N, Van Zanten SV, Kahrilas P, Dent J, Jones R, Global Consensus Group. The Montreal definition and classification of gastroesophageal reflux disease (GERD) – a global evidence-based consensus. Am J Gastroenterol. 2006;101:1900–20.
2. Richter JE, Rubenstein JH. Presentation and epidemiology of gastroesophageal reflux disease. Gastroenterology. 2018;154:267.

3. Dent J, El-Serag HB, Wallander MA, Johansson S. Epidemiology of gastro-oesophageal reflux disease: a systematic review. Gut. 2005;54:710–7.
4. Chung KF, Pavord ID. Prevalence, pathogenesis, and causes of chronic cough. Lancet. 2008;371(9621):1364–74.
5. Morice AH, Fontana GA, Sovijarvi AR, et al. The diagnosis and management of chronic cough. Eur Respir J. 2004;24:481–92.
6. Irwin RS. Chronic cough due to gastroesophageal reflux disease: ACCP evidence-based clinical practice guidelines. Chest. 2006;129:80S–94S.
7. Morice AH, McGarvey L, Pavord I, British Thoracic Society Cough Guideline Group. Recommendations for the management of cough in adults. Thorax. 2006;61(Suppl 1):i1–24.
8. Locke GR 3rd, Talley NJ, Fett SL, Zinsmeister AR, Melton LJ 3rd. Prevalence and clinical spectrum of gastroesophageal reflux: a population-based study in Olmsted County, Minnesota. Gastroenterology. 1997;112:1448–56.
9. Stanghellini V. Relationship between upper gastrointestinal symptoms and lifestyle, psychosocial factors and comorbidity in the general population: results from the domestic/international gastroenterology surveillance study (DIGEST). Scand J Gastroenterol Suppl. 1999;231:29–37.
10. Merati AL. Reflux and cough. Otolaryngol Clin N Am. 2010;43(1):97–110.
11. Peery AF, Dellon ES, Lund J, et al. Burden of gastrointestinal disease in the United States: 2012 update. Gastroenterology. 2012;143(5):1179–87.e3.
12. Aguero GC, Lemme EM, Alvariz A, Carvalho BB, Schechter RB, Abrahao L Jr. Prevalence of supraesophageal manifestations in patients with gastroesophageal erosive and non-erosive reflux disease. Arq Gastroenterol. 2007;44:39–43.
13. McGarvey LP, Heaney LG, Lawson JT, et al. Evaluation and outcome of patients with chronic non-productive cough using a comprehensive diagnostic protocol. Thorax. 1998;53:738–43.
14. Rafferty G, Mainie I, McGarvey LPA. Respiratory and laryngeal symptoms secondary to gastro-oesophageal reflux. Frontline Gastroenterol. 2011;2(4):212–7.
15. Irwin RS, Curley FJ, French CL. Chronic cough. The spectrum and frequency of causes, key components of the diagnostic evaluation, and outcome of specific therapy. Am Rev Respir Dis. 1990;141:640–7.
16. Everett CF, Morice AH. Clinical history in gastroesophageal cough. Respir Med. 2007;101(2):345–8.
17. Dent J, Dodds WJ, Friedman RH, Sekiguchi T, Hogan WJ, Arndorfer RC, Petrie DJ. Mechanism of gastroesophageal reflux in recumbent asymptomatic human subjects. J Clin Invest. 1980;65(2):256–67.
18. Moayyedi P, Preston C. Antacids and lifestyle advice for reflux oesophagitis and endoscopy negative reflux disease. Cochrane Database Syst Rev. 2001;(4).
19. Kahrilas PJ. Smoking and oesophageal reflux disease. Eur J Gastroenterol Hepatol. 2000;12:837–42.
20. Phua SY, McGarvey LP, Ngu MC, Ing AJ. Patients with gastro-oesophageal reflux disease and cough have impaired laryngopharyngeal mechanosensitivity. Thorax. 2005;60:488–91.
21. Stovold R, Forrest IA, Corris PA, Murphy DM, Smith JA, Decalmer S, Johnson GE, Dark JH, Pearson JP, Ward C. Pepsin, a biomarker of gastric aspiration in lung allografts: a putative association with rejection. Am J Respir Crit Care Med. 2007;175:1298–303.
22. Grabowski M, Kasran A, Seys S, Pauwels A, Medrala W, Dupont L, Panaszek B, Bullens D. Pepsin and bile acids in induced sputum of chronic cough patients. Respir Med. 2011;105:1257–61.
23. Ing AJ, Ngu MC, Breslin AB. Pathogenesis of chronic persistent cough associated with gastroesophageal reflux. Am J Respir Crit Care Med. 1994;149:160–7.
24. Patterson RN, Johnston BT, Ardill JE, Heaney LG, McGarvey LP. Increased tachykinin levels in induced sputum from asthmatic and cough patients with acid reflux. Thorax. 2007;62:491–5.
25. Chang AB, Gibson PG, Ardill J, McGarvey LP. Calcitonin gene-related peptide relates to cough sensitivity in children with chronic cough. Eur Respir J. 2007;30:66–72.
26. Field SK, Evans JA, Price LM. The effects of acid perfusion of the esophagus on ventilation and respiratory sensation. Am J Respir Crit Care Med. 1998;157:1058–62.

27. Javorkova N, Varechova S, Pecova R, et al. Acidification of the oesophagus acutely increases the cough sensitivity in patients with gastro-oesophageal reflux and chronic cough. Neurogastroenterol Motil. 2008;20(2):119–24.
28. Houghton LA, Lee AS, Badri H, DeVault KR, Smith JA. Respiratory disease and the oesophagus: reflux, reflexes and microaspiration. Nat Rev Gastroenterol Hepatol. 2016;13(8):445–60.
29. Smith JA, Decalmer S, Kelsall A, McGuinness K, Jones H, Galloway S, Woodcock A, Houghton LA. Acoustic cough-reflux associations in chronic cough: potential triggers and mechanisms. Gastroenterology. 2010;139(3):754–62.
30. Kahrilas PJ, Altman KW, Chang AB, Field SK, Harding SM, Lane AP, Lim K, McGarvey L, Smith J, Irwin RS, CHEST Expert Cough Panel. Chronic cough due to gastroesophageal reflux in adults: CHEST guideline and expert panel report. Chest. 2016;150(6):1341–60.
31. Kastelik JA, Redington AE, Aziz I, Buckton GK, Smith CM, Dakkak M, Morice AH. Abnormal oesophageal motility in patients with chronic cough. Thorax. 2003;58(8):699–702.
32. Patterson RN, Johnston BT, MacMahon J, Heaney LG, McGarvey LP. Oesophageal pH monitoring is of limited value in the diagnosis of "reflux-cough". Eur Respir J. 2004;24:724–7.
33. Sifrim D, Dupont L, Blondeau K, et al. Weakly acidic reflux in patients with chronic unexplained cough during 24 hour pressure, pH, and impedance monitoring. Gut. 2005;54:449–54.
34. Patterson N, Mainie I, Rafferty G, McGarvey L, Heaney L, Tutuian R, Castell D, Johnston BT. Nonacid reflux episodes reaching the pharynx are important factors associated with cough. J Clin Gastroenterol. 2009;43(5):414–9.
35. Herregods TV, Pauwels A, Jafari J, Sifrim D, Bredenoord AJ, Tack J, Smout AJ. Determinants of reflux-induced chronic cough. Gut. 2017;66:2057.
36. Ours TM, Kavuru MS, Schilz RJ, Richter JE. A prospective evaluation of oesophageal testing and a double-blind, randomized study of omeprazole in a diagnostic and therapeutic algorithm for chronic cough. Am J Gastroenterol. 1999;94(11):3131–8.
37. Kiljander TO, Salomaa ERM. Chronic cough and gastro-oesophageal reflux: a double-blind placebo-controlled study with omeprazole. Eur Respir J. 2000;16:633–8.
38. Baldi F, Cappiello R, Cavoli C, Ghersi S, Torresan F, Roda E. Proton pump inhibitor treatment of patients with gastroesophageal reflux-related chronic cough: a comparison between two different daily doses of lansoprazole. World J Gastroenterol. 2006;12(1):82–8.
39. Faruqi S, Molyneux ID, Fathi H, Wright C, Thompson R, Morice AH. Chronic cough and esomeprazole: a double-blind placebo-controlled parallel study. Respirology. 2011;16:1150–6.
40. Chang AB, Lasserson TJ, Gaffney J, Connor FL, Garske LA. Gastro-oesophageal reflux treatment for prolonged non-specific cough in children and adults. Cochrane Database Syst Rev. 2011;(1):CD004823.
41. Kahrilas PJ, Howden CW, Hughes N, Molloy-Bland M. Response of chronic cough to acid-suppressive therapy in patients with gastroesophageal reflux disease. Chest. 2013;143(3):605–12.
42. Shaheen NJ, et al. Randomised clinical trial: high-dose acid suppression for chronic cough - a double-blind, placebo-controlled study. AlimentPharmacolTher. 2011;33(2):225–34.

# Reflux and Aspiration: Their Presumed Role in Chronic Cough and the Development of End-Stage Lung Disease

Jacob A. Klapper, Brian Gulack, and Matthew G. Hartwig

## Introduction

Amongst patients with end-stage lung disease (ESLD), symptoms and diagnostic evidence of gastroesophageal reflux disease (GERD) are extremely common. In fact, roughly two-thirds of all patients with ESLD have documentable gastroesophageal reflux [1]. The presence of significant reflux is not limited to one pulmonary disease, but is seen in patients with ESLD secondary to COPD, cystic fibrosis and idiopathic pulmonary fibrosis (IPF) [2, 3]. While the pathophysiology of COPD and cystic fibrosis are well understood, it remains unknown what leads to the eventual development of IPF. Interestingly, evidence has continued to mount over the last 20 years that reflux is not just prevalent in patients with IPF, but may in fact be contributing to its development.

The increasing interest in patients with GERD and concomitant pulmonary disease is not just limited to establishing its cause-and-effect relationship with IPF. Since the first successful lung transplants in the early 1980s, many investigators have noted that reflux tends to worsen after lung transplant [4, 5]. Mechanisms for why this occurs have been proposed. More importantly, there is a growing body of evidence suggesting that laryngopharyngeal reflux, or LPR, contributes greatly to chronic lung allograft disease, also known as bronchiolitis obliterans syndrome (BOS) [6].

The purpose of this chapter is to first examine the evidence that exists to support the contention that reflux contributes to chronic cough, and, over a lifetime, may lead to the development of IPF and other lung diseases. Second, it will examine how prevalent reflux is across the spectrum of ESLD patients. At the same time, the chapter will address the questions that remain in definitively linking reflux and lung

J. A. Klapper · B. Gulack · M. G. Hartwig (✉)
Division of Cardiovascular and Thoracic Surgery, Department of Surgery,
Duke University Medical Center, Durham, NC, USA
e-mail: jacob.klapper@duke.edu; brian.gulack@duke.edu; matthew.hartwig@duke.edu

disease. To conclude, the focus of the chapter will transition to evaluating the prevalence of GERD in lung recipients, how reflux potentially contributes to graft dysfunction, and what measures have been taken to reduce the risk that chronic reflux can lead to BOS.

## Reflux and Chronic Cough

If one were to consider the development of ESLD to be the final result of repeated insults to the airway from reflux, it would make intuitive sense to conclude that one of the earliest potential manifestations of the effects of GERD would be cough. In fact, for years, an association between GERD and the development of chronic cough has been hinted at in the literature. Establishing a cause-and-effect relationship between the two has been more difficult as there exists a multitude of causes of chronic cough, and GERD, either asymptomatic or symptomatic, afflicts many otherwise healthy adults. Along these same lines, no diagnostic algorithm has been developed that can reliably correlate a patient's GERD with cough. For instance, endoscopy and barium esophagoscopy while useful in defining esophageal dysfunction and disease are of no crossover utility in terms of the patient's respiratory symptoms. More advanced diagnostic techniques, such as pH monitoring and manometry, have also been applied to patients with chronic cough but again have limitations in definitively establishing an association between the two disease processes. In the end, identifying those patients whose cough is related to their reflux essentially comes down to more traditional methods of diagnosis; consultation and physical examination [7].

In lieu of a test that can prove a patient's cough is related to their reflux, clinicians have instead turned to the application of medications in those individuals for whom high levels of suspicion exist. Fathi et al. randomized 50 adult non-smokers with chronic cough to 20 mg twice daily esomeprazole versus placebo. All patients included in this study were assessed for the likelihood that their cough was reflux related based on an administered questionnaire and the elicitation of symptoms, such as cough after eating and with subsequent bending at the waist. The authors of this small study found no difference in cough scores between the two groups and thus concluded that PPIs were of no utility in the treatment of chronic cough [8]. In a comparable study published by the American Lung Association, but one in which the patient cohort consisted of individuals with poorly controlled asthma, the authors again found that PPIs did not positively impact asthma control despite the high incidence of reflux amongst the study participants [9].

Interestingly, current recommendations from the American College of Chest Physicians suggest surgical therapy for patients with chronic cough and poorly controlled GERD [10]. Unlike the two randomized studies presented above, there have been no such studies produced in the surgical literature, and in truth with the steady decline in referrals for Nissen fundoplication, it is unlikely that a well-designed trial will ever be completed. Thus, much remains unknown regarding the association between cough and reflux.

## Reflux Prevalence in Patients with ESLD

Reflux in patients who present with ESLD is now well characterized. D'Ovidio et al. were some of the first to thoroughly assess its prevalence in patients presenting for evaluation for lung transplantation. In an analysis of 78 consecutive patients, with a variety of presenting disease processes (i.e. COPD, CF, IPF, scleroderma), GERD related symptoms were noted in 63% of the patients [1]. Similarly, Sweet noted in 109 patient evaluations for lung transplantation that at least one typical symptom of GERD could be found in 69% of patients [2]. Although Sweet et al. reported on the common nature of GERD symptoms in some of these patients, one of the lessons from these studies and others like them is that relying on the patients' description of symptoms is likely to miss a subset of individuals who have significant reflux. Again, D'Ovidio et al. found that 14% of asymptomatic patients had pathologic lower esophageal acid reflux and 7% had pathologic proximal acid reflux. Similarly, when comparing a patient's symptom profile to their ambulatory pH monitoring, Sweet found that symptoms had a sensitivity and specificity for accurately detecting distal and proximal reflux of 67% and 26% and 62% and 26% respectively. As will be discussed later in the chapter, the impact of abnormal acid exposure and impaired lung function appear to be intimately related to one another thus capturing all patients with reflux, whether symptomatic or not, is imperative.

In an attempt to further characterize the reflux seen in these patients, studies such as the ones mentioned above and multiple others have documented the impressive degree to which these patients suffer esophageal dysmotility and documented reflux [3]. Thirty-three percent of the patients in the D'Ovidio et al. study had abnormal peristalsis, 38% had abnormal proximal pH testing, and 72% had diminished LES tone [1]. Comparably, Sweet found that 55% of patients with GERD had a reduced LES tone. In addition, it was noted that patients with GERD had a significantly higher DeMeester score and incidence of proximal reflux then patients without GERD [2]. Finally, in a study of 18 consecutive patients with IPF, investigators from UCSF noted reflux symptoms in two-thirds of patients, which correlated with manometric findings of a hypotensive LES, and pH monitoring that documented abnormal proximal reflux in 50% of patients [11].

## GERD and IPF

While the etiology of idiopathic pulmonary fibrosis is not well understood, the prevalence of GERD amongst patients with this disease has led many to ponder whether IPF may be caused by chronic GERD and/or aspiration [12]. A number of studies utilizing animals demonstrated very clearly that acidic aspiration can cause significant damage and eventual fibrosis in the lungs [13–15]. During this same time, additional evidence in human subjects drew a correlation between esophagitis and the eventual development of pulmonary disease [16, 17]. As a direct extension of these pre-clinical and clinical studies, a number of more recent studies have utilized modern diagnostic modalities (i.e. manometry and pH monitoring) in order to further characterize how GERD may contribute to IPF [12, 18].

The prevailing theory on how GERD may lead to the development of IPF is that over an extended period of time chemical burn from gastrointestinal contents results in the release of inflammatory cytokines, that then recruit neutrophils and macrophages to the site of injury. In time, fibroblasts arrive leading to fibrosis and the clinical development of disease processes such as diffuse aspiration bronchiolitis [19–21]. As mentioned above, decades of animal research have repeatedly demonstrated that the instillation of acid or gastric juice leads to epithelial damage, pulmonary edema, eventual fibrosis, and diminished gas exchange [22]. More recent experimental evidence has even elucidated the transcriptional mechanisms involved in acid-induced lung inflammation [23]. While suggestive of the degree to which acute aspiration can induce lung injury, experimental evidence is less abundant when it comes to the effects of chronic aspiration. To address this, Appel et al. created a rodent model in which gastric fluid or saline were instilled into the left lung of rats weekly for 4, 8, 12, or 16 weeks. Treated rats (i.e. gastric fluid) had bronchoalveolar lavage specimens that exhibited increased CD4:CD8 counts, high levels of inflammatory cytokines, and most importantly histologic evidence of lymphocytic bronchiolitis and obliterative bronchiolitis. These autopsy findings from the rats were comparable to what would be seen in the lung of a human patient with pulmonary fibrosis and thus further supports the cause-and-effect relationship of reflux and fibrosis [24].

Despite these highly suggestive pre-clinical studies, the onus remains on proving that some of the human subjects who develop pulmonary fibrosis do so secondary to reflux. As we know, the signs and symptoms of GERD in patients with ESLD are not only limited to those with IPF. With that in mind it would seem prudent to establish that there is something unique about the reflux seen in IPF patients. To that end, the group at the University of Washington compared 17 patients with newly diagnosed IPF to eight patients with other forms of interstitial lung disease. Notably the patients with IPF had much higher rates of not only distal acid exposure but, perhaps more importantly, proximal acid exposure (particularly in the supine position). This fact, the authors claim, suggests that patients with IPF may develop the disease secondary to nocturnal aspiration of acidic contents [25]. In expansion of this previous study Raghu et al. evaluated 65 patients with newly diagnosed IPF using a pH probe; once again demonstrating a high incidence of abnormal acid exposure which eclipsed that seen in a separate group of asthmatic patients [26]. In a similar cohort of 30 IPF patients, Sweet et al., relying on both manometry and pH monitoring, found that two-thirds of IPF patients had abnormal reflux, poor peristalsis, and a hypotensive lower esophageal sphincter [18].

Taken at face value, the data from these studies is very suggestive of a causal relationship between IPF and GERD. Upon deeper examination, however, there remains much to be reconciled before such a correlation can be definitively drawn. First, in the studies mentioned above, none were able to demonstrate an association between lung function and acid exposure. In fact, somewhat perplexingly, Sweet et al. found that patients with reflux actually had better pulmonary function testing. Along these same lines, it would be expected, in keeping with the presumed pathophysiology, that patients with IPF would have a high incidence of proximal acid exposure. Contrary to Tobin et al., Raghu et al. found no difference in this measured variable between patients with IPF or asthma and only 30% of the patients in Sweet's cohort had abnormal proximal acid exposure. Another issue is the discrepancy in the histopathology that exists in the lungs of patients with aspiration-related lung injury and what is seen in IPF. As an example, IPF patients typically have a usual interstitial pneumonia pattern that is marked by heterogeneous fibrosis at the lung periphery. In comparison, patients with aspiration related injury have more airway damage with granulomatous inflammation [27].

These contradictions are not the only ones that raise doubt. While many assume that it is the GERD that causes IPF, the reverse may actually be true. It is known, for instance, that the fibrosis that results from IPF has a significant impact on normal chest wall physiology and it is therefore not a radical departure to assume that these changes can distort mediastinal structures such as the esophagus. In fact, evidence does exist, especially in patients with fibrotic lung disease (cystic fibrosis and IPF) that a shortened esophagus is an anatomic reality coexistent with abnormal peristalsis and diminished lower esophageal sphincter tone [2]. Finally, if one hypothesizes that GERD accelerates the development of IPF, strong evidence should exist establishing that early treatment with anti-reflux medications or surgery can halt disease progression and preserve lung function. While some studies have suggested that this is the case, indisputable evidence does not exist and current treatment guidelines do not mandate such therapies [26, 28, 29]. Additionally, given the prevalence of symptomatic reflux within the general American population, one might expect a much higher incidence of IPF. Thus, it only seems logical to conclude that reflux, while contributory, is by no means solely responsible for the development of IPF.

## Reflux and Lung Allograft Dsyfunction

In the last 20 years, as the number of patients, with and without GERD, who have received lung transplants has steadily increased, clinicians have come to realize that reflux not only persists post-transplant, but in many cases progressively worsens. In addition, even those recipients who never had GERD develop evidence of reflux postoperatively [30]. Given what is known about the effects of reflux on native lungs and that bronchiolitis obliterans syndrome (BOS) is clearly life-limiting, many have surmised that reflux post-transplant contributes to the development of BOS. Li et al. tested this hypothesis with a mouse model designed to assess the effects of chronic aspiration. In this study, transplanted mice were given either a gastric fluid aspiration or not over a period of 8 weeks after which the allografts were harvested and examined. In 67% of the mice that were subjected to induced aspiration, the investigators discovered evidence of obliterative bronchiolitis [31].

The above study was the first animal model to draw a direct correlation between gastric acid aspiration and the development of obliterative bronchiolitis. In humans,

GERD has been recognized as a possible contributing factor in the development of BOS. The basis for this theory is heavily influenced by observations that patients with reflux have persistent, if not worse, reflux after transplant and that patients who did not have reflux pre-transplant develop it after surgery [4, 5, 30, 32]. While some of the evidence for this is based on abnormal pH exposure times, studies published in the last 10 years have elected to measure levels of pepsin and bile acids in the BAL specimens of transplanted patients. Considered to be strong markers of aspiration, it is felt that the repeated exposure of the bronchial epithelium to these gastric products instigates a cycle of repeated inflammation that leads to BOS. Indeed, multiple investigators have found that transplanted patients, as compared to normal controls, have significantly higher pepsin and bile acid levels in their BAL specimens [33–36].

With elevated acid exposure times post-transplant along with high quantities of pepsin and bile acid in BAL specimens it seems logical to assume that these factors are detrimental to immediate allograft function and possibly contributory to BOS. Shah et al. evaluated 60 transplant patients with pH probes to ascertain how reflux impacted the incidence of acute rejection episodes. Notably, they found that patients with GERD had a higher unadjusted rate of acute rejection episodes compared to those without GERD, earlier onset of acute rejection and more frequent rejection episodes [37]. Meanwhile, Fisichella noted that the BAL specimens of patients with acute rejection contained much higher levels of pepsin than those with no evidence of rejection [34, 35]. Stovold and Ward in two additional studies of pepsin in the BAL specimens of recipients also discovered high pepsin levels correlated with acute rejection episodes [36, 38].

In terms of the development of BOS, the data available can best be termed highly suggestive, but not quite definitive. Blondeau et al., for instance, studied 63 lung transplant patients who were all out from transplant greater than a year. The purpose of the study was to assess the degree of gastric aspiration in patients with BOS. The conclusions are somewhat conflicted with the authors finding that patients with BOS did not have a higher prevalence of reflux while at the same time noting that patients with BOS had an increased presence of bile acids in their BAL specimens [33]. Blondeau et al., however, are not the only ones to publish this seemingly contradictory finding. Fisichella et al. also found that GERD patients did not develop BOS more rapidly than those without reflux, but progression to BOS was indeed more rapid in those with detectable pepsin levels in their BAL specimens [34, 35]. Finally, in contradiction to both of the above studies, D'Ovidio et al. found lung transplant patients with abnormal acid exposure (based on pH studies) did indeed have a significantly reduced freedom from BOS. In addition, like Blondeau, the presence of bile acids in the BAL specimens was associated with the development of BOS (pepsin levels were not measured) [39]. So how to resolve these apparent discrepancies and make logical sense of how reflux or its various contents contribute to BOS? Perhaps, as Blondeau states, the development of chronic rejection is related more to the specific content of the reflux (i.e. bile acids) than the actual frequency or volume of reflux (i.e. pH probe analysis). Also, the lung recipient's own immune system likely plays a role as non-alloimmune injury stimulants such as aspiration may lead to alloimmune injury. It is likely that future research will help delineate how reflux contributes to lung injury after lung transplantation. To this end, the RESULT study (Reflux Surgery in Lung Transplantation) is a retrospective study designed to recruit multiple centers in hopes of identifying specific aspiration markers that correlate with adverse clinical outcomes post-transplant (www.clinicaltrials.gov, NCT014406210).

Regardless of exactly what role chronic reflux plays in acute and chronic rejection, it is very clearly present in the majority of transplant patients. Presumed mechanisms abound as to why it is so common. Likely the development of reflux is multifactorial. Many have proposed that the operation itself induces reflux secondary to trauma to the vagal nerves at the time of surgery and that this postoperatively explains the esophageal dysmotility and delayed gastric emptying that is so common in the lung transplant population [40]. Other investigators have suggested that the effects of vagal nerve damage impact mucociliary transport in the post-transplant patient. In theory, this impaired vagal nerve function serves to create a situation in which patients not only have more reflux and aspiration but also lack the ability to protect the tracheobronchial tree from these toxic exposures. Bhashayam et al. developed a murine model that nicely elucidates this hypothesis. In their study they ligated the right vagus in multiple consecutive mice; first finding that vagotomy had little effect on mucociliary clearance (MCC) at baseline. They then compared the impact on MCC when these same mice (and non-vagotomized controls) were exposed to the nociceptor agent capsaicin. Interestingly, as compared to the control group, the vagotomized mice had no increase in MCC thus suggesting that denervation negatively impacts the ability to clear the airway of damaging aspirate [41].

While the idea of increased reflux being a byproduct of vagal injury is intuitive, it is unlikely that so many lung recipients are subject to vagal injury during transplantation. Young, for instance, in a review of 23 lung transplant patients found that 65% had abnormal acid contact times post-transplant and that this did not correlate with esophageal dysmotility and gastroparesis. Other possible explanations for such increases in acid exposure may be due to immunosuppression medications, as steroids are known contributors to reflux [42]. Other common post transplant medications, such as azathioprine or mycophenolate, are commonly associated with gastrointestinal complaints. As another possibility, Young mentions that changes in "diaphragm mechanics" postoperatively may have an adverse effect on competence of the lower esophageal sphincter [30].

Independent of how reflux develops in lung transplant patients, investigators have focused on what changes are occurring at the cellular level at the site of the injury. As we know from the BAL aspirates of these individuals, pepsin and bile acids are present to varying degrees and are presumably injurious to the bronchial epithelium. For example, researchers at the University of Toronto were able to demonstrate reduced levels of pulmonary surfactant in transplanted patients who had elevated bile acids in their BAL specimens [39]. The function of these surfactants includes the opsonization of bacteria, fungi and viruses as well as the regulation of macrophage and neutrophil cytokine production. In theory, a lack of surfactant creates a cycle of immune cell proliferation with varying cytokine production that over time will lead to the deposition of fibrocytes that are a hallmark of chronic rejection [43].

## Reflux Management and Chronic Rejection

While it seems unlikely that reflux is the sole contributor to chronic allograft rejection, many practitioners take an aggressive approach to treating reflux in post-transplant patients. Options consist of medical management with antacid therapy and surgical management with a full or partial fundoplication. The former offers the patient the opportunity to avoid another operation by utilizing a widely available and inexpensive class of medications. Whether these drugs are really of any true benefit seems debatable. Blondeau, for instance, found that while transplant patients on proton-pump inhibitors (PPIs) had less esophageal acid exposure there were no differences in terms of acid reflux events and volume of exposure as compared to controls. In addition, pepsin and bile acid levels in BAL specimens were similar in transplant patients both on and off PPIs [33]. Likewise, Stovold reported that PPI therapy had no impact on the pepsin levels measured in the BAL specimens of post-transplant patients [36].

What these studies point to is that PPIs and other related classes of medications may be effective at reducing acidic reflux but they do nothing to prevent mildly acidic, neutral or alkaline reflux which potentially can be just as damaging. In other words, these patients still have reflux and thus are still prone to possible aspiration. With that in mind, it only makes sense that a surgical option that would create a physical barrier to refluxate and the potential for aspiration would be preferred. In support of this notion, Fisichella demonstrated that pepsin levels in the BAL specimens of transplant patients with GERD were higher than in those with GERD who underwent an anti-reflux procedure. While there was no difference in the time to BOS between patients who underwent a fundoplication and those who did not, it was notable that detectable pepsin levels were associated with more severe rejection episodes and a quicker progression to BOS [34, 35].

The group at Duke University was among the first to define the benefit and safety of early fundoplication and have continued to demonstrate its merits [34, 35, 44, 45]. In a review of 457 transplant patients, of which 14 had reflux and underwent early fundoplication, the authors found a significant improvement in freedom from BOS and actuarial survival. Impressively, many of these patients underwent a fundoplication just over a month from their transplant with no 30-day mortality. In an even larger study of 297 recipients, patients with GERD who underwent a fundoplication (n = 165) had significantly higher $FEV_1$ as compared to those with GERD who did not (n = 65). In addition, those with GERD who did not undergo a fundoplication had a significant reduction in their mean percent predicted peak $FEV_1$ as compared to those undergoing surgical correction [6].

## Conclusions

Whether they demonstrate classic symptoms or not, objectively measured reflux clearly predominates in patients with various forms of severe pulmonary disease. Although there is considerable circumstantial evidence linking GERD to pulmonary disease, a direct causal relationship has still not been delineated. Considerable work linking the two diseases remains to be done. Likewise, the most efficacious treatment modality for GERD in these patients remains to be determined. However, it appears from the experience of the lung transplant community that a physical barrier to GERD is optimal, as compared to medical antacid therapy [46]. What role newer reflux treatment options play in this area, such as STRETTA or LINX remains to be seen, but these newer technologies will almost certainly play an important part of managing these patients in the near future.

## References

1. D'Ovidio F, Singer L, Hadjiliadis D, et al. Prevalence of gastroesophageal reflux in end-stage lung disease candidates for lung transplant. Ann Thorac Surg. 2005;80:1254–61.
2. Sweet M, Herbella F, Leard L, et al. The prevalence of distal and proximal gastroesophageal reflux in patients awaiting lung transplantation. Ann Surg. 2006;244:491–7.
3. Gasper W, Sweet M, Golden J, et al. Lung transplantation in patients with connective tissue disorders and esophageal dysmotility. Dis Esophagus. 2008;21:650–5.
4. Reid K, McKenzie F, Menkis A, et al. Importance of chronic aspiration in recipients of heart-lung transplants. Lancet. 1990;336:206–8.
5. Rinaldi M, Martinelli L, Volpato G, et al. Gastroesophageal reflux as a cause of obliterative bronchiolitis: a case report. Transplant Proc. 1995;27:2006–7.
6. Hartwig M, Anderson D, Onaitis M, et al. Fundoplication after lung transplantation prevents the allograft dysfunction associated with reflux. Ann Thorac Surg. 2011;92:462–9.
7. Birring S. Controversies in the evaluation and management of chronic cough. Am J Respir Crit Care Med. 2010;183:709–15.
8. Fathi H, Wright C, Thompson R, et al. Chronic cough and esomeprazole: a double-blind placebo-controlled parallel study. Respirology. 2011;16:1150–6.
9. Mastronarde J, Anthonisen N, Castro M, et al. Efficacy of esomeprazole for treatment of poorly controlled asthma. N Engl J Med. 2009;360:1487–99.
10. Irwin R, Baumann M, Bolser D, et al. Diagnosis and management of cough executive summary: ACCP evidence-based clinical practice guidelines. Chest. 2006;129:1S–23S.
11. Patti M, Tedesco P, Golden J, et al. Idiopathic pulmonary fibrosis: how often is it really idiopathic? J Gastrointest Surg. 2005;9:1053–8.
12. Raghu G. The role of gastroesophageal reflux in idiopathic pulmonary fibrosis. Am J Med. 2003;115:60S–4S.
13. Glauser FL, Millen JE, Falls R, et al. Increased alveolar epithelial permeability with acid aspiration: the effects of high-dose steroids. Am Rev Respir Dis. 1970;120:1119–23.
14. Salley S, Santo G, Barnhart M, et al. Immediate histopathology of hydrocholoric acid aspiration. Scan Electron Microsc. 1970;3:911–20.
15. Schwartz D, Wynne J, Gibbs C, et al. The pulmonary consequences of aspiration of gastric contents at pH values greater than 2.5. Am Rev Respir Dis. 1980;121:119–26.
16. el-Serag HB, Sonnenberg A. Comorbid occurrence of laryngeal or pulmonary disease with esophagitis in United States military veterans. Gastroenterology. 1997;113:755–60.
17. Mays E, Dubois J, Hamilton G, et al. Pulmonary fibrosis associated with tracheobronchial aspiration: a study of the frequency of hiatal hernia and gastroesophageal reflux in interstitial pulmonary fibrosis of obscure etiology. Chest. 1976;69:512–5.

18. Sweet M, Patti M, Leard L, et al. Gastroesophageal reflux in patients with idiopathic pulmonary fibrosis referred for lung transplantation. J Thorac Cardiovasc Surg. 2007;133:1078–84.
19. Beck-Schimmer B, Bonvini J. Bronchoaspiration: incidence, consequences and management. Eur J Anaesthesiol. 2011;28:78–84.
20. Hu X, Lee J, Pianosi P, et al. Aspiration-related pulmonary syndromes. Chest. 2015;147:815–23.
21. Marik P. Pulmonary aspiration syndromes. Curr Opin Pulm Med. 2011;17:148–54.
22. Kennedy T, Johnson K, Kunkel R, et al. Acute acid aspiration lung injury in the rat: biphasic pathogenesis. Anesth Analg. 1989;69:87–92.
23. Madjdpour L, Kneller S, Booy C, et al. Acid-induced lung injury: role of nuclear factor-κB. Anesthesiology. 2003;99:1323–32.
24. Appel J, Lee S, Hartwig M, et al. Characterization of the innate response to chronic aspiration in a novel rodent model. Respir Res. 2007;8:87.
25. Tobin R, Pope C, Pellegrini C, et al. Increased prevalence of gastroesophageal reflux in patients with idiopathic pulmonary fibrosis. Am J Respir Crit Care Med. 1998;158:1804–8.
26. Raghu G, Freudenberger T, Yang S, et al. High prevalence of abnormal acid gastro-oesophageal reflux in idiopathic pulmonary fibrosis. Eur Respir J. 2006;27:136–42.
27. Lee J, Collard H, Raghu G, et al. Does chronic microaspiration cause idiopathic pulmonary fibrosis. Am J Med. 2010;123:304–11.
28. Lee J, Ryu J, Elicker B, et al. Gastroesophageal reflux therapy is associated with longer survival in patients with idiopathic pulmonary fibrosis. Am J Respir Crit Care Med. 2011;184:1390–4.
29. Linden P, Gilbert R, Yeap B, et al. Laparoscopic fundoplication in patients with end-stage lung disease awaiting transplantation. J Thorac Cardiovasc Surg. 2006;131:438–46.
30. Young L, Hadjiliadis D, Davis D, et al. Lung transplantation exacerbates gastroesophageal reflux disease. Chest. 2003;124:1689–93.
31. Li B, Hartwig M, Appel J, et al. Chronic aspiration of gastric fluid induces the development of obliterative bronchiolitis in rat lung transplants. Am J Transplant. 2008;8:1614–21.
32. Palmer S, Miralles A, Howell D, et al. Gastresophageal reflux as a reversible cause of allograft dysfunction after lung transplantation. Chest. 2000;118:1214–7.
33. Blondeau K, Mertens V, Vanaudenaerde B, et al. Gastro-oesophageal reflux and gastric aspiration in lung transplant patients with or without chronic rejection. Eur Respir J. 2008;31:707–13.
34. Fisichella P, Davis C, Gagermeier J, et al. Laparoscopic antireflux surgery for gastroesophageal reflux disease after lung transplantation. J Surg Res. 2011;170:e279–86.
35. Fisichella P, Davis C, Lundberg P, et al. The protective role of laparoscopic antireflux surgery against aspiration of pepsin after lung transplantation. Surgery. 2011;150:598–606.
36. Stovold R, Forrest I, Corris P, et al. Pepsin, a biomarker of gastric aspiration in lung allografts. Am J Respir Crit Care Med. 2007;175:1298–303.
37. Shah N, Force S, Mitchell P, et al. Gastroesophageal reflux disease is associated with an increased rate of acute rejection in lung transplant allografts. Transplant Proc. 2010;42:2702–6.
38. Ward C, Forrest I, Brownlee I, et al. Pepsin like activity in bronchoalveolar lavage fluid is suggestive of gastric aspiration in lung allografts. Thorax. 2005;60:872–4.
39. D'Ovidio F, Mura M, Ridsdale R, et al. The effect of reflux and bile acid aspiration on the lung allograft and its surfactant and innate immunity molecules of SP-A and SP-D. Am J Transplant. 2006;6:1930–8.
40. Berkowitz N, Shulman L, McGregor C, et al. Gastroparesis after lung transplantation: potential role in postoperative respiratory complications. Chest. 1995;108:1602–7.
41. Bhashyam A, Mogayzel P, Cleary J, et al. Vagal control of mucociliary clearance in murine lungs: a study in a chronic preparation. Auton Neurosci. 2010;154:74–8.
42. Pazetti R, Pêgo-Fernandes P, Jatene F. Adverse effects of immunosuppressant drugs upon airway epithelial and mucociliary clearance: implications for lung transplant recipients. Drugs. 2013;73:1157–69.
43. Fisichella P, Davis C, Lowery E, et al. Pulmonary immune changes early after laparoscopic antireflux surgery in lung transplant patients with gastroesophageal reflux disease. J Surg Res. 2012;177:e65–73.

44. Cantu E, Appel J, Hartwig M, et al. Early fundoplication prevents chronic allograft dysfunction in patients with gastroesophageal reflux disease. Ann Thorac Surg. 2004;78:1142–51.
45. Robertson A, Krishman A, Ward C, et al. Anti-reflux in lung transplant recipients: outcomes and effects on quality of life. Eur Respir J. 2012;39:691–7.
46. Hoppo T, Jarido V, Pennathur A, et al. Antireflux surgery preserves lung function in patients with gastroesophageal reflux disease and end-stage lung disease before and after lung transplantation. Arch Surg. 2011;146:1041–7.

# Part IV

# Reflux Aspiration in Specific Circumstances

# Reflux and Aspiration in the Intensive Care Unit

## Peter V. Dicpinigaitis

**Abstract**

Critical illness often involves multisystem organ dysfunction and/or failure. Therapeutic interventions aimed at one source of illness may have undesired consequences elsewhere. Gastroesophageal reflux is common in critically ill patients, and is promoted or further exacerbated by the initiation of mechanical ventilation necessitated by respiratory failure. Prophylaxis against stress ulcers of the gastrointestinal mucosa may promote bacterial overgrowth and perhaps ventilator-associated pneumonia (VAP) by eliminating protective gastric acidity. Identification of which subgroups of critically ill patients should receive stress-ulcer prophylaxis, and which pharmacological agents should be used for this purpose, are areas of ongoing investigation. Provision of enteral nutrition is an essential therapeutic intervention for critically ill patients; however, risk of aspiration of oropharyngeal and gastric contents is increased by the administration of feeds to the gastrointestinal tract. Delivery of enteral feeds beyond the gastric pylorus directly into the small intestine has been supported as a strategy to decrease the incidence of aspiration and to optimize the amount of nutrition delivered to the patient, however supportive data are not robust and debate continues. The severe consequences of VAP have stimulated the development of multi-component patient care "bundles" (including head-of-bed elevation and oral care with chlorhexidine) that have shown some success in decreasing occurrence of VAP and other unwanted iatrogenic consequences in the intensive care unit (ICU), but outcomes to date have been mixed, and individual components of the bundle have shown discordant effects on patient-centered outcomes.

P. V. Dicpinigaitis
Albert Einstein College of Medicine and Montefiore Medical Center, Bronx, NY, USA

## Introduction

Critical illness often results in multiorgan dysfunction and/or failure, regardless of the nature and origin of the initial trigger. Playing a prominent role in the critically-ill patient are disorders of gastrointestinal function, including hypoperfusion of the gastrointestinal mucosa resulting in gut ischemia; gastroesophageal reflux (GER); dysmotility; loss of normal gastrointestinal flora; and, aspiration potentially resulting in pneumonia. Further contributing to and exacerbating these issues are the effects of mechanical ventilation that is often required in this patient population.

## Reflux in Critically-Ill Patients

Gastroesophageal reflux (GER) is a common phenomenon among patients in the intensive care unit (ICU), with potential complications including erosive esophagitis and/or gastritis and risk of gastrointestinal (GI) bleeding. In nonventilated patients, transient lower esophageal sphincter (LES) relaxations are the most common mechanism underlying reflux [1]. Mechanical ventilation introduces extrinsic positive pressure to the thorax with subsequent effects on cardiopulmonary as well as GI function. Thus, GER in the mechanically ventilated patient is common and may be predominantly due to very low or absent LES pressure, with elevated intrathoracic pressure further exacerbated by cough and/or strain [1, 2] (patient-ventilator asynchrony or dyssynchrony) [3, 4].

Gastrointestinal motility disorders including GER are common in critically ill patients [5, 6] and are predictors of increased mortality and ICU length of stay [5]. Factors promoting GI motility disorders in this patient population include sepsis, mechanical ventilation, and commonly-used pharmacologic agents such as vasopressors, opioids and anticholinergic agents [5]. Relevant implications of GI motility disorders, besides promotion of GER, include malnutrition due to intolerance and malabsorption of enteral feeds, bacterial overgrowth, and aspiration [6], discussed further below. Furthermore, recent studies have demonstrated that the presence of GER in ICU patients is an important risk factor for recurrent acute lung injury [7], and that the presence of GER significantly and independently increased the risk of admission to an ICU and need for mechanical ventilation among patients with chronic obstructive pulmonary disease (COPD) [8].

## Stress Ulcer Prophylaxis

With GER being common in critically ill patients, and its complications potentially severe, proactive suppression of gastric acid gained widespread use in ICUs worldwide. However, this intervention carries possible negative consequences, as gastric acidity provides an environment preventing bacterial colonization and overgrowth. Thus, elimination of gastric acid may promote the occurrence of pneumonia as a result of aspiration, especially in mechanically-ventilated patients (see section on ventilator-associated pneumonia below). Thus, current recommendations limit the use of routine stress-ulcer prophylaxis to patients considered to be at high risk for clinically important bleeding, including: those on mechanical ventilation for greater than 48 h, and patients with coagulopathy [9, 10].

The decision to initiate stress ulcer prophylaxis raises the question of which type of pharmacological agent to employ. Although proton pump inhibitors (PPIs) are frequently used for this purpose, concerns have arisen that the potent acid suppression of PPIs may promote aspiration pneumonia [11–13], however other studies have failed to arrive at this conclusion and thus the area remains controversial. Recent data also suggest that PPI use may be associated with increased likelihood of developing enterocolitis due to *Clostridium difficile* [11, 14, 15].

Other agents used for stress ulcer prophylaxis in the ICU include histamine-2 receptor antagonists (H2RAs) and sucralfate. Two recent analyses evaluating the comparative efficacies of PPIs and H2RAs for stress ulcer prophylaxis in critically ill patients reached differing conclusions. One group of authors, limiting their review to trials at low risk for bias, concluded that the evidence does not clearly support lower bleeding rates with PPIs over H2RAs [9], whereas another analysis evaluating 19 trials enrolling 2117 patients concluded that PPIs were superior to H2RAs in preventing clinically important and overt GI bleeding, without significantly increasing the risk of pneumonia or mortality [16]. Few studies have directly compared sucralfate with other agents for stress ulcer prophylaxis. One randomized controlled trial found no difference in the occurrence of clinically important bleeding between groups treated with sucralfate, omeprazole, famotidine and placebo [17]. One recent study observed no benefit or harm with the prophylactic administration of the PPI pantoprazole, relative to placebo, in mechanically ventilated critically ill patients anticipated to receive enteral nutrition [18].

## Aspiration in Critically-Ill Patients

As noted above, mechanisms promoting reflux and thus risk of aspiration in the ICU include transient lower esophageal sphincter (LES) relaxations in nonventilated patients, and very low or absent LES pressure in mechanically ventilated patients [1, 2]. Aspiration of oropharyngeal or gastric contents into the lower respiratory tract is a common occurrence in critically ill patients and can result in pneumonia or pneumonitis, with progression to acute lung injury [19].

Provision of enteral nutrition is a vital component of the care of the critically ill patient. Unfortunately, delivery of feeds to the gastrointestinal tract increases the risk of aspiration. Specific factors increasing the risk of aspiration in critically ill patients include: inability to protect the airway and/or reduced level of consciousness (in nonventilated patients), presence of a nasoenteric enteral access device, mechanical ventilation, age >70 years, poor oral care, inadequate nurse/patient ratio, supine positioning, neurological deficits, GER, transport out of ICU, and provision of enteral nutrition in the form of intermittent bolus feeds [20].

## Enteral Feeding: Gastric Versus Post-Pyloric

The question of whether delivery of enteral nutrition beyond the gastric pylorus (into the duodenum or jejunum) reduces the incidence of aspiration and pneumonia, and whether it increases the amount of nutrition delivered to critically ill patients relative to gastric feeding, has been an area of controversy for decades. A recently published Cochrane Database Systematic Review evaluated 14 trials including 1109 patients in a meta-analysis [21]. The reviewers found moderate-quality evidence of a 30% lower rate of pneumonia associated with post-pyloric feeding, and low-quality evidence suggesting an increase in the amount of nutrition delivered. The 2016 guidelines for provision and assessment of nutrition support therapy in adult critically ill patients, published jointly by the Society of Critical Care Medicine (SCCM) and the American Society for Parenteral and Enteral Nutrition (A.S.P.E.N.) recommend diverting the level of feeding by post-pyloric enteral access device placement in patients deemed to be at high risk for aspiration, citing moderate-to-high quality of evidence [20].

## Aspiration and Ventilator-Associated Pneumonia

Perhaps the most serious consequence of aspiration of oropharyngeal and/or gastric contents in a critically ill patient is the development of ventilator-associated pneumonia (VAP). In the ICU, VAP is associated with prolonged ventilator dependence, increased ICU length of stay, cost, and mortality [22]. Thus, strategies to prevent the occurrence of VAP comprise a vital component of the management of mechanically-ventilated, critically ill patients [23, 24].

Concern that suppression or elimination of gastric acid may promote the occurrence of VAP has stimulated significant effort to establish guidelines for the use of stress ulcer prophylaxis in the ICU, and to determine whether the agent chosen affects the incidence of VAP. As discussed above, the question of whether PPIs are more likely to induce VAP compared with H2RAs remains unsettled [9]. Two recent studies suggest that the use of sucralfate for stress ulcer prophylaxis results in fewer cases of VAP compared with PPIs and H2RAs [25, 26].

One strategy aimed at reducing VAP occurrence is subglottic secretion drainage in mechanically ventilated patients. A recent analysis of 17 randomized controlled trials, with a total of 3369 adult patients, comparing subglottic secretion drainage versus no subglottic secretion drainage, concluded that subglottic secretion drainage is associated with lower VAP rates but does not clearly decrease duration of mechanical ventilation, ICU length of stay, ventilator-associated events, mortality or antibiotic usage [27]. Thus further work is needed in this area.

Because aspiration of oropharyngeal contents can lead to VAP, oral hygiene care in critically ill patients as a strategy to reduce occurrence of VAP has received considerable attention. A recent Cochrane Database Systematic Review [28] evaluated 38 randomized, controlled trials including 6016 patients. Four main comparisons comprised the analysis: chlorhexidine mouthrinse or gel versus placebo/usual care;

tooth brushing versus no tooth brushing; powered versus manual tooth brushing; and, comparisons of oral care solutions. The authors concluded that oral hygiene care including chlorhexidine mouthwash or gel reduced the risk of developing VAP from 25% to 19%, with the number needed to treat for an additional beneficial outcome (NNTB) of 17. No evidence of a difference in the outcomes of mortality, duration of mechanical ventilation or duration of ICU stay was discerned. It should be noted that two recent meta-analyses of randomized clinical trials [29, 30] as well as a recent large, single-center, retrospective analysis [31] reported a paradoxical observation of lower VAP rates yet potentially higher mortality rates, in patients receiving oral care with chlorhexidine. The reason for such a possible increase in mortality remains to be elucidated.

Given the importance of preventing VAP, standard ICU care now entails the implementation of a patient care "ventilator bundle" containing most or all of the following components: head-of-bed elevation; sedative infusion interruption; spontaneous breathing trials; oral care with chlorhexidine; thromboprophylaxis; and stress ulcer prophylaxis [31–34]. Some studies have documented a positive effect of the VAP-prevention bundle [33, 34] whereas others have demonstrated the individual components of the bundle to vary in their associations with patient-centered outcomes [31, 35].

## References

1. Nind G, Chen WH, Protheroe R, Iwakiri K, Fraser R, Young R, et al. Mechanisms of gastroesophageal reflux in critically ill mechanically ventilated patients. Gastroenterology. 2005;128:600–6.
2. Schallom M, Orr J, Metheny N, Pierce J. Gastroesophageal reflux in critically ill patients. Dimens Crit Care Nurs. 2013;32:69–77.
3. Murias G, Lucangelo U, Blanch L. Patient-ventilator asynchrony. Curr Opin Crit Care. 2016;22:53–9.
4. Beitler JR, Sands SA, Loring SH, Owens RL, Malhotra A, Spragg RG, et al. Quantifying unintended exposure to high tidal volumes from breath stacking dyssynchrony in ARDS: the BREATHE criteria. Intensive Care Med. 2016;42:1427–36.
5. Adike A, Quigley EM. Gastrointestinal motility problems in critical care: a clinical perspective. J Dig Dis. 2014;15:335–44.
6. Chapman MJ, Nguyen NQ, Deane AM. Gastrointestinal dysmotility: clinical consequences and management of the critically ill patient. Gastroenterol Clin N Am. 2011;40:725–39.
7. Bice T, Li G, Malinchoc M, Lee AS, Gajic O. Incidence and risk factors of recurrent acute lung injury. Crit Care Med. 2011;39:1069–73.
8. Tsai CL, Lin YH, Wang MT, Chien LN, Jeng C, Chian CF, et al. Gastro-oesophageal reflux disease increases the risk of intensive care unit admittance and mechanical ventilation use among patients with chronic obstructive pulmonary disease: a nationwide population-based cohort study. Crit Care. 2015;19:110.
9. Barletta JF, Bruno JJ, Buckley MS, Cook DJ. Stress ulcer prophylaxis. Crit Care Med. 2016;44:1395–405.
10. Buendgens L, Koch A, Tacke F. Prevention of stress-related ulcer bleeding at the intensive care unit: risks and benefits of stress ulcer prophylaxis. World J Crit Care Med. 2016;5:57–64.
11. MacLaren R, Reynolds PM, Allen RR. Histamine-2 receptor antagonists vs proton pump inhibitors on gastrointestinal tract hemorrhage and infectious complications in the intensive care unit. JAMA Intern Med. 2014;174:564–74.

12. Bateman BT, Bykov K, Choudhry NK, Schneeweiss S, Gagne JJ, Polinski JM, et al. Types of stress ulcer prophylaxis and risk of nosocomial pneumonia in cardiac surgical patients: cohort study. BMJ. 2013;347:f5416.
13. Herzig SJ, Howell MD, Ngo LH, Marcantonio ER. Acid-suppressive medication use and the risk for hospital-acquired pneumonia. JAMA. 2009;301:2120–8.
14. Barletta JF, Sclar DA. Proton pump inhibitors increase the risk for hospital-acquired *Clostridium difficile* infection in critically ill patients. Crit Care. 2014;18:714.
15. Buendgens L, Bruensing J, Matthes M, Duckers H, Luedde T, Trautwein C, et al. Administration of proton pump inhibitors in critically ill medical patients is associated with increased risk of developing *Clostridium difficile*-associated diarrhea. J Crit Care. 2014;29:696.e11–5.
16. Alshamsi F, Belley-Cote E, Cook D, Almenawer SA, Alqahtani Z, Perri D, et al. Efficacy and safety of proton pump inhibitors for stress ulcer prophylaxis in critically ill patients: a systematic review and meta-analysis of randomized trials. Crit Care. 2016;20:120.
17. Kantorova I, Svoboda P, Scheer P, Doubek J, Rehorkova D, Bosakova H, et al. Stress ulcer prophylaxis in critically ill patients: a randomized controlled trial. Hepato-Gastroenterology. 2004;51:757–61.
18. Selvanderan SP, Summers MJ, Finnis ME, Plummer MP, Ali Abdelhamid Y, Anderson MB, et al. Pantoprazole or placebo for stress ulcer prophylaxis (POP-UP): randomized double-blind exploratory study. Crit Care Med. 2016;44:1842–50.
19. Raghavendran K, Nemzek J, Napolitano LM, Knight PR. Aspiration-induced lung injury. Crit Care Med. 2011;39:818–26.
20. Taylor BE, McClave SA, Martindale RG, Warren MM, Johnson DR, Braunschweig C, et al. Guidelines for the provision and assessment of nutrition support therapy in the adult critically ill patient: Society of Critical Care Medicine (SCCM) and American Society for Parenteral and Enteral Nutrition (A.S.P.E.N.). Crit Care Med. 2016;44:390–438.
21. Alkhawaja S, Martin C, Butler RJ, Gwadry-Sridhar F. Post-pyloric versus gastric tube feeding for preventing pneumonia and improving nutritional outcomes in critically ill adults. Cochrane Database Syst Rev. 2015;(8):CD008875.
22. Mehta A, Bhagat R. Preventing ventilator-associated infections. Clin Chest Med. 2016;37:683–92.
23. Cocoros NM, Klompas M. Ventilator-associated events and their prevention. Infect Dis Clin N Am. 2016;30:887–908.
24. Li Bassi G, Senussi T, Xiol EA. Prevention of ventilator-associated pneumonia. Curr Opin Infect Dis. 2017;30:214. https://doi.org/10.1097/QCO.0000000000000358.
25. Khorvash F, Abbasi S, Meidani M, Dehdashti F, Ataei B. The comparison between proton pump inhibitors and sucralfate in incidence of ventilator associated pneumonia in critically ill patients. Adv Biomed Res. 2014;3:52.
26. Grindlinger GA, Cairo SB, Duperre CB. Pneumonia prevention in intubated patients given sucralfate versus proton-pump inhibitors and/or histamine II receptor blockers. J Surg Res. 2016;206:398–404.
27. Caroff DA, Li L, Muscedere J, Klompas M. Subglottic secretion drainage and objective outcomes: a systematic review and meta-analysis. Crit Care Med. 2016;44:830–40.
28. Hua F, Xie H, Worthington HV, Furness S, Zhang Q, Li C. Oral hygiene care for critically ill patients to prevent ventilator-associated pneumonia. Cochrane Database Syst Rev. 2016;10:CD008367.
29. Price R, MacLennan G, Glen J, SuDDICU Collaboration. Selective digestive or oropharyngeal decontamination and topical oropharyngeal chlorhexidine for prevention of death in general intensive care: systematic review and network meta-analysis. BMJ. 2014;348:g2197.
30. Klompas M, Speck K, Howell MD, Greene LR, Berenholtz SM. Reappraisal of routine oral care with chlorhexidine gluconate for patients receiving mechanical ventilation: systematic review and meta-analysis. JAMA Intern Med. 2014;174:751–61.
31. Klompas M, Li L, Kleinman K, Szumita PM, Massaro AF. Associations between ventilator bundle components and outcomes. JAMA Intern Med. 2016;176:1277–83.

32. Rello J, Chastre J, Cornaglia G, Masterton R. A European care bundle for management of ventilator-associated pneumonia. J Crit Care. 2011;26:3–10.
33. Morris AC, Hay AW, Swann DG, Everingham K, McCulloch C, McNulty J, et al. Reducing ventilator-associated pneumonia in intensive care: impact of implementing a care bundle. Crit Care Med. 2011;39:2218–24.
34. Okgun AA, Demir KF, Uyar M. Prevention of ventilator-associated pneumonia: use of the care bundle approach. Am J Infect Control. 2016;44:e173–6.
35. O'Horo JC, Lan H, Thongprayoon C, Schenck L, Ahmed A, Dziadzko M. "Bundle" practices and ventilator-associated events: not enough. Infect Control Hosp Epidemiol. 2016;37:1453–7.

# 20. Incidence and Risk of Aspiration in Mechanically Ventilated Patients

Miles J. Klimara, Rahul Nanchal, and Nikki Johnston

## Abstract

Mechanical ventilation is essential for many patients with critical illness and respiratory failure, but places patients at risk of life-threatening complications termed ventilator-associated events (VAEs). VAEs occur in approximately 25% of mechanically ventilated patients. These increase duration of mechanical ventilation, intensive care unit (ICU) and hospital length of stay, healthcare costs, and risk of disability and death. Many VAEs are aspiration-associated events such as pneumonia and Acute Lung Injury (ALI); aspiration pneumonia in particular is the second most common diagnosis among hospitalized adult patients. However, the lack of standardized diagnostic methods to confirm suspicion of aspiration poses a barrier to diagnosis of aspiration-related events in mechanically ventilated patients. Therefore, development of biomarkers to detect the early occurrence of aspiration in mechanically ventilated patients is a national priority in the United States. These biomarkers would enable development of novel therapies and allow clinicians to institute such therapies early to attenuate the incidence of adverse events. Ongoing research aims to assess the sensitivity and specificity of specific biomarkers to detect occurrence of early aspiration events in adult and pediatric patients receiving mechanical ventilation. To this end, our research group is

---

M. J. Klimara
Department of Otolaryngology and Communication Sciences,
Medical College of Wisconsin, Milwaukee, WI, USA

R. Nanchal
Department of Medicine, Medical College of Wisconsin, Milwaukee, WI, USA

N. Johnston (✉)
Department of Otolaryngology and Communication Sciences,
Medical College of Wisconsin, Milwaukee, WI, USA

Department of Microbiology and Immunology, Medical College of Wisconsin,
Milwaukee, WI, USA
e-mail: njohnston@mcw.edu

actively measuring pepsin and salivary amylase in tracheal aspirates from mechanically ventilated individuals as markers of gastric and oropharyngeal aspiration respectively. We hypothesize that aspiration events, identified by these markers, will correlate with incidence/time to VAEs and ICU outcomes including mortality, ventilator days, ICU days and hospital days. Accurate estimation of the incidence of aspiration and its impact on outcomes in mechanically ventilated patients will enable future trials of interventions to decrease morbidity/mortality from aspiration-associated pulmonary complications.

## Introduction

Acute respiratory failure is a complex syndrome that occurs from a variety of etiologies including pulmonary disease, neuromuscular disease and sepsis [1]. Invasive mechanical ventilation (ventilation provided via an artificial airway) is an essential life-saving intervention for patients with acute respiratory failure and in most circumstances this therapy is provided in an intensive care unit (ICU) environment. Although mechanical ventilation is the most frequent modality of organ support therapy, more than half of all complications that occur during ICU admission are related to ventilator support, particularly if its use is prolonged [2]. Acute respiratory failure requiring mechanical ventilation continues to contribute to mortality and adversely affects long-term functional outcomes in patients admitted to the ICU. Ventilator associated events (VAEs) and in particular ventilator associated pneumonia (VAP) is amongst the most dreaded complications associated with mechanical ventilation. Development of VAP heralds a complicated clinical course independently associated with excess mortality and morbidity [3–6]. In addition to these associated risks, mechanical ventilation is also labor intensive and very costly. Many quality improvement initiatives in the United States that endeavor to reduce ventilator associated events (VAEs), improve outcomes and lower costs are centered on persons receiving invasive mechanical ventilation [7–9]. Moreover, because studies in adults far out-number those conducted in the pediatric population, pediatric intensivists frequently extrapolate relevant adult data for their patient population [10]. Therefore, accurate information about the incidence, characteristics and outcomes of complications associated with invasive mechanical ventilation in both adult and pediatric populations is important from a clinical and health policy perspective.

Aspiration has been proposed by many as a key factor in the development and worsening of numerous VAEs (Fig. 20.1) [11, 12]. Overt or macro-aspiration is clearly linked to the development of aspiration pneumonitis and acute lung injury (ALI), however micro-aspiration of sterile oro-gastric contents and/or pathogenic micro-organisms that colonize the upper aero-digestive tract during critical illness likely contributes to the risk of VAEs. Within hours after establishment of an artificial airway, pathogenic micro-organisms colonize the upper aero-digestive tract. Subsequently oro-pharyngeal secretions colonized with these organisms

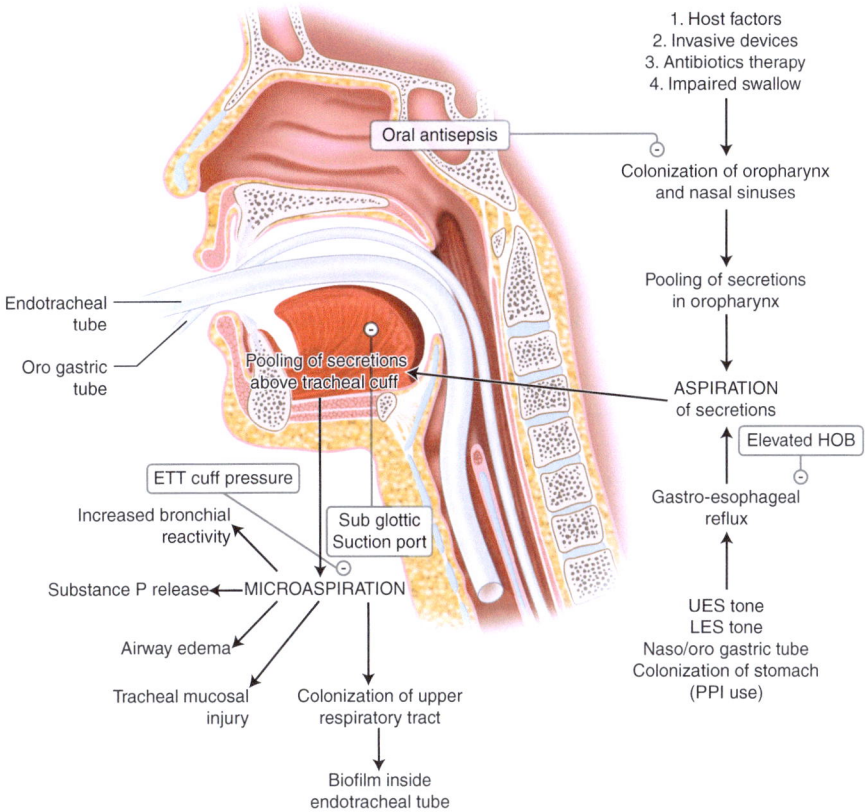

**Fig. 20.1** Framework of aspiration in patients with endotracheal tubes receiving mechanical ventilation

accumulate above the cuff of the artificial airway. Thereafter micro-aspiration of these subglottic secretions occurs through underinflated cuffs or through longitudinal folds in high-volume low pressure cuffs. Micro-aspiration of these organisms or even sterile oro-gastric secretions likely provokes inflammation and development of VAEs. Little consensus exists on the frequency of aspiration in patients receiving mechanical ventilation, because the accuracy of diagnosis has been problematic. However, a well-controlled study by Torres et al. [13] reported that aspiration occurred in 32% of semirecumbent patients receiving mechanical ventilation, but in 68% of patients who were supine [13]. Diagnosis of micro-aspiration using tracheo-bronchial colonization is often confounded by the use of antimicrobial agents, newer biomarkers such as gastric pepsin and salivary amylase show promise in refining the diagnosis but have yet to be rigorously validated in multi-center trials. Pulmonary aspiration can cause Acute Lung Injury (ALI), transient hypoxemia, and pneumonia. Such complications in turn increase the duration of mechanical ventilation, length of hospital stay, and use of medical resources [3, 14, 15]. For example, in studies of critically ill patients receiving mechanical ventilation, relative to patients without pneumonia, those with ventilator associated pneumonia (VAP) required on average 16 additional days in the hospital, resulting in per patient costs that were $30,000–40,000 greater [3, 14–16].

Aspiration of both gastric contents (gastric aspiration) and of oropharyngeal secretions (salivary aspiration) has been described. The relative contribution of either type of aspiration on the development of VAEs is unknown, because recognizing and distinguishing between these different types of aspiration remains challenging. Clinicians need to detect aspiration early so that interventions targeted towards gastric aspiration, oropharyngeal aspiration, or both can be implemented to prevent further aspiration events, complications and poor outcomes.

Salivary amylase, which is not normally found in the lungs, has recently been proposed as a biomarker for oropharyngeal aspiration. Weiss et al. reported that bronchoalveolar lavage amylase is not only associated with risk factors for aspiration, but may also be useful as an early screening tool to guide management of patients suspected of aspiration [17].

A prior attempt to detect gastric aspiration by measuring glucose in tracheal secretions as a marker of aspiration proved inadequate [18]. Flexible bronchoscopy is typically used to assess the airway in children with severe pulmonary conditions, and frequently a bronchoalveolar lavage (BAL) is performed to evaluate for possible aspiration. Measurement of lipid laden alveolar macrophages (LLM) from BAL is currently the most widely used test to identify aspiration in children. However, this test lacks both sensitivity and specificity. The premise of the test is that refluxate will be phagocytosed by alveolar macrophages, and that staining for these in the BAL should verify gastric aspiration [19]. Unfortunately, since LLMs are not necessarily exogenous, they may simply reflect measurements of phospholipid degradation from pulmonary inflammation and damage. While Ahrens et al. demonstrated higher levels of LLM in BAL samples in patients with lung disease and gastroesophageal reflux (GER) [20], other studies also found LLM in patients without GER and in control participants, suggesting that LLM is not a suitable marker [20, 21]. Moreover, the diagnostic utility of LLM is severely limited because studies used different methods for obtaining measurements (including the LLM index or measurements of the amount of lipid per cell) producing variable and inconclusive results [22–24]. Our findings, similarly, suggest that analysis of LLM has substantial potential for false positive tests (Table 20.1) [25]. In our study, not all controls were negative for this test. Additionally, our data suggest that analysis of LLM

**Table 20.1** Pepsin and lipid-laden macrophage (LLM) results from bronchoalveolar lavage fluid specimens from control subjects and patients undergoing bronchoscopy and tracheostomy [25]

|  | Total (n = 76) | Control (n = 11) | Bronchoscopy group (n = 34) | Tracheostomy group (n = 31) |
|---|---|---|---|---|
| Pepsin positive samples | 47 (62%) | 0 (0%) | 25 (74%) | 22 (71%) |
| LLM positive samples | 54 (71%) | 7 (64%) | 31 (91%) | 16 (52%) |

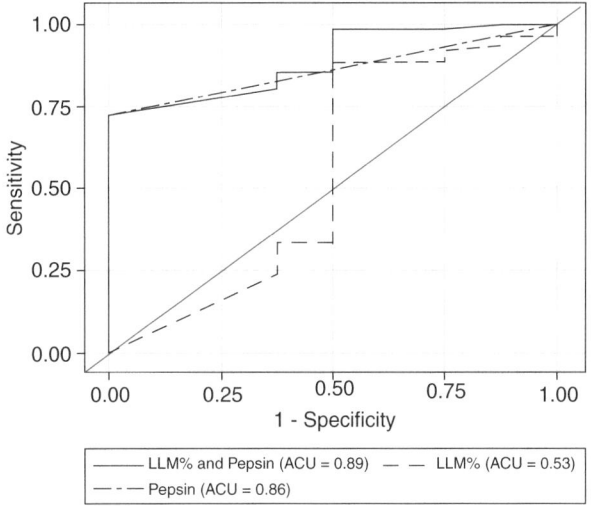

**Fig. 20.2** Predictive power of pepsin vs lipid-laden macrophages (LLMs) [25]. Receiver operating characteristic (ROC) analysis was performed to evaluate the ability of pepsin and LLMs (as quantified as percentage of LLMs among all macrophages) to predict the at-risk group compared with the control group

misses true positive patients with gastric aspiration. As such, the positive predictive value of the LLM test appears to be quite poor (Fig. 20.2).

Our preliminary observations also suggest that the performance of pepsin to reliably detect aspiration may be far superior to LLM. Unlike LLM, pepsin is purely exogenous in origin. Prior studies have also supported the use of pepsin as a measurement of aspiration [18, 19, 26]. Pepsin, an exogenous protein secreted only in the stomach, was introduced as a biomarker of gastric aspiration in animal studies [27]. More recently pepsin was implicated in acute exacerbations of idiopathic pulmonary fibrosis [28]. It was also detected in patients requiring mechanical ventilation who were at risk for aspiration [18]. Anticipating pepsin as a suitable biomarker of gastric aspiration, Stovold et al. reported elevated levels of pepsin in BAL of lung allografts, the highest levels found in patients with acute rejection [29]. Fisichella et al., 2011, who also used pepsin in the BAL as a biomarker for aspiration, concluded that laparoscopic anti-reflux surgery was an effective means to prevent aspiration [30]. We investigated the prevalence of gastric aspiration in a cohort of pediatric patients with chronic respiratory symptoms and in patients with tracheostomies by assessing the presence of pepsin in BAL specimens (Table 20.1) [25]. Pepsin-positive BAL specimens were identified in 25 patients who underwent bronchoscopy (74%) and 22 patients with tracheostomy (71%). All specimens from controls (n = 11) were negative for pepsin. Additionally, in order to confirm the utility of pepsin as a biomarker, we compared the results of pepsin detection in the BAL specimens with LLM analysis of the same tracheal aspirate [25]. Lipid-laden macrophages were found in the BAL fluid samples from 7 (64%) patients in the control group, 31 (91%) patients in the bronchoscopy group, and 16 (52%) patients in the tracheostomy group. We are currently further investigating the use of pepsin as a biomarker for aspiration and VAEs. To this end we have obtained tracheal lavage samples and clinical data including demographic data, incidence of VAEs, and time to VAEs from mechanically ventilated patients. Correlation of presence and levels with incidence of and time to VAEs will reveal the utility of pepsin as a predictive tool.

Tracheal cuff shape is posited to play a protective role in preventing aspiration and other complications in ventilated patients, as a conical (tapered) cuff might improve the seal between the external surface of the cuff and the internal surface of the trachea. This theory has been supported by in vitro models of endotracheal cuffs which showed decreased air or fluid leakage with use of a conical cuff. However, a recent clinical study found no significant difference in tracheobronchial colonization in patients ventilated with conical as opposed to standard cylindrical cuffs [31]. Recognizing that tracheobronchial colonization is a poor marker for microaspiration, Jaillette et al. performed a multicenter randomized control study evaluating the impact of tracheal cuff shape on the development of gastric and oropharyngeal aspiration, ventilator associated pneumonia, and other VAEs [32]. In their study, both abundant microaspiration of gastric contents as measured by gastric pepsin and abundant microaspiration of oropharyngeal secretions measured by salivary amylase were similar between the tapered and standard cuff cohorts. They concluded that tapered tracheal cuffs should not be used in the ICU to prevent microaspiration or VAP [32].

Proton pump inhibitor (PPI) therapy is routinely administered as prophylaxis for stress-related mucosal damage (SRMD) in critically ill patients and hence prevent gastric bleeding, but there have been few clinical trials to examine their efficacy for preventing SRMD compared to less costly alternatives such as $H_2$ receptor antagonists [30]. Given their superior acid-suppressive effects and the risk of tachyphylaxis with H2RAs, PPIs might be expected to more substantially reduce the risk of SRMD and decrease further complications such as blood transfusion that increase ICU costs and length of stay. However, there is currently insufficient pharmacoeconomic data to support this proposed benefit [33]. In light of the large cost differential between H2RAs and PPIs, future research should attempt to determine the cost-effectiveness of these acid suppression therapies for SRMD prevention in critical care settings.

While PPI therapy is a mainstay in the treatment of gastro-esophageal reflux disease (GERD), its efficacy for the treatment of airway reflux remains doubtful [34]. Multiple placebo-controlled trials have failed to demonstrate any therapeutic benefit of PPIs in long term treatment of airway reflux—laryngopharyngeal reflux (LPR) [35–40]. Approximately $26 billion per year is currently being spent on PPIs for the treatment of laryngopharyngeal reflux (LPR), despite their poor efficacy for this patient population [41]. It has been suggested that PPI therapy may even be detrimental due to inhibition of gastric acid's anti-microbial activity and continued reflux of non-acidic gastric contents. Pauwels et al. examined the effects of gastric juices obtained from cystic fibrosis patients on cytokine expression in bronchial epithelial cells, and found that gastric juice from patients taking PPIs induced a much greater IL-8 response than juice from patients who were not taking PPIs [42]. In light of IL-8's potent chemoattractant properties it is possible that this paradoxically increased inflammation in patients on PPIs might play a role in furthering pathogenesis of lung disease, particularly in vulnerable patients. Given pepsin's role in nonacidic airway reflux associated symptoms and mucosal injury, it has been proposed as a novel therapeutic target. The promise of irreversible inhibitors of peptic activity and/or receptor antagonists as potential new therapeutics for airway reflux has been discussed [43–47]. It has been proposed that extra-esophageal reflux (EER) is much more dependent on pepsin-mediated damage in the laryngeal and airway mucosa than acid-mediated damage. In this regard, our research group is currently leading an international drug discovery program to develop a drug that specifically targets pepsin. This might be used either alone or as an adjunct to PPIs to provide more effective treatment for non-acidic airway reflux. Such an advance would be particularly helpful in highly vulnerable patient populations such as patients with cystic fibrosis and patients receiving PPIs to prevent stress-related mucosal bleeding.

In summary, aspiration is a significant contributor to VAEs. The risks and costs associated with these complications are considerable [3, 14, 15]. Pepsin and salivary amylase are sensitive and specific biomarkers for the detection of gastric reflux and aspiration, and oropharyngeal aspiration, respectively. Both measurements are practical in the clinical setting. Testing for pepsin and salivary amylase should improve recognition of gastric and oropharyngeal aspiration in this high-risk patient population, subsequently leading to earlier institution of preventive management. Moreover, airway reflux-related symptoms and injury are known to occur despite acid suppression therapy and are associated with non-acid reflux events. Unlike GER, proximal reflux into the airway is predominantly non-acidic, and our studies have demonstrated pepsin-mediated damage in such an environment [44–46, 48]. In addition to using pepsin as a biomarker for reflux and aspiration, a therapy which specifically targets pepsin may be more effective against non-acid reflux/aspiration in patients receiving mechanical ventilation.

## References

1. Esteban A, Anzueto A, Frutos F, Alia I, Brochard L, Stewart TE, Benito S, Epstein SK, Apezteguia C, Nightingale P, Arroliga AC, Tobin MJ, Mechanical Ventilation International Study Group. Characteristics and outcomes in adult patients receiving mechanical ventilation: a 28-day international study. JAMA. 2002;287(3):345–55.
2. Manczur TI, Greenough A, Pryor D, Rafferty GF. Comparison of predictors of extubation from mechanical ventilation in children. Pediatr Crit Care Med. 2000;1(1):28–32.
3. Kollef MH, Hamilton CW, Ernst FR. Economic impact of ventilator-associated pneumonia in a large matched cohort. Infect Control Hosp Epidemiol. 2012;33(3):250–6. https://doi.org/10.1086/664049.
4. Blot S. Infection prevention in the ICU: more than just picking one or another preventive measure. Aust Crit Care. 2013;26(4):151–2. https://doi.org/10.1016/j.aucc.2013.07.004.
5. Timsit JF, Zahar JR, Chevret S. Attributable mortality of ventilator-associated pneumonia. Curr Opin Crit Care. 2011;17(5):464–71. https://doi.org/10.1097/MCC.0b013e32834a5ae9.

6. Safdar N, Dezfulian C, Collard HR, Saint S. Clinical and economic consequences of ventilator-associated pneumonia: a systematic review. Crit Care Med. 2005;33(10):2184–93.
7. Berwick DM, Calkins DR, McCannon CJ, Hackbarth AD. The 100,000 lives campaign: setting a goal and a deadline for improving health care quality. JAMA. 2006;295(3):324–7. https://doi.org/10.1001/jama.295.3.324.
8. Chelluri L, Im KA, Belle SH, Schulz R, Rotondi AJ, Donahoe MP, Sirio CA, Mendelsohn AB, Pinsky MR. Long-term mortality and quality of life after prolonged mechanical ventilation. Crit Care Med. 2004;32(1):61–9. https://doi.org/10.1097/01.CCM.0000098029.65347.F9.
9. Wunsch H, Linde-Zwirble WT, Angus DC, Hartman ME, Milbrandt EB, Kahn JM. The epidemiology of mechanical ventilation use in the United States. Crit Care Med. 2010;38(10):1947–53. https://doi.org/10.1097/CCM.0b013e3181ef4460.
10. Mehta NM, Arnold JH. Mechanical ventilation in children with acute respiratory failure. Curr Opin Crit Care. 2004;10(1):7–12.
11. Metheny NA, Chang YH, Ye JS, Edwards SJ, Defer J, Dahms TE, Stewart BJ, Stone KS, Clouse RE. Pepsin as a marker for pulmonary aspiration. Am J Crit Care. 2002;11(2):150–4.
12. Nseir S, Zerimech F, Fournier C, Lubret R, Ramon P, Durocher A, Balduyck M. Continuous control of tracheal cuff pressure and microaspiration of gastric contents in critically ill patients. Am J Respir Crit Care Med. 2011;184(9):1041–7. https://doi.org/10.1164/rccm.201104-0630OC.
13. Torres A, Serra-Batlles J, Ros E, Piera C, Puig de la Bellacasa J, Cobos A, Lomena F, Rodriguez-Roisin R. Pulmonary aspiration of gastric contents in patients receiving mechanical ventilation: the effect of body position. Ann Intern Med. 1992;116(7):540–3.
14. Klompas M, Magill S, Robicsek A, Strymish JM, Kleinman K, Evans RS, Lloyd JF, Khan Y, Yokoe DS, Stevenson K, Samore M, Platt R, CDC Prevention Epicenters Program. Objective surveillance definitions for ventilator-associated pneumonia. Crit Care Med. 2012;40(12):3154–61. https://doi.org/10.1097/CCM.0b013e318260c6d9.
15. Restrepo MI, Anzueto A, Arroliga AC, Afessa B, Atkinson MJ, Ho NJ, Schinner R, Bracken RL, Kollef MH. Economic burden of ventilator-associated pneumonia based on total resource utilization. Infect Control Hosp Epidemiol. 2010;31(5):509–15. https://doi.org/10.1086/651669.
16. Byers JF, Sole ML. Analysis of factors related to the development of ventilator-associated pneumonia: use of existing databases. Am J Crit Care. 2000;9(5):344–9; quiz 51.
17. Weiss CH, Moazed F, DiBardino D, Swaroop M, Wunderink RG. Bronchoalveolar lavage amylase is associated with risk factors for aspiration and predicts bacterial pneumonia. Crit Care Med. 2013;41(3):765–73. https://doi.org/10.1097/CCM.0b013e31827417bc.
18. Meert KL, Daphtary KM, Metheny NA. Detection of pepsin and glucose in tracheal secretions as indicators of aspiration in mechanically ventilated children. Pediatr Crit Care Med. 2002;3(1):19–22.
19. Farrell S, McMaster C, Gibson D, Shields MD, McCallion WA. Pepsin in bronchoalveolar lavage fluid: a specific and sensitive method of diagnosing gastro-oesophageal reflux-related pulmonary aspiration. J Pediatr Surg. 2006;41(2):289–93. https://doi.org/10.1016/j.jpedsurg.2005.11.002.
20. Ahrens P, Noll C, Kitz R, Willigens P, Zielen S, Hofmann D. Lipid-laden alveolar macrophages (LLAM): a useful marker of silent aspiration in children. Pediatr Pulmonol. 1999;28(2):83–8.
21. Kitz R, Boehles HJ, Rosewich M, Rose MA. Lipid-laden alveolar macrophages and pH monitoring in gastroesophageal reflux-related respiratory symptoms. Pulm Med. 2012;2012:673637. https://doi.org/10.1155/2012/673637.
22. Boesch RP, Daines C, Willging JP, Kaul A, Cohen AP, Wood RE, Amin RS. Advances in the diagnosis and management of chronic pulmonary aspiration in children. Eur Respir J. 2006;28(4):847–61. https://doi.org/10.1183/09031936.06.00138305.
23. Furuya ME, Moreno-Cordova V, Ramirez-Figueroa JL, Vargas MH, Ramon-Garcia G, Ramirez-San Juan DH. Cutoff value of lipid-laden alveolar macrophages for diagnosing aspiration in infants and children. Pediatr Pulmonol. 2007;42(5):452–7. https://doi.org/10.1002/ppul.20593.
24. Reilly BK, Katz ES, Misono AS, Khatwa U, Didas A, Huang L, Haver K, Rahbar R. Utilization of lipid-laden macrophage index in evaluation of aerodigestive disorders. Laryngoscope. 2011;121(5):1055–9. https://doi.org/10.1002/lary.21467.

25. Kelly EA, Parakininkas DE, Werlin SL, Southern JF, Johnston N, Kerschner JE. Prevalence of pediatric aspiration-associated extraesophageal reflux disease. JAMA Otolaryngol Head Neck Surg. 2013. https://doi.org/10.1001/jamaoto.2013.4448.
26. Krishnan U, Mitchell JD, Messina I, Day AS, Bohane TD. Assay of tracheal pepsin as a marker of reflux aspiration. J Pediatr Gastroenterol Nutr. 2002;35(3):303–8.
27. Badellino MM, Buckman RF Jr, Malaspina PJ, Eynon CA, O'Brien GM, Kueppers F. Detection of pulmonary aspiration of gastric contents in an animal model by assay of peptic activity in bronchoalveolar fluid. Crit Care Med. 1996;24(11):1881–5.
28. Lee JS, Song JW, Wolters PJ, Elicker BM, King TE Jr, Kim DS, Collard HR. Bronchoalveolar lavage pepsin in acute exacerbation of idiopathic pulmonary fibrosis. Eur Respir J. 2012;39(2):352–8. https://doi.org/10.1183/09031936.00050911.
29. Stovold R, Forrest IA, Corris PA, Murphy DM, Smith JA, Decalmer S, Johnson GE, Dark JH, Pearson JP, Ward C. Pepsin, a biomarker of gastric aspiration in lung allografts: a putative association with rejection. Am J Respir Crit Care Med. 2007;175(12):1298–303. https://doi.org/10.1164/rccm.200610-1485OC.
30. Fisichella PM, Davis CS, Lundberg PW, Lowery E, Burnham EL, Alex CG, Ramirez L, Pelletiere K, Love RB, Kuo PC, Kovacs EJ. The protective role of laparoscopic antireflux surgery against aspiration of pepsin after lung transplantation. Surgery. 2011;150(4):598–606. https://doi.org/10.1016/j.surg.2011.07.053.
31. Philippart F, Gaudry S, Quinquis L, Lau N, Ouanes I, Touati S, Nguyen JC, Branger C, Faibis F, Mastouri M, Forceville X, Abroug F, Ricard JD, Grabar S, Misset B. Randomized intubation with polyurethane or conical cuffs to prevent pneumonia in ventilated patients. Am J Respir Crit Care Med. 2015;191(6):637–45. https://doi.org/10.1164/rccm.201408-1398OC.
32. Jaillette E, Girault C, Brunin G, Zerimech F, Behal H, Chiche A, Broucqsault-Deirdre C, Fayolle C, Minacori F, Alves I, Barrailler S, Labreuche J, Robriquet L, Tamion F, Delaporte E, Thellier D, Delcourte C, Duhamel A, Nseir S. Impact of tapered-cuff tracheal tube on microaspiration of gastric contents in intubated critically ill patients: a multicenter cluster-randomized cross-over controlled trial. Intensive Care Med. 2017. https://doi.org/10.1007/s00134-017-4736-x.
33. Brett S. Science review: the use of proton pump inhibitors for gastric acid suppression in critical illness. Crit Care. 2005;9(1):45–50. https://doi.org/10.1186/cc2980.
34. Martinucci I, et al. Optimal treatment of laryngopharyngeal reflux disease. Ther Adv Chronic Dis. 2013;4:287–301. https://doi.org/10.1177/2040622313503485.
35. Eherer AJ, Habermann W, Hammer HF, Kiesler K, Friedrich G, Krejs GJ. Effect of pantoprazole on the course of reflux-associated laryngitis: a placebo-controlled double-blind crossover study. Scand J Gastroenterol. 2003;38:462–7.
36. El-Serag HB, Lee P, Buchner A, Inadomi JM, Gavin M, McCarthy DM. Lansoprazole treatment of patients with chronic idiopathic laryngitis: a placebo-controlled trial. Am J Gastroenterol. 2001;96:979–83. https://doi.org/10.1111/j.1572-0241.2001.03681.x.
37. Noordzij JP, Khidr A, Evans BA, Desper E, Mittal RK, Reibel JF, Levine PA. Evaluation of omeprazole in the treatment of reflux laryngitis: a prospective, placebo-controlled, randomized, double-blind study. Laryngoscope. 2001;111:2147–51. https://doi.org/10.1097/00005537-200112000-00013.
38. Steward DL, Wilson KM, Kelly DH, Patil MS, Schwartzbauer HR, Long JD, Welge JA. Proton pump inhibitor therapy for chronic laryngo-pharyngitis: a randomized placebo-control trial. Otolaryngol Head Neck Surg. 2004;131(4):342–50. https://doi.org/10.1016/j.otohns.2004.03.037.
39. Wo JM, Koopman J, Harrell SP, Parker K, Winstead W, Lentsch E. Double-blind, placebo-controlled trial with single-dose pantoprazole for laryngopharyngeal reflux. Am J Gastroenterol. 2006;101(9):1972–8; quiz 2169. https://doi.org/10.1111/j.1572-0241.2006.00693.x.
40. Vaezi MF, Richter JE, Stasney CR, Spiegel JR, Iannuzzi RA, Crawley JA, Hwang C, Sostek MB, Shaker R. Treatment of chronic posterior laryngitis with esomeprazole. Laryngoscope. 2006;116(2):254–60. https://doi.org/10.1097/01.mlg.0000192173.00498.ba.
41. Francis DO, Rymer JA, Slaughter JC, Choksi Y, Jiramongkolchai P, Ogbeide E, Tran C, Goutte M, Gaelyn Garrett C, Hagaman D, Vaezi MF. High economic burden of caring for patients

41. with suspected extraesophageal reflux. Am J Gastroenterol. 2013;108:905–11. https://doi.org/10.1038/ajg.2013.69.
42. Pauwels A, Verleden S, Farre R, Vanaudenaerde BM, Van Raemdonck D, Verleden G, Sifrim D, Dupont LJ. The effect of gastric juice on interleukin-8 production by cystic fibrosis primary bronchial epithelial cells. J Cyst Fibros. 2013;12:700–5. https://doi.org/10.1016/j.jcf.2013.03.006.
43. Johnston N, Dettmar PW, Bishwokarma B, et al. Activity/stability of human pepsin: implications for reflux attributed laryngeal disease. Laryngoscope. 2007;117:1036–9. https://doi.org/10.1097/MLG.0b013e31804154c3.
44. Johnston N, Wells CW, Samuels TL, Blumin JH. Pepsin in nonacidic refluxate can damage hypopharyngeal epithelial cells. Ann Otol Rhinol Laryngol. 2009;118:677–85. https://doi.org/10.1177/000348940911800913.
45. Johnston N, Wells CW, Samuels TL, Blumin JH. Rationale for targeting pepsin in the treatment of reflux disease. Ann Otol Rhinol Laryngol. 2010;119:547–58. https://doi.org/10.1177/000348941011900808.
46. Samuels TL, Johnston N. Pepsin as a causal agent of inflammation during nonacidic reflux. Otolaryngol Head Neck Surg. 2009;141:559–63. https://doi.org/10.1016/j.otohns.2009.08.022.
47. Bardhan KD, Strugala V, Dettmar PW. Reflux revisited: advancing the role of pepsin. Int J Otolaryngol. 2012;2012:646901. https://doi.org/10.1155/2012/646901.
48. Dettmar PW, Castell DO, Heading RC, Eds. Reflux and its consequences - The Laryngeal, Pulmonary and Oesophageal Manifestations. Aliment Pharmacol Ther. 2011;33(Suppl 1):1–71. https://doi.org/10.1111/j.1365-2036.2011.04581.x.

# Reflux in Pediatrics

## 21

Nina Gluchowski and Rachel Rosen

## Abbreviations

| | |
|---|---|
| AHR | Airway hyper-responsiveness |
| AR | Anti regurgitation |
| BAL | Broncho-alveolar lavage |
| COPD | Chronic obstructive pulmonary disease |
| GER | Gastroesophageal reflux |
| GERD | Gastroesophageal reflux disease |
| H2 | Histamine2 |
| LARS | Laparoscopic anti-reflux surgery |
| LES | Lower esophageal sphincter |
| LPR | Laryngo-pharyngeal reflux |
| MII | Multiple intraluminal impedance |
| NASPGHAN | North American Society of Gastroenterology, Hepatology and Nutrition |
| OSA | Obstructive sleep apnea |
| pH-MII | Multiple intraluminal impedance with pH |
| PPI | Proton pump inhibitor |
| SIDS | Sudden infant death syndrome |
| TLESR | Transient lower esophageal sphincter relaxation |
| tLESRs | Transient lower esophageal sphincter relaxations |
| VCD | Vocal cord dysfunction |

N. Gluchowski · R. Rosen (✉)
Division of Gastroenterology, Hepatology and Nutrition, Aerodigestive Center,
Boston Children's Hospital, Boston, MA, USA
e-mail: Nina.Gluchowski@childrens.harvard.edu; Rachel.Rosen@childrens.harvard.edu

## Reflux in Pediatrics

Gastroesophageal reflux (GER) is the passage of gastric contents into the esophagus with or without regurgitation or vomiting. This process occurs multiple times a day in healthy infants and children and most episodes cause few or no symptoms. When the refluxate reaches the mouth, the reflux is caused regurgitation. GER becomes gastroesophageal reflux disease (GERD) when the passage of gastric contents into the esophagus is associated with troublesome symptoms and/or complications. However, deciding what symptoms are troublesome is often difficult in children who are non-verbal or who are unable to accurately convey symptoms [1, 2].

## Prevalence

Reflux is especially common in infants. Up to half of infants, ages 0–3 months, experience at least one episode of regurgitation daily, the prevalence peaks at 67% of infants by 4 months of age with complete resolution of symptoms in most infants by 12–13 months of age [3]. Another report indicates that 12% of infants ages 0–12 months old fit Rome II criteria for infant regurgitation defined as at least two episodes of regurgitation daily for at least 3 weeks, with most symptomatic infants younger than 5 months old [4]. There is some evidence that the peak of infant regurgitation occurs earlier in non-Western infants and is between 1 and 2 months of age [5–7].

Prevalence for GER vary widely for older children and adolescents. Children ages 8–11 years are more likely to have symptoms of GER if they had symptoms of regurgitation for more than 90 days during infancy [8]. Anywhere from 6 to 40% of adolescents report symptoms of GER with increased prevalence reported among those with asthma and obesity. Cigarette smoking, use of non-steroidal anti-inflammatory medications and alcohol are also associated with increased reported GER symptoms [9–12]. It is estimated that only a quarter of adolescents with symptoms of GER see a physician for this complaint [12].

Prevalence may be increased in certain subpopulations of infants and children including patients with respiratory diseases such as asthma, laryngomalacia and/or tracheomalacia, neurologic impairment, congenital esophageal disease including esophageal atresia, cystic fibrosis, hiatal hernia, achalasia after myotomy or balloon dilation, lung transplantation, and those with a family history of GERD, Barrett's esophagus or esophageal adenocarcinoma [1, 13].

## Pathophysiology

The primary mechanism of GER in infants and children is similar to that in adults with spontaneous transient lower esophageal sphincter relaxation (TLESR) allowing gastric contents to enter the esophagus [14–17]. Manometric studies show this process accounts for up to 82% of reflux episodes [15, 18]. TLESR is also the primary mechanism of GER in patients predisposed to severe GERD including those with repaired esophageal atresia [19]. The rate of TLESR is the same in infants with and without symptoms of GER, however patients with symptoms were more likely to have acidic reflux at the time of a TLESR. Furthermore, certain triggers such as increased intra-abdominal pressure, body positioning, and proximity to meals, may make reflux at the time of a TLESR more likely [17, 20].

Other mechanisms of reflux have also been proposed including hypotonic LESs, and abnormal gastric emptying. However, gastric emptying rates are similar between infants and children with GERD and controls [17, 21] and studies in adults and infants as young as 31 weeks gestational age indicate that low LES tone accounts only for a minority of reflux episodes and is more likely to occur in patients with severe esophagitis [15, 18]. The esophageal sphincter is competent even in premature infants and reflux clearance mechanisms including swallow-induced peristalsis are also intact. There seems to be no difference in resting LES tone in formula fed versus breast fed infants or those receiving caffeine when compared to controls. Despite this, infants receiving caffeine may have more episodes of acidic GER [18].

## Diagnosis

### History and Physical Examination

The diagnosis of GERD is often clinical and the presentation varies by age [1, 2]. The main role of the history and physical exam is to evaluate for more serious conditions and complications of GERD. Features that may indicate a more worrisome condition include gastrointestinal bleeding, bilious emesis, onset of emesis after 6 months old, hepatosplenomegaly, and neurologic signs or symptoms [1]. The diagnosis of GERD in infants can be particularly challenging because gastroesophageal reflux can be a normal physiologic process and the symptoms ascribed to reflux by parents are often symptoms of other diseases or normal physiologic signs of infancy and early childhood. Symptoms include crying, fussiness, arching, poor sleep, feeding difficulties, vomiting and cough. Because of the overlap of symptoms between children with reflux and other diagnoses or normal physiologic variants, questionnaires have been developed and revised and can help differentiate healthy babies from those with GERD [22–24]. In children ages 1–17 years old abdominal pain, vomiting and cough are the most common symptoms found in at least 60% of children with esophagitis or abnormal pH monitoring. The prevalence of symptoms in non-erosive and erosive esophagitis is similar with the exception of anorexia and food refusal, which are more common in children with erosive esophagitis [25]. In patients ages 9–18 years old, an adult GERD questionnaire showed similar sensitivity and specificity as that in adults, 65.5 and 80% respectively, with heartburn, reflux, epigastric pain, nausea, sleep disturbance and use of over-the-counter medications as the greatest indicators of pathologic reflux as measured by esophagitis on upper endoscopy [26].

## Esophageal pH Monitoring

Continuous esophageal pH monitors can be used to record esophageal pH using a catheter placed through the nose of infants and children or a wireless capsule that attaches to the distal esophagus in children older than 4 years old [27, 28]. The reflux index (RI) is the percentage of time that the measured pH is <4 and adult studies suggest that typical reflux symptoms occur when the esophageal pH is <4 for at least 4% of time [29]. Pediatric studies suggest an abnormal RI if the pH is <4 for >6% of the time for children older than 1 year old or >12% of time for infants through the age of 12 months [1]. Unfortunately, the reproducibility of these tests in children can be as low as 69% so results should be interpreted in the clinical context and not in isolation [30]. The pH probe can only reliably detect reflux with a pH <4 because the ambient pH of the esophagus is 5–7 so when the pH prove reads ≥5, the probe could be detecting weakly acidic reflux or ambient esophageal pH so reflux will be missed. Since up to 89% of reflux is non-acidic in children, the sensitivity of the pH probe has been questioned in this population. In children with a greater non-acid reflux burden, the sensitivity of the pH probe is reduced [31]. This is particularly true in children taking acid suppression, patients who are continuously fed by gastrostomy tube, or infants who are fed every 2–3 h. While adult consensus guidelines support the use of pH testing for the diagnosis of reflux, the data in children suggest that pH probe testing correlates poorly with therapeutic outcomes and may not represent the "true" reflux burden since nonacid reflux is so common in children [32, 33]. pH-metry in children is useful in differentiating causes of esophagitis, eosinophilic esophagitis versus gastroesophageal reflux disease, to assess medication efficacy or to correlate acid reflux events with typical symptoms of GERD such as chest pain or heartburn.

## Combined Multiple Intraluminal Impedance and pH Monitoring

Multiple Intraluminal Impedance (MII) measures changes in electrical impedance between channel electrodes along a catheter and can detect movement of acidic and non-acidic fluid and air along the length of the esophagus. It allows for detection of direction, velocity and the height of retrograde boluses as small as 0.1 mL [34]. As with pH-metry, there are varying reports of reproducibility [35]. When used in combination with pH monitoring (pH-MII), reflux can be classified into three groups: acidic reflux (pH < 4), weakly acidic (pH 5–7), and alkaline (pH > 7) though by convention in the literature many paper classify and any refluxate with a pH > 4 as nonacidic. Using this catheter, there are also episodes that are only detected by pH probe, but not impedance that are called pH only reflux episodes [1, 31, 36]. In infants, most reflux episodes were undetectable by pH probe as only 14.9% of episodes were associated with decreases in pH to <4 [37]. In older children the sensitivity of pH monitoring and MII is similar if patients stop their acid suppression prior to testing, but the sensitivity of pH monitoring is much lower in patients taking acid suppression therapy. This suggests that MII is useful to assess reflux burden in patients with persistent symptoms despite acid suppression therapy, to evaluate the efficacy of acid suppression, or to correlate symptoms with reflux in patients predisposed to non-acidic gastric contents such as infants or continuously or frequently fed children [31]. One of the limitations of all catheter based testing is that the success of interpretation depends on the accuracy with which patients and their families record symptoms during their 24-h study. Both adult and pediatric studies have shown that patients fail to record up to 50% of symptoms and new technologies have been used, such as intraesophageal pressure monitoring and acoustic recording to improve symptoms detection by creating an electronic record of when a symptom occurs thereby eliminating the need for patient recording of symptoms [38, 39].

## Endoscopy and Biopsies

Upper gastrointestinal endoscopy allows for direct visualization of the esophageal mucosa to evaluate for reflux esophagitis, breaks in the esophageal mucosa or non-erosive reflux disease (NERD), symptoms associated with gastroesophageal reflux without associated mucosal breaks [1, 2]. In the patients with aerodigestive symptoms, the primary role of upper endoscopy in reflux is to evaluate for other conditions on the differential including eosinophilic esophagitis in patients not responding to pharmacologic therapy or to administer therapies such as Botulinum toxin for the treatment of gastroparesis and severe vomiting [40]. In children with respiratory symptoms undergoing upper GI endoscopy, 32% had abnormal esophageal biopsies including 8% which had a diagnosis of eosinophilic esophagitis [41].

## Additional Diagnostic Tests

Other imaging of the gastrointestinal tract is indicated in patients with symptoms of reflux-related lung disease. Upper gastrointestinal contrast radiography, while not routinely recommended in the diagnosis of GERD, is helpful in the patient with respiratory symptoms in evaluating for tracheoesophageal fistula. Similarly, videofluoroscopic swallow studies not only evaluate for oropharyngeal dysphagia and aspiration during swallowing (both of which present with identical symptoms to gastroesophageal reflux), but can also identify high tracheoesophageal fistulae. Finally, nuclear medicine gastric emptying scans, also known in some institutions as milk scans, can evaluate for gastroparesis as a cause for gastroesophageal reflux disease and, at some institutions, can evaluate for pulmonary aspiration with delayed imaging [42].

## Reflux Biomarkers

Because catheter based reflux testing only measures esophageal reflux, additional reflux biomarkers have been studied to diagnose extra-esophageal reflux symptoms.

The most commonly studied have been pepsin and bile acids, both of which are found in the gastrointestinal tract and should not be found in the lung unless aspiration was occurring. There have been several studies looking at the relationship between the presence of pepsin or bile acids and the presence of gastroesophageal reflux in the esophagus. Unfortunately, using esophageal reflux as the gold standard, the sensitivity of these biomarkers is low, but whether esophageal reflux burden is the correct standard to measure extraesophageal reflux is not known [43–46].

## Treatment

### Non-Pharmacologic Treatment in Infants

There are multiple non-pharmacologic therapies suggested in the treatment of GERD in infants. While infant seats are not shown to have any benefit in decreasing GER [47], several studies using pH probes and MII-pH in term and preterm infants have shown the benefit of prone and left lateral positioning when compared to right lateral and supine positions [48–50]. The prone position offers an anatomic benefit placing the LES above the gastric body and the left lateral position confers a decrease in the number of TLESRs by placing the stomach contents in the body and greater curvature which together act like a reservoir [51]. Interestingly, while the right lateral position is associated with more rapid gastric emptying, this benefit is not sufficient to overcome the benefit of the TLESR reduction in the left lateral decubitus position so while one study recommends the right lateral position for the first post-prandial hour, others suggest the left lateral position is preferred [17, 50]. It is important to note that the American Academy of Pediatrics recommends the supine position for sleeping infants in order to decrease the risk of sudden infant death syndrome (SIDS) [52]. Therefore, recommendations suggesting prone positioning should only be applied to awake and observed infants, infants with certain upper airway disorders in which the risk of death from GERD is greater than that from SIDS, or children over the age of 1 year [1]. Formula thickening is another proposed treatment of GER in infants. In the United States, rice cereal is the most common agent used to thicken formula and studies have used 1 teaspoon of cereal for every ounce of formula [1, 53]. While studies show no significant decreases in acid GER in term and preterm infants fed thickened formula or breast milk [54–58], thickened feeds have been shown to decrease regurgitation and emesis witnessed by caretakers [54, 57, 59, 60]. Infants taking thickened feeds also may sleep more and cry less which may also be helpful for caretakers [59]. Formula with added thickener is more calorie dense and may provide more energy than necessary whereas antiregurgitation (AR) formulas are available and are similar in caloric density to standard infant formulas and also do not require increased sucking effort [1]. However, it is important to note that the addition of cereal (not formulas with added thickening where the benefits of thickening do not occur until the formula reaches acidic gastric contents) can reduce aspiration in patients with oropharyngeal dysphagia and may serve two benefits, for GER and swallowing dysfunction.

Another potential feeding intervention for GERD symptoms is change of formula to hypoallergenic formulas. This formula intolerance presents with identical symptoms to reflux including crying, regurgitation, vomiting. Multiple studies have shown that hypoallergenic formulas and maternal dietary restrictions in breast fed infants lead to decreased crying time [61–63]. There is also increasing evidence that GERD and esophagitis may be caused by food hypersensitivites [64] and infants with cow's milk allergy that are challenged with cow's milk protein have increased total GER and weakly acidic GER [65]. Lastly, modifying feeding patterns by giving smaller volume and more frequent feedings reduces acid reflux, but increases the relative amount of non-acid reflux [17].

## Lifestyle Changes in the Treatment in Children and Adolescents

Non-pharmacologic interventions for the treatment of GERD that have been studied in adults are potentially useful in children and adolescents, however their applicability to children of all ages is uncertain and there are few studies in children addressing non-pharmacologic interventions [1]. While positioning has been studied extensively in infants, there are no studies in older children. In adults, elevation the head of the bed may decrease full column reflux as measured by pharyngeal pH monitoring, which may have implication for the treatment of extra-esophageal symptoms [66]. There is very little data on dietary modification in children. In adults, patients who ate dinner closer to bedtime had more nocturnal reflux than patients who ate earlier in the evening [67]. The relationship between reflux burden and obesity has been debated though current recommendations are that weight loss should be encouraged as a method of reflux control [1, 68]. While avoidance of caffeine, alcohol and spicy foods has been recommended if they provoke symptoms, no data exists to support these recommendations in children. Smoking should be avoided for many reasons including the link between cigarette smoking and adenocarcinoma of the esophagus in adults [1].

## Pharmacologic Treatment

Histamine2 (H2) antagonists and proton pump inhibitors (PPI) have been studied in infants and children with GERD and clearly have been shown to block acid production and to result in mucosal healing [69–76]. H2 blockers have been shown to decrease esophageal acid exposure and regurgitation frequency in infants [75, 77], but this improvement in acid control does not always equate with symptom resolution. Studies of H2 antagonists have not been shown in randomized trials to reduce crying [78]. Similarly, randomized trials of proton pump inhibitors in infants have failed to show any benefit of PPIs for the control of symptoms of crying, fussiness, wheezing and cough [71–73, 78–80], despite multiple studies showing proton pump inhibitors reduce gastric acid production. In older children, proton pump inhibitors showed no benefit in the treatment of poorly controlled asthma in terms of lung function, medication usage, hospitalization, and symptom control [33]. This effective acid control, however, does result in mucosal healing in the esophagus with 89% of esophageal erosions healing within 8 weeks of starting PPIs [69]. While there are documented benefits to taking acid suppression therapy, there are some notable risks of which to be aware, particularly in the care of the aerodigestive patient. Acid suppression use has been associated with an increased risk of infections including community-acquired pneumonia, upper respiratory tract infections, gastroenteritis, and Clostridium difficile infections [33, 81, 82]. the possible mechanism of which is changes in the gastric and lung flora resulting from bacterial overgrowth in a non-acidic environment [79]. The use of PPI therapy is also associated with increased incidence of food allergies [83]. Therefore, in the aerodigestive patient who experiences frequent respiratory infections and is treated with multiple antibiotic courses, acid suppression should be used with close monitoring for both worsening infections and the development of C. difficile colitis. Current NASPGHAN guidelines recommend a short trial of acid suppression in infants only after other treatments including hypoallergenic formula have been tried. A short trial of PPI therapy may be useful in older children with classic symptoms of GERD and is recommended for those with endoscopy proven esophagitis. While other pharmacologic therapies have been pursued, there is insufficient evidence to support the routine use of metoclopramide, erythromycin, bethanechol, cisapride and domperidone for the reduction of reflux in infants and children [1]. However, in the aerodigestive population, macrolide use is often utilized to improve gastric motility, to reduce lung inflammation, and to provide antibiotic coverage in patients with concurrent immune deficiency [84].

## Surgical Treatment

Surgical options for the treatment of GERD in infants and children include Nissen fundoplication and jejunal or post-pyloric feeding. Nissen fundoplication involves wrapping the gastric fundus around the distal esophagus. This procedure corrects hiatal herniation if present, lengthens the intra-abdominal portion of the esophagus, tightens the crura, increases the pressure of the LES and decreases the number of TLESR events [1, 85]. It was shown early on in case series of infants and children to decrease the mean time the esophagus is exposed to acid and result in complete resolution of GER in most patients [86, 87]. While randomized controlled studies in adults have shown that fundoplication outcomes are comparable to acid suppression outcomes in terms of symptoms control and rates of Barrett's esophagus [88], rates of extraesophageal symptom control with both acid suppression and fundoplication are less encouraging, largely because proving causality between atypical symptoms of reflux is difficult [89–91]. From an aerodigestive perspective, while fundoplication may control gastroesophageal reflux, obstruction the lower esophagus with the surgical wrap may result in worsening of aspiration symptoms. Between 25 and 50% of children undergoing fundoplication for recurrent aspiration pneumonia have worsening of pneumonias after surgery compared to before, suggesting that esophageal obstruction can compromise pulmonary function [89, 91]. Esophageal obstruction may be even more compromising from a pulmonary perspective in patients with poor esophageal motility such as esophageal atresia, where stasis is already a significant concern, even before distal esophageal obstruction with a fundoplication. In another high-risk population, patients with cystic fibrosis, who underwent Nissen fundoplication, there was no change in body mass index or FEV1 and 48% had recurrence of GERD post-operatively [92]. In the lung transplant population, fundoplication is safe in adult patients with lung transplantation and may improve survival but no pediatric data is available [93]. At this time fundoplication should be reserved for select patients who have failed optimal medical treatment [1, 94].

Jejunal or post-pyloric feeds have been proposed as an alternative treatment for GER and is a less invasive option than fundoplication in patients requiring tube feeds. It is thought that with less volume in the stomach the likelihood of reflux is reduced and rates of reflux with post-pyloric feeds are similar to the rates in the post-fundoplication patient [95]. It is important to note that jejunal feeds do not eliminate reflux completely. One study looked at adult patients on mechanical ventilation in the intensive care unit randomized to gastric or jejunal feeds with technetium added to the feeds several hours each day. The patients that received jejunal feeds had less episodes of GER, although not zero, and trended toward less aspiration of feeds [96]. In a single pediatric study, rates of respiratory complication including pneumonia were equivalent between children who received post-pyloric feeds compared to patients who received a fundoplication [97]. Adults fed formula via jejunal tube had more episodes of reflux than those who received saline, concluding that nutrient infusion into the jejunum can induce GER [98]. In a single pediatric study of children with GJ tubes, more reflux occurred during feed versus non-feed periods [32]. In a study of patients with neurologic impairment, 8% failed jejunal feeds and went on to fundoplication whereas 14.5% spontaneously improved and the tube was removed without further surgical intervention suggesting the GJ tube feeding can be effective in buying time until reflux is outgrown without more invasive surgeries [99]. Apnea in premature infants is often attributed to GER and of 15 babies trialed on post-pyloric feeds, 12 had significant improvement in the number of apneic events. That said, 9 of the 12 had continued improvement after discontinuation of jejunal feeds suggesting that perhaps gestational age and maturity played a role [100]. Jejunal feeds may be helpful in determining if a patient's symptoms are reflux related and if that patient is a candidate for anti-reflux surgery [1, 95].

## References

1. Vandenplas Y, Rudolph CD, Di Lorenzo C, et al. Pediatric gastroesophageal reflux clinical practice guidelines: joint recommendations of the North American Society for Pediatric Gastroenterology, Hepatology, and Nutrition (NASPGHAN) and the European Society for Pediatric Gastroenterology, Hepatology, and Nutrition (ESPGHAN). J Pediatr Gastroenterol Nutr. 2009;49(4):498–547. https://doi.org/10.1097/MPG.0b013e3181b7f563.
2. Sherman PM, Hassall E, Fagundes-Neto U, et al. A global, evidence-based consensus on the definition of gastroesophageal reflux disease in the pediatric population. Am J Gastroenterol. 2009;104:1278–95; quiz1296. https://doi.org/10.1038/ajg.2009.129.

3. Nelson SP, Chen EH, Syniar GM, Christoffel KK. Prevalence of symptoms of gastroesophageal reflux during infancy: a pediatric practice-based survey. Arch Pediatr Adolesc Med. 1997;151(6):569–72. https://doi.org/10.1001/archpedi.1997.02170430035007.
4. Campanozzi A, Boccia G, Pensabene L, et al. Prevalence and natural history of gastroesophageal reflux: pediatric prospective survey. Pediatrics. 2009;123(3):779–83. https://doi.org/10.1542/peds.2007-3569.
5. Miyazawa R, Tomomasa T, Kaneko H, Tachibana A, Ogawa T, Morikawa A. Prevalence of gastro-esophageal reflux-related symptoms in Japanese infants. Pediatr Int. 2002;44(5):513–6.
6. Osatakul S, Sriplung H, Puetpaiboon A, Junjana C-O, Chamnongpakdi S. Prevalence and natural course of gastroesophageal reflux symptoms: a 1-year cohort study in Thai infants. J Pediatr Gastroenterol Nutr. 2002;34(1):63–7.
7. Hegar B, Boediarso A, Firmansyah A, Vandenplas Y. Investigation of regurgitation and other symptoms of gastroesophageal reflux in Indonesian infants. World J Gastroenterol. 2004;10(12):1795–7.
8. Martin AJ, Pratt N, Kennedy JD, et al. Natural history and familial relationships of infant spilling to 9 years of age. Pediatrics. 2002;109(6):1061–7.
9. Chen J-H, Wang H-Y, Lin HH, Wang C-C, Wang L-Y. Prevalence and determinants of gastroesophageal reflux symptoms in adolescents. J Gastroenterol Hepatol. 2014;29(2):269–75. https://doi.org/10.1111/jgh.12330.
10. Koebnick C, Getahun D, Smith N, Porter AH, Der-Sarkissian JK, Jacobsen SJ. Extreme childhood obesity is associated with increased risk for gastroesophageal reflux disease in a large population-based study. Int J Pediatr Obes. 2011;6(2-2):e257–63. https://doi.org/10.3109/17477166.2010.491118.
11. Debley JS, Carter ER, Redding GJ. Prevalence and impact of gastroesophageal reflux in adolescents with asthma: a population-based study. Pediatr Pulmonol. 2006;41(5):475–81. https://doi.org/10.1002/ppul.20399.
12. Gunasekaran TS, Dahlberg M, Ramesh P, Namachivayam G. Prevalence and associated features of gastroesophageal reflux symptoms in a Caucasian-predominant adolescent school population. Dig Dis Sci. 2008;53(9):2373–9. https://doi.org/10.1007/s10620-007-0150-5.
13. Woodley FW, Machado RS, Hayes D, et al. Children with cystic fibrosis have prolonged chemical clearance of acid reflux compared to symptomatic children without cystic fibrosis. Dig Dis Sci. 2014;59(3):623–30. https://doi.org/10.1007/s10620-013-2950-0.
14. Werlin SL, Dodds WJ, Hogan WJ, Arndorfer RC. Mechanisms of gastroesophageal reflux in children. J Pediatr. 1980;97(2):244–9. https://doi.org/10.1111/j.1572-0241.2001.03865.x.
15. Dent J, Holloway RH, Toouli J, Dodds WJ. Mechanisms of lower oesophageal sphincter incompetence in patients with symptomatic gastrooesophageal reflux. Gut. 1988;29(8):1020–8. https://doi.org/10.1136/gut.29.8.1020.
16. Cucchiara S, Bortolotti M, Minella R, Auricchio S. Fasting and postprandial mechanisms of gastroesophageal reflux in children with gastroesophageal reflux disease. Dig Dis Sci. 1993;38(1):86–92.
17. Omari TI, Barnett CP, Benninga MA, et al. Mechanisms of gastro-oesophageal reflux in preterm and term infants with reflux disease. Gut. 2002;51(4):475–9.
18. Omari TI, Barnett C, Snel A, et al. Mechanisms of gastroesophageal reflux in healthy premature infants. J Pediatr. 1998;133(5):650–4. https://doi.org/10.1016/s0022-3476(98)70106-4.
19. van Wijk M, Knüppe F, Omari T, de Jong J, Benninga M. Evaluation of gastroesophageal function and mechanisms underlying gastroesophageal reflux in infants and adults born with esophageal atresia. J Pediatr Surg. 2013;48(12):2496–505. https://doi.org/10.1016/j.jpedsurg.2013.07.024.
20. Jadcherla SR, Chan CY, Moore R, Malkar M, Timan CJ, Valentine CJ. Impact of feeding strategies on the frequency and clearance of acid and nonacid gastroesophageal reflux events in dysphagic neonates. J Parenter Enter Nutr. 2012;36(4):449–55. https://doi.org/10.1177/0148607111415980.
21. Knatten CK, Åvitsland TL, Medhus AW, et al. Gastric emptying in children with gastroesophageal reflux and in healthy children. J Pediatr Surg. 2013;48(9):1856–61. https://doi.org/10.1016/j.jpedsurg.2013.03.076.

22. Orenstein SR, Cohn JF, Shalaby TM, Kartan R. Reliability and validity of an infant gastroesophageal reflux questionnaire. Clin Pediatr. 1993;32(8):472–84. https://doi.org/10.1177/000992289303200806.
23. Orenstein SR, Shalaby TM, Cohn JF. Reflux symptoms in 100 normal infants: diagnostic validity of the infant gastroesophageal reflux questionnaire. Clin Pediatr. 1996;35(12):607–14. https://doi.org/10.1177/000992289603501201.
24. Aggarwal S, Mittal SK, Kalra KK, Rajeshwari K, Gondal R. Infant gastroesophageal reflux disease score: reproducibility and validity in a developing country. Trop Gastroenterol. 2004;25(2):96–8.
25. Gupta SK, Hassall E, Chiu Y-L, Amer F, Heyman MB. Presenting symptoms of nonerosive and erosive esophagitis in pediatric patients. Dig Dis Sci. 2006;51(5):858–63. https://doi.org/10.1007/s10620-006-9095-3.
26. Chiu J-Y, Wu J-F, Ni Y-H. Correlation between gastroesophageal reflux disease questionnaire and erosive esophagitis in school-aged children receiving endoscopy. Pediatr Neonatol. 2014;55(6):439–43. https://doi.org/10.1016/j.pedneo.2014.01.004.
27. Hochman JA, Favaloro-Sabatier J. Tolerance and reliability of wireless pH monitoring in children. J Pediatr Gastroenterol Nutr. 2005;41(4):411–5.
28. Croffie JM, Fitzgerald JF, Molleston JP, et al. Accuracy and tolerability of the Bravo catheter-free pH capsule in patients between the ages of 4 and 18 years. J Pediatr Gastroenterol Nutr. 2007;45(5):559–63. https://doi.org/10.1097/MPG.0b013e3180dc9349.
29. Wenner J, Johansson J, Johnsson F, Öberg S. Optimal thresholds and discriminatory power of 48-h wireless esophageal pH monitoring in the diagnosisof GERD. Am J Gastroenterol. 2007;102(9):1862–9. https://doi.org/10.1111/j.1572-0241.2007.01269.x.
30. Mahajan L, Wyllie R, Oliva L, Balsells F, Steffen R, Kay M. Reproducibility of 24-hour intraesophageal pH monitoring in pediatric patients. Pediatrics. 1998;101(2):260–3. https://doi.org/10.1542/peds.101.2.260.
31. Rosen R, Lord C, Nurko S. The sensitivity of multichannel intraluminal impedance and the pH probe in the evaluation of gastroesophageal reflux in children. Clin Gastroenterol Hepatol. 2006;4(2):167–72. https://doi.org/10.1053/S1542-3565(05)00854-2.
32. Rosen R, Hart K, Warlaumont M. Incidence of gastroesophageal reflux during transpyloric feeds. J Pediatr Gastroenterol Nutr. 2011;52(5):532–5. https://doi.org/10.1097/MPG.0b013e31820596f8.
33. Holbrook JT, Wise RA, Gold BD, Blake K. Randomized clinical trial of lansoprazole for poorly controlled asthma in children: the American Lung Association Asthma Clinical Research Centers. JAMA. 2012;307:373. https://doi.org/10.1001/jama.2011.2035.
34. Peter CS, Wiechers C, Bohnhorst B, Silny J, Poets CF. Detection of small bolus volumes using multiple intraluminal impedance in preterm infants. J Pediatr Gastroenterol Nutr. 2003;36(3):381–4.
35. Dalby K, Nielsen RG, Markoew S, Kruse-Andersen S, Husby S. Reproducibility of 24-hour combined multiple intraluminal impedance (MII) and pH measurements in infants and children. Evaluation of a diagnostic procedure for gastroesophageal reflux disease. Dig Dis Sci. 2007;52(9):2159–65. https://doi.org/10.1007/s10620-006-9731-y.
36. Wenzl TG. Investigating esophageal reflux with the intraluminal impedance technique. J Pediatr Gastroenterol Nutr. 2002;34(3):261–8.
37. Wenzl TG, Moroder C, Trachterna M, et al. Esophageal pH monitoring and impedance measurement: a comparison of two diagnostic tests for gastroesophageal reflux. J Pediatr Gastroenterol Nutr. 2002;34(5):519–23.
38. Rosen R, Amirault J, Giligan E, Khatwa U, Nurko S. Intraesophageal pressure recording improves the detection of cough during multichannel intraluminal impedance testing in children. J Pediatr Gastroenterol Nutr. 2014;58(1):22–6. https://doi.org/10.1097/MPG.0b013e3182a80059.
39. Rosen R, Amirault J, Heinz N, Litman H, Khatwa U. The sensitivity of acoustic cough recording relative to intraesophageal pressure recording and patient report during reflux testing. Neurogastroenterol Motil. 2014;26(11):1635–41. https://doi.org/10.1111/nmo.12445.

40. Arbizu RA, Rodriguez L. Use of Clostridium botulinum toxin in gastrointestinal motility disorders in children. World J Gastrointest Endosc. 2015;7(5):433–7. https://doi.org/10.4253/wjge.v7.i5.433.
41. Rosen R, Amirault J, Johnston N, et al. The utility of endoscopy and multichannel intraluminal impedance testing in children with cough and wheezing. Pediatr Pulmonol. 2014;49(11):1090–6. https://doi.org/10.1002/ppul.22949.
42. Ravelli AM, Panarotto MB, Verdoni L, Consolati V, Bolognini S. Pulmonary aspiration shown by scintigraphy in gastroesophageal reflux-related respiratory disease. Chest. 2006;130(5):1520–6. https://doi.org/10.1378/chest.130.5.1520.
43. Starosta V, Kitz R, Hartl D, Marcos V, Reinhardt D, Griese M. Bronchoalveolar pepsin, bile acids, oxidation, and inflammation in children with gastroesophageal reflux disease. Chest. 2007;132(5):1557–64. https://doi.org/10.1378/chest.07-0316.
44. Grabowski M, Kasran A, Seys S, et al. Pepsin and bile acids in induced sputum of chronic cough patients. Respir Med. 2011;105(8):1257–61. https://doi.org/10.1016/j.rmed.2011.04.015.
45. Hayat JO, Gabieta-Somnez S, Yazaki E, et al. Pepsin in saliva for the diagnosis of gastro-oesophageal reflux disease. Gut. 2015;64(3):373–80. https://doi.org/10.1136/gutjnl-2014-307049.
46. Rosen R, Johnston N, Hart K, Khatwa U, Nurko S. The presence of pepsin in the lung and its relationship to pathologic gastro-esophageal reflux. Neurogastroenterol Motil. 2012;24(2):129–33, e84-5. https://doi.org/10.1111/j.1365-2982.2011.01826.x.
47. Orenstein SR, Whitington PF, Orenstein DM. The infant seat as treatment for gastroesophageal reflux. N Engl J Med. 1983;309(13):760–3. https://doi.org/10.1056/NEJM198309293091304.
48. Vandenplas Y, Sacre-Smits L. Seventeen-hour continuous esophageal pH monitoring in the newborn. J Pediatr Gastroenterol Nutr. 1985;4(3):356–61. https://doi.org/10.1097/00005176-198506000-00006.
49. Ewer AK, James ME, Tobin JM. Prone and left lateral positioning reduce gastro-oesophageal reflux in preterm infants. Arch Dis Child Fetal Neonatal Ed. 1999;81(3):F201–5.
50. van Wijk MP, Benninga MA, Dent J, et al. Effect of body position changes on postprandial gastroesophageal reflux and gastric emptying in the healthy premature neonate. J Pediatr. 2007;151(6):585–90, 590.e1-2. https://doi.org/10.1016/j.jpeds.2007.06.015.
51. Corvaglia L, Rotatori R, Ferlini M, Aceti A, Ancora G, Faldella G. The effect of body positioning on gastroesophageal reflux in premature infants: evaluation by combined impedance and pH monitoring. J Pediatr. 2007;151(6):591–6, 596.e1. https://doi.org/10.1016/j.jpeds.2007.06.014.
52. American Academy of Pediatrics Task Force on Sudden Infant Death Syndrome. The changing concept of sudden infant death syndrome: diagnostic coding shifts, controversies regarding the sleeping environment, and new variables to consider in reducing risk. Pediatrics. 2005;116(5):1245–55. https://doi.org/10.1542/peds.2005-1499.
53. Chao HC, Vandenplas Y. Comparison of the effect of a cornstarch thickened formula and strengthened regular formula on regurgitation, gastric emptying and weight gain in infantile regurgitation. Dis Esophagus. 2007;20(2):155–60. https://doi.org/10.1111/j.1442-2050.2007.00662.x.
54. Khoshoo V, Ross G, Brown S, Edell D. Smaller volume, thickened formulas in the management of gastroesophageal reflux in thriving infants. J Pediatr Gastroenterol Nutr. 2000;31(5):554–6.
55. Corvaglia L, Ferlini M, Rotatori R, et al. Starch thickening of human milk is ineffective in reducing the gastroesophageal reflux in preterm infants: a crossover study using intraluminal impedance. J Pediatr. 2006;148(2):265–8. https://doi.org/10.1016/j.jpeds.2005.09.034.
56. Bailey DJ, Andres JM, Danek GD, Pineiro-Carrero VM. Lack of efficacy of thickened feeding as treatment for gastroesophageal reflux. J Pediatr. 1987;110(2):187–9. https://doi.org/10.1016/S0022-3476(87)80151-8.
57. Wenzl TG, Schneider S, Scheele F, Silny J, Heimann G, Skopnik H. Effects of thickened feeding on gastroesophageal reflux in infants: a placebo-controlled crossover study using intraluminal impedance. Pediatrics. 2003;111(4):e355–9. https://doi.org/10.1542/peds.111.4.e355.

58. Xinias I, Mouane N, Le Luyer B, et al. Cornstarch thickened formula reduces oesophageal acid exposure time in infants. Dig Liver Dis. 2005;37(1):23–7. https://doi.org/10.1016/j.dld.2004.07.015.
59. Orenstein SR, Magill HL, Brooks P. Thickening of infant feedings for therapy of gastroesophageal reflux. J Pediatr. 1987;110(2):181–6. https://doi.org/10.1016/s0022-3476(87)80150-6.
60. Chao H-C, Vandenplas Y. Effect of cereal-thickened formula and upright positioning on regurgitation, gastric emptying, and weight gain in infants with regurgitation. Nutrition. 2007;23(1):23–8. https://doi.org/10.1016/j.nut.2006.10.003.
61. Hill DJ, Hudson IL, Sheffield LJ, Shelton MJ, Menahem S, Hosking CS. A low allergen diet is a significant intervention in infantile colic: results of a community-based study. J Allergy Clin Immunol. 1995;96(6 Pt 1):886–92.
62. Jakobsson I, Lothe L, Ley D, Borschel MW. Effectiveness of casein hydrolysate feedings in infants with colic. Acta Paediatr. 2000;89(1):18–21.
63. Lucassen PLBJ, Assendelft WJJ, Gubbels JW, van Eijk JT, Douwes AC. Infantile colic: crying time reduction with a whey hydrolysate: a double-blind, randomized, placebo-controlled trial. Pediatrics. 2000;106(6):1349–54. https://doi.org/10.1542/peds.106.6.1349.
64. Heine RG. Gastroesophageal reflux disease, colic and constipation in infants with food allergy. Curr Opin Allergy Clin Immunol. 2006;6(3):220–5. https://doi.org/10.1097/01.all.0000225164.06016.5d.
65. Borrelli O, Mancini V, Thapar N, et al. Cow's milk challenge increases weakly acidic reflux in children with cow's milk allergy and gastroesophageal reflux disease. J Pediatr. 2012;161(3):476–481.e1. https://doi.org/10.1016/j.jpeds.2012.03.002.
66. Scott DR, Simon RA. Supraesophageal reflux: correlation of position and occurrence of acid reflux; effect of head-of-bed elevation on supine reflux. J Allergy Clin Immunol Pract. 2015. https://doi.org/10.1016/j.jaip.2014.11.019.
67. Piesman M, Hwang I, Maydonovitch C, Wong RKH. Nocturnal reflux episodes following the administration of a standardized meal. Does timing matter? Am J Gastroenterol. 2007;102(10):2128–34. https://doi.org/10.1111/j.1572-0241.2007.01348.x.
68. Kaltenbach T, Crockett S, Gerson LB. Are lifestyle measures effective in patients with gastroesophageal reflux disease? An evidence-based approach. Arch Intern Med. 2006;166(9):965–71. https://doi.org/10.1001/archinte.166.9.965.
69. Tolia V, Youssef NN, Gilger MA, Traxler B, Illueca M. Esomeprazole for the treatment of erosive esophagitis in children: an international, multicenter, randomized, parallel-group, double-blind (for dose) study. BMC Pediatr. 2010;10(1):41. https://doi.org/10.1186/1471-2431-10-41.
70. Faure C, Michaud L, Shaghaghi EK, et al. Lansoprazole in children: pharmacokinetics and efficacy in reflux oesophagitis. Aliment Pharmacol Ther. 2001;15(9):1397–402. https://doi.org/10.1046/j.1365-2036.2001.01076.x.
71. Omari TI, Haslam RR, Lundborg P, Davidson GP. Effect of omeprazole on acid gastroesophageal reflux and gastric acidity in preterm infants with pathological acid reflux. J Pediatr Gastroenterol Nutr. 2007;44(1):41–4. https://doi.org/10.1097/01.mpg.0000252190.97545.07.
72. Omari T, Davidson G, Bondarov P, Nauclér E, Nilsson C, Lundborg P. Pharmacokinetics and acid-suppressive effects of esomeprazole in infants 1-24 months old with symptoms of gastroesophageal reflux disease. J Pediatr Gastroenterol Nutr. 2007;45(5):530–7. https://doi.org/10.1097/MPG.0b013e31812e012f.
73. Moore DJ, Tao B, Lines DR, Hirte C, Heddle ML. Double-blind placebo-controlled trial of omeprazole in irritable infants with gastroesophageal reflux. J Pediatr. 2003. https://doi.org/10.1067/S0022-3476(03)00207-5.
74. Orenstein SR, Blumer JL, Faessel HM, et al. Ranitidine, 75 mg, over-the-counter dose: pharmacokinetic and pharmacodynamic effects in children with symptoms of gastro-oesophageal reflux. Aliment Pharmacol Ther. 2002;16(5):899–907. https://doi.org/10.1046/j.1365-2036.2002.01243.x.
75. Sutphen JL, Dillard VL. Effect of ranitidine on twenty-four-hour gastric acidity in infants. J Pediatr. 1989;114(3):472–4. https://doi.org/10.1016/s0022-3476(89)80576-1.

76. Hyman PE, Garvey TQ, Abrams CE. Tolerance to intravenous ranitidine. J Pediatr. 1987;110(5):794–6.
77. Orenstein SR, Shalaby TM, Devandry SN, et al. Famotidine for infant gastro-oesophageal reflux: a multi-centre, randomized, placebo-controlled, withdrawal trial. Aliment Pharmacol Ther. 2003;17(9):1097–107. https://doi.org/10.1046/j.1365-2036.2003.01559.x.
78. Jordan B, Heine RG, Meehan M, Catto-Smith AG, Lubitz L. Effect of antireflux medication, placebo and infant mental health intervention on persistent crying: a randomized clinical trial. J Paediatr Child Health. 2006;42(1-2):49–58. https://doi.org/10.1111/j.1440-1754.2006.00786.x.
79. Rosen R, Amirault J, Liu H, et al. Changes in gastric and lung microflora with acid suppression. JAMA Pediatr. 2014;168(10):932–7. https://doi.org/10.1001/jamapediatrics.2014.696.
80. Orenstein SR, Hassall E, Furmaga-Jablonska W, Atkinson S, Raanan M. Multicenter, double-blind, randomized, placebo-controlled trial assessing the efficacy and safety of proton pump inhibitor lansoprazole in infants with symptoms of gastroesophageal reflux disease. J Pediatr. 2009;154(4):514–520.e514. https://doi.org/10.1016/j.jpeds.2008.09.054.
81. Canani RB, Cirillo P, Roggero P, et al. Therapy with gastric acidity inhibitors increases the risk of acute gastroenteritis and community-acquired pneumonia in children. Pediatrics. 2006;117(5):e817–20. https://doi.org/10.1542/peds.2005-1655.
82. Dial S, Delaney JAC, Barkun AN, Suissa S. Use of gastric acid–suppressive agents and the risk of community-acquired Clostridium difficile–associated disease. JAMA. 2005;294(23):2989–95. https://doi.org/10.1001/jama.294.23.2989.
83. Trikha A, Baillargeon JG, Kuo Y-F, et al. Development of food allergies in patients with gastroesophageal reflux disease treated with gastric acid suppressive medications. Pediatr Allergy Immunol. 2013;24(6):582–8. https://doi.org/10.1111/pai.12103.
84. Wagner T, Burns JL. Anti-inflammatory properties of macrolides. Pediatr Infect Dis J. 2007. https://doi.org/10.1097/01.inf.0000253037.90204.9f.
85. Di Lorenzo C, Orenstein S. Fundoplication: friend or foe? J Pediatr Gastroenterol Nutr. 2002;34(2):117–24.
86. Berquist WE, Fonkalsrud EW, Ament ME. Effectiveness of Nissen fundoplication for gastroesophageal reflux in children as measured by 24-hour intraesophageal pH monitoring. J Pediatr Surg. 1981;16(6):872–5.
87. Fung KP, Seagram G, Pasieka J, Trevenen C, Machida H, Scott B. Investigation and outcome of 121 infants and children requiring Nissen fundoplication for the management of gastroesophageal reflux. Clin Invest Med. 1990;13(5):237–46.
88. Lundell L, Attwood S, Ell C, et al. Comparing laparoscopic antireflux surgery with esomeprazole in the management of patients with chronic gastro-oesophageal reflux disease: a 3-year interim analysis of the LOTUS trial. Gut. 2008;57(9):1207–13. https://doi.org/10.1136/gut.2008.148833.
89. Lee SL, Shabatian H, Hsu J-W, Applebaum H, Haigh PI. Hospital admissions for respiratory symptoms and failure to thrive before and after Nissen fundoplication. J Pediatr Surg. 2008;43(1):59–63; discussion 63-5. https://doi.org/10.1016/j.jpedsurg.2007.09.020.
90. Barnhart DC, Hall M, Mahant S, et al. Effectiveness of fundoplication at the time of gastrostomy in infants with neurological impairment. JAMA Pediatr. 2013;167(10):911–8. https://doi.org/10.1001/jamapediatrics.2013.334.
91. Goldin AB, Sawin R, Seidel KD, Flum DR. Do antireflux operations decrease the rate of reflux-related hospitalizations in children? Pediatrics. 2006;118(6):2326–33. https://doi.org/10.1542/peds.2006-2212.
92. Boesch RP, Acton JD. Outcomes of fundoplication in children with cystic fibrosis. J Pediatr Surg. 2007;42(8):1341–4. https://doi.org/10.1016/j.jpedsurg.2007.03.030.
93. Pegna V, Mickevičius A, Tsang C. How useful is antireflux surgery in lung transplant patients with gastroesophageal reflux? Medicina (Kaunas). 2014;50(6):318–22. https://doi.org/10.1016/j.medici.2014.11.006.
94. Vakil N. Review article: the role of surgery in gastro-oesophageal reflux disease. Aliment Pharmacol Ther. 2007;25(12):1365–72. https://doi.org/10.1111/j.1365-2036.2007.03333.x.

95. Rosen R. Gastroesophageal reflux in infants. JAMA Pediatr. 2014;168(1):83–9. https://doi.org/10.1001/jamapediatrics.2013.2911.
96. Heyland DK, Drover JW, MacDonald S, Novak F, Lam M. Effect of postpyloric feeding on gastroesophageal regurgitation and pulmonary microaspiration: results of a randomized controlled trial. Crit Care Med. 2001;29(8):1495–501.
97. Srivastava R, Downey EC, O'Gorman M, et al. Impact of fundoplication versus gastrojejunal feeding tubes on mortality and in preventing aspiration pneumonia in young children with neurologic impairment who have gastroesophageal reflux disease. Pediatrics. 2009;123(1):338–45. https://doi.org/10.1542/peds.2007-1740.
98. Lien HC, Chang CS, Yeh HZ. The effect of jejunal meal feeding on gastroesophageal reflux. Scand J Gastroenterol. 2001;36(4):343–6. https://doi.org/10.1080/00365520121289.
99. Wales PW, Diamond IR, Dutta S, et al. Fundoplication and gastrostomy versus image-guided gastrojejunal tube for enteral feeding in neurologically impaired children with gastroesophageal reflux. J Pediatr Surg. 2002;37(3):407–12. https://doi.org/10.1053/jpsu.2002.30849.
100. Misra S, Macwan K, Albert V. Transpyloric feeding in gastroesophageal-reflux-associated apnea in premature infants. Acta Paediatr. 2007;96(10):1426–9. https://doi.org/10.1111/j.1651-2227.2007.00442.x.

# Aspiration in the Elderly

## 22

Midori Miyagi and Satoru Ebihara

**Abstract**

In the elderly, even though many antibiotics were developed, pneumonia has still been one of the major causes of mortality. Especially aspiration pneumonia which is the main problem. Aspiration pneumonia whose onset mechanism is not only dysphagia but also the depression of the cough reflex. There are six main causes of dysphagia, one of them is discordance between respiration and swallowing. It is important problem in aspiration pneumonia. Respiration and swallowing have common points in anatomy and function. By the common points, if swallowing was detached from respiration, discordance between respiration and swallowing would occur, and then dysphagia would be caused immediately. Moreover swallowing and cough reflexes are recognized as airway protective reflexes and these are related with various brain functions. Brain functions are depressed by aging. Therefore in the elderly, swallowing and cough reflexes are depressed. When we think about the reactivation of swallowing and cough reflexes, it is important to think about the relationship between these reflex and brain functions. These days, anti-aspiration drugs are found by research focusing on the relationship between brain function and airway protective reflexes.

## Aspiration Pneumonia and the Onset Mechanism in the Elderly

In the elderly, even though many antibiotics were developed, pneumonia still has been one of the major causes of mortality [1]. Pneumonia is ranked highly as the cause of death in the countries with an aging population. The elderly show the delay

M. Miyagi · S. Ebihara (✉)
Department of Rehabilitation Medicine, Toho University Graduate School of Medicine, Tokyo, Japan
e-mail: satoru.ebihara@med.toho-u.ac.jp

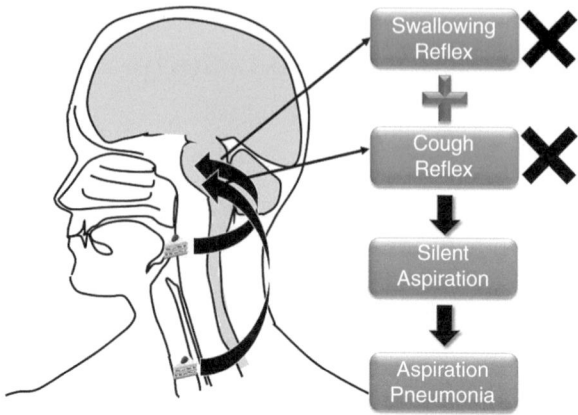

**Fig. 22.1** The crisis mechanism of aspiration pneumonia in the elderly. The elderly show the delay in swallowing reflex and impairment of cough reflex. The depression of both reflexes lead to aspiration pneumonia

in swallowing reflex and impairment of cough reflex. Both swallowing and cough reflexes are recognized as airway protective reflexes. The onset mechanism is not only dysphagia but also depression of cough reflex leading to aspiration pneumonia in the elderly [2] (Fig. 22.1).

## The Mechanism of Dysphagia in the Elderly

In the elderly, some difficulties lead to aspiration. There are six main difficulties. Firstly, shortage of larynx elevation leads to dysphagia. This phenomenon caused by fall of larynx position. Secondly, saliva and some bolus of food stay in the pharynx because of depression of constrictors of pharynx contraction power. Thirdly, dysfunction of pharyngeal constrictor leads failure of closing function of oropharynx. Fourthly, lack of teeth. The fifth, the depression of oropharynx sensory input is a factor of the sensory nerve [3]. Sixth, discordance between respiration and swallowing. This problem is very important in dysphagia.

## Discordance Between Respiration and Swallowing

Respiration and swallowing have common points in anatomy and function. On the anatomical structure, respiration central pattern generator (CPG) and swallowing CPG overlap in spinal cord and they have common sensory pathway in the pharynx [4]. If swallowing was detached from respiration, discordance between respiration and swallowing is seen, and then dysphagia is caused immediately. Normally when young people swallow something, they exhale [5]. But in the elderly, they inhale after swallowing. This discordance between respiration and swallowing leads to dysphagia. Respiration is stopped by swallowing in respiration phases. However the length until the onset of next inhalation phase becomes maximum is when the swallowing reflex occurs around switching over from inhalation phase to exhalation phase and the minimum when swallowing reflex occurred just before switching over from exhalation phase to inhalation phase [6]. The shorter the length until the onset of next inhalation phase, then the more danger of dysphagia. That is why dysphagia tends to start by the swallowing reflex occurring just before switching over from exhalation phase to inhalation phase.

## The Mechanism of Depression of Cough Reflex in the Elderly

In older people who have dysfunction of the insular cortex, primary sensory cortex, supplementary motor area, anterior midcingulate cortex, cerebellum, and orbitofrontal cortex, we observed depression of the cough reflex [7]. It suggests that the cough reflex is controlled by the cortex. In the previous study, the cough reflex is recognized as the medullary reflex. But nowadays we know about a new controller of the cough reflex. It is called 'urge-to-cough': going before the cough reflex which is a sensory signal input to the cortex and controls the cough reflex. The older people who depress the cough reflex show almost zero level of cough reflex sensitivity [8]. Moreover the cough reflex sensitivity is not depressed by only aging but also the urge-to-cough is depressed by aging [9].

These results disclose the mechanism of aspiration pneumonia. The mechanism has three steps which correspondence to depression of brain function with aging. First step is dysphagia, second step is lack of urge-to-cough and the third step is depression of cough reflex.

## Methods Against Aspiration Pneumonia in the Elderly

Reactivation of cough and swallowing reflexes is important in the treatment of aspiration pneumonia. Oral care is the most famous treatment for aspiration pneumonia. Bacteria locate around the teeth. If we clean this up, we can prevent the elderly getting aspiration pneumonia. Brushing stimulates oropharynx sensory inputs and this enhances efferent pathways of the swallowing reflex [10]. We can improve the elderly's swallowing reflex when adding a bolus of food and temperature stimulation to oropharynx [11]. Because elderly people who depress swallowing reflex also depress temperature sensitive function. For that reason there is a swallowing function delay when the elderly swallow the food with near to body temperature (30–40°). So meals have to be served at a variety of temperatures which is far from body temperatures [11]. Moreover, spices as the temperature-sensitive transient receptor potential (TRP) channel the agonist improved swallowing reflex. Because TRP is stimulated by spices [12] and TRP has six kinds of receptors and 4–6 are involved with the swallowing reflex [12]. The 4 receptors are TRPV1, TRPV2, TRPV8, and TRPA1. Especially TRPA1, if we give chronic or acute stimulation, the swallowing reflex is improved. Capsaicin gives chronic stimulation to TRPA1 [8, 13, 14].

However, there is no compensation for loss of consciousness or severe ADL depression in people with aspiration pneumonia. For these people, aroma-therapy using black pepper oil stimulate olfactory will improve the insular cortex function which is associated with the swallowing reflex, and increase in substance P which is the neurotransmitter of swallowing. As a result of these effects, the swallowing reflex is improved [15]. But it is difficult to have a smell of black pepper oil before every meal. Recently, black pepper oil aroma tips were developed which hang around the neck and the effect can last for a week. There are four other anti-aspiration drugs.

Cilostazol is usually used as an anti-platelet drug and shows increasing substance P and improvement of the swallowing reflex [16]. Amantadine is recognized for its improvement of dopaminergic system located in the basal ganglia and it also improves the swallowing reflex [17]. Theophylline is known as an adenosine A2 receptor antagonist. The adenosine A2 receptor is located in the dopaminergic nerve. Moreover it improves the dopaminergic system located in the basal ganglia and then the improvement of the swallowing reflex [18]. Angiotensin-converting Enzyme (ACE) Inhibitor increases not only angiotensin 1 but also substance P and improves the swallowing reflex [19–26].

## References

1. Ebihara S. Thermal taste and anti-aspiration drugs: a novel drug discovery against pneumonia. Curr Pharm Des. 2014;20:2755.
2. Nakajoh K, Nakagawa T, Sekizawa K, Matsui T, Arai H, Sasaki H. Relation between incidence of pneumonia and protective reflexes in poset-stroke patients with oral or tube feeding. J Intern Med. 2000;247:39–42.
3. Ebihara S. Frontiers in molecular therapy for aspiration pneumonia: from pharyngeal sensory receptor to lymphangiogenic factors. Folia Pharmacol Jpn. 2015;145:283.
4. Oku Y. Deglutition. Physiol Rev. 2013;2(Pt 1):47–52.
5. Shaker R, et al. Coordination of deglutition and phases of respiration: effect of sging, tachypnea, bolus volume, and chronic obstructive pulmonary disease. Am J Physiol. 1992;263:G750–5.
6. Paydarfar D, et al. Respiratory phase resetting and airflow changes induced by swallowing in humans. J Physiol. 1995;483(Pt 1):273–88.
7. Ebihara S, Ebihara T, Kanezaki M, Gui P, Yamasaki M, Arai H, Kohzuki M. Aging deterionated perception of urge-to-cough without changing cough reflex threshold to citric acid in female never-smokers. Cough. 2011;7:3.
8. Ebihara T, Sekizawa K, Nakazawa H, Sasaki H. Capsaicin and swallowing reflex. Lancet. 1993;341(8842):432.
9. Yamanda S, Ebihara S, Ebihara T, Yamasaki M, Asamura T, Asada M, Une K, Arai H. Impaired urge-to-cough in elderly patients with aspiration pneumonia. Cough. 2008;4:11.
10. Yoshino A, Ebihara T, Ebihara S, Fuji H, Sasaki H. Daily oral care and risk factors for pneumonia among elderly nursing home patients. JAMA. 2001;286(18):2235–6.
11. Ebihara S, Ebihara T. Cough in the elderly: a novel strategy for preventing aspiration pneumonia. Pulm Pharmacol Ther. 2011;24:318–23.
12. Ebihara S, Ebihara T, Masahiro K. Effect of aging on cough and swallowing reflexes: implications for aspiration pneumonia. Lung. 2012;190:29–33.
13. Watando A, Ebihara S, Ebihara T, Okazaki T, Takahashi H, Asada M, et al. Daily oral care and cough reflex sensitivity in elderly nursing home patients. Chest. 2004;126(4):1066–70.

14. Ebihara T, Takahashi H, Ebihara S, Okazaki T, Sasaki T, Watando A, Nemoto M, Sasaki H. Capsaicin troch for swalloing dysfunction in older people. J Am Geriatr Soc. 2005;53:824–8.
15. Ebihara T, Ebihara S, Maruyama M, Kobayashi M, Itou A, Takahashi H, Arai H, Sasaki H. A randomized trial of olfactory stimulation using black pepper oil in older people with swallowing dysfunction. J Am Geriatr Soc. 2006;54:1401–6.
16. Teramoto S, Yamamoto H, Yamaguchi Y, et al. Antiplatelet cilostazol, an inhibitor of type III phosphodiesterase, improves swallowing function in patients with a history of stroke. J Am Geriatr Soc. 2008;56:1153–4.
17. Kobayashi H, Nakagawa T, Sekizawa K, Arai H, Sasaki H. Levodopa and swallowing reflex. Lancet. 1996;348:1320–1.
18. Ebihara T, Ebihara S, Okazaki T, et al. Theophylline-improved swallowing reflex in elderly nursing home patients. J Am Geriatr Soc. 2004;52:1787–8.
19. Yamaya M, Yanai M, Ohrui T, Arai H, Sasaki H. Interventions to prevent pneumonia among older adults. J Am Geriatr Soc. 2001;49:85–90.
20. Kaplan R, Psaty B. ACE-inhibitor therapy and nosocomial pneumonia. Am J Hypertens. 1999;12:1161–2.
21. Sekizawa K, Matsui T, Nakagawa T, Nakayama K, Sasaki H. ACE inhibitors and pneumonia. Lancet. 1998;352:1069.
22. Arai T, Yasuda Y, Takaya T, et al. ACE inhibitors and reduction of the risk of pneumonia in elderly people. Am J Hypertens. 2000;13:1050–1.
23. Arai T, Yasuda Y, Takaya T, et al. Angiotensin-converting enzyme inhibitors, angiotensin-II receptor antagonists, and pneumonia in elderly hypertensive patients with stroke. Chest. 2001;119:660–1.
24. Arai T, Yasuda Y, Toshima S, Yoshimi N, Kashiki Y. ACE inhibitors and pneumonia in elderly people. Lancet. 1998;352:1937–8.
25. Okaishi K, Morimoto S, Fukuo K, et al. Reduction of risk of pneumonia associated with use of angiotensin I converting enzyme inhibitors in elderly inpatients. Am J Hypertens. 1999;12:778–83.
26. Ohkubo T, Chapman N, Neal B, Woodward M, Omae T, Chalmers J, Perindopril Protection Against Recurrent Stroke Study Collaborative Group. Effects of an angiotensin-converting enzyme inhibitor-based regimen on pneumonia risk. Am J Respir Crit Care Med. 2004;169:1041–5.

# Part V
# Therapy of Airway Reflux

# Acid Suppression for Management of Gastroesophageal Reflux Disease: Benefits and Risks

## 23

Carmelo Scarpignato and Luigi Gatta

## Introduction

Gastro-esophageal reflux (i.e. the reflux of gastric contents into the esophagus, GER) is a physiological phenomenon, occurring in everybody, especially after large and fat meals. Under physiologic conditions, efficient esophageal clearing mechanisms return most of the refluxed material to the stomach and symptoms do not occur [1]. However, when the reflux of gastric contents is large or aggressive enough, it causes symptoms and/or complications and impairs quality of life, giving rise to GER disease (GERD) [2]. According to the Montreal definition [3], GERD is a chronic condition which develops when the reflux of stomach contents causes troublesome and recurrent symptoms (which could be typical, i.e. esophageal or/and atypical, i.e. extra-esophageal), and/or complications, which include esophagitis, ulcer, stricture and Barrett's esophagus.

GERD is a highly prevalent disorder in Western Europe, North and South America, as its predominant symptom, heartburn, can occur once a week in up to 26% of the general population [4]. Despite geographical variations (Fig. 23.1), the prevalence of GERD is increasing worldwide.

Over the past decade, it has been realized that there are two different phenotypes of the disease. Some patients present esophageal mucosal lesions (i.e. erosive esophagitis), but the majority (up to 70%) have a macroscopically normal mucosa

---

C. Scarpignato (✉)
Clinical Pharmacology and Digestive Pathophysiology Unit, Department of Clinical and Experimental Medicine, University of Parma, Parma, Italy
e-mail: scarpi@tin.it

L. Gatta
Clinical Pharmacology and Digestive Pathophysiology Unit, Department of Clinical and Experimental Medicine, University of Parma, Parma, Italy

Gastroenterology and Endoscopy Unit, Versilia Hospital, Azienda USL Toscana Nord Ovest, Lido di Camaiore, Italy

© Springer International Publishing AG, part of Springer Nature 2018
A. H. Morice, P. W. Dettmar (eds.), *Reflux Aspiration and Lung Disease*,
https://doi.org/10.1007/978-3-319-90525-9_23

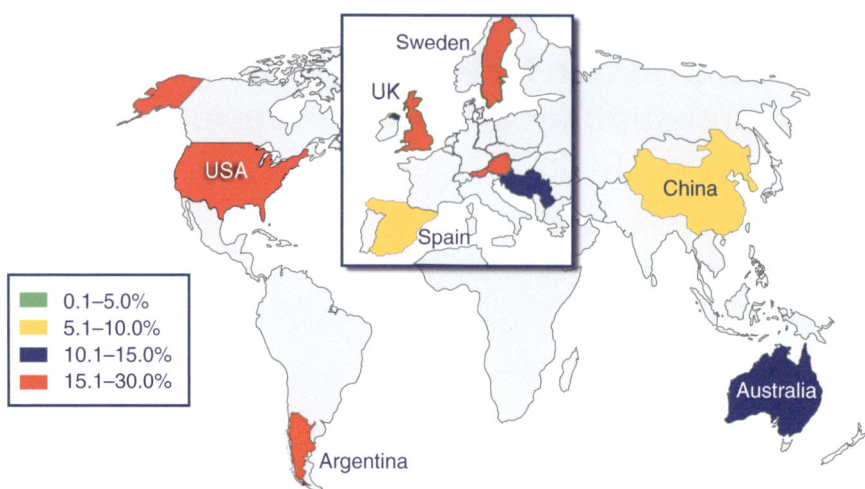

**Fig. 23.1** Global variation in the prevalence of GERD, defined as occurrence of at least weakly heartburn and/or regurgitation (from El-Serag et al. [4])

at endoscopy. Such patients are usually considered to have non-erosive reflux disease (NERD) [3, 5].

## Medical Management of GERD

Symptoms are crucial to the diagnosis of typical GERD and represent the main therapeutic target. Despite the symptom pattern does not allow to differentiate the erosive disease from NERD [6], patients seek medical assistance because of symptoms and ask for quick symptom relief.

The aims of GERD therapy are therefore the following [7, 8]:

- Symptom relief, with consequent improvement of quality of life
- Healing of esophageal lesions
- Prevention of recurrences (both symptomatic and endoscopic) and of complications

GERD is primarily a motor disorder and its pathogenesis is multifactorial (Fig. 23.2) [9]. The main motility abnormalities include an impaired function of the lower esophageal sphincter (LES), an abnormal esophageal clearance, and a delayed gastric emptying in up to 40% of cases. The presence of hiatal hernia favors reflux, but this association is not mandatory. The ultimate consequence of the above motor abnormalities is the presence of acid in the wrong place (i.e. in contact with the esophageal mucosa) [10]. In addition, the amount of reflux increases markedly after meals both in healthy subjects and GERD patients, an event almost exclusively due to the increase of transient (inappropriate) LES relaxations by meal-induced gastric

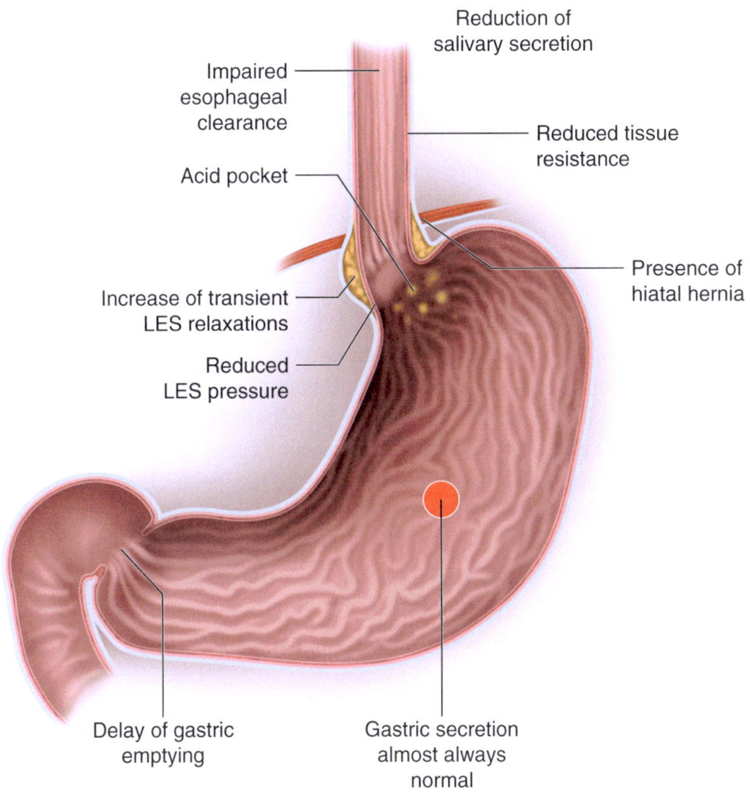

**Fig. 23.2** Pathophysiology of GERD (modified from Scarpignato and Savarino [9])

accommodation. Despite the buffering content of food, the pH of the material refluxed into the distal esophagus is very acidic due to the presence of an "acid pocket", which occurs in both healthy subjects and GERD patients. It represents an area of unbuffered gastric acid that accumulates in the proximal stomach after meals and serves as a reservoir for acid reflux [11]. The abnormal esophageal exposure to acid, on the other hand, is not secondary to gastric acid hypersecretion, which has been documented in only a small subset of GERD patients [10]. All the above pathophysiological mechanisms are exaggerated in obese subjects [12, 13].

Current pharmacologic approaches to address this clinically challenging condition are limited. Reflux inhibitors represent a promise unfulfilled, effective prokinetics are lacking and antidepressants, despite being effective in selected patients, give rise to adverse events in up to 32% of patients [14–17]. Antisecretory drugs ($H_2$-receptor antagonists, $H_2$RAs, and proton pump inhibitors, PPIs) remain

**Table 23.1** Antisecretory drugs: pharmacology and safety of H2RAs and PPIs (from Scarpignato et al. [18])

|  | H$_2$RAs | PPIs |
|---|---|---|
| Target cell | Parietal cell | Parietal cell |
| Target receptor | H$_2$-receptor | H$^+$/K$^+$-ATPase |
| Pharmacodynamic effects | ↓ GAS & ↓ EEA | ↓ GAS & ↓ EEA |
| Onset of action | Quick | Delayed |
| Duration of action | Short | Long |
| Tolerance development | Yes | No |
| Safety | Excellent | Excellent |

*GAS* gastric acid secretion, *EEA* esophageal exposure to acid

therefore the mainstay of medical treatment for GERD. They act indirectly by reducing the amount and concentration of gastric secretion available for reflux (Table 23.1), thus lessening the aggressive power of the refluxed material [7, 18]. PPIs also reduce the size of the acid pocket and increase the pH (from 1 to 4) of its content [11]. The clinical efficacy of these drugs has been clearly shown in many studies and the superiority of PPIs over H$_2$RAs has been established beyond doubt [19]. The greater pharmacodynamic effect of PPIs depends on their ability to block the final step in the production of acid, regardless the secretory stimulus. Moreover, PPIs are relatively more effective during the daytime than the nighttime and this leads to a better control of post-prandial reflux events [19].

## Efficacy of PPIs in GERD

Eight-week therapy with standard (once daily) dose PPIs can achieve healing of reflux esophagitis in more than 80% of patients [20], a rate depending on the severity of mucosal lesions [21, 22]. This healing rate can be further improved by doubling the PPI dose (NNT = 25) [20]. Meta-analyses have shown that—when compared to omeprazole, lansoprazole and pantoprazole—esomeprazole achieves the highest healing rates of reflux esophagitis in the short-term [21–23]. The more favorable clinical benefit of esomeprazole appears negligible in less severe esophagitis (A & B according to the Los Angeles classification [24, 25]), but it might be important in more severe disease [22]. Vonoprazan, a member of the new generation *reversible* PPIs (called potassium-competitive acid blockers, P-CABs), is able to achieve higher intragastric pH, effectively controlling both daytime and nighttime acid secretion [26], As a consequence, it proved to be capable of healing almost 100% of severe (C & D) esophagitis [27], a benefit also maintained during the remission phase [28].

It is worth mentioning that currently available PPI regimens do not provide the same control of intragastric pH, evaluated both in terms of mean pH over the 24 h and percentage time spent at pH >4. This has been repeatedly demonstrated in patients with GERD or taking NSAIDs [29]. A large meta-analysis [30], including 57 studies measuring intragastric pH after different PPI regimens, found that the relative potencies of the five compounds, compared to omeprazole, were 0.23, 0.90, 1.60, and 1.82 for pantoprazole, lansoprazole, esomeprazole, and rabeprazole, respectively. This lack of pharmacodynamic equivalence should be taken into account when switching from a given PPI to another.

PPIs are effective in obtaining symptom relief in both erosive and non-erosive disease [31]. Their efficacy for the relief of regurgitation is however modest, and considerably lower than that achieved for heartburn [32]. The myth that PPIs are less effective in NERD has recently been dispelled by a meta-analysis [33], showing that—when a functional investigation (pH-metry or pH-impedance-recording) is added to a negative endoscopy to objectively confirm this condition—the estimated complete symptom response rate after PPI therapy is comparable to that observed in patients with erosive disease.

NERD is however an umbrella term, including at least 4 different patient subgroups [34], of whom only those where acid is implicated in symptom generation (i.e. true NERD and patients with acid hypersensitive esophagus) are clearly responsive to PPIs (Fig. 23.3) [35]. This is not the case of patients who are hypersensitive to nonacidic reflux or those with functional heartburn. According to Rome IV criteria [36], both acid hypersensitive esophagus (now called *reflux hypersensitivity*) and functional heartburn are functional GI disorders, which should be no longer included in GERD. The lack of abnormal acid exposure and symptom-reflux association makes patients with functional heartburn not responsive to PPIs. This subgroup of subjects may benefit of visceral analgesics (e.g. antidepressants) [16].

Although not as frequent as previously suggested, PPI-refractory heartburn, occurring more commonly in NERD than in erosive disease, does exist however. Some 20% (range 15–27%) of correctly diagnosed and *appropriately* treated

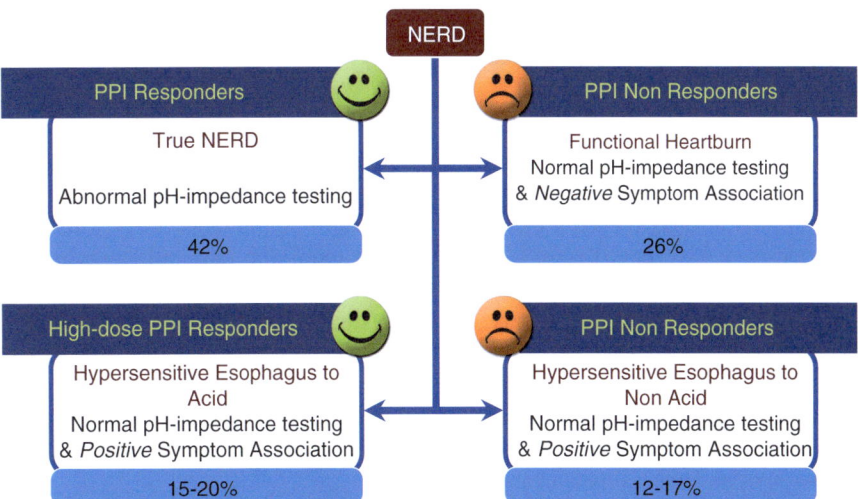

**Fig. 23.3** Subgroups of NERD patients and their response to PPIs: lessons from pH-impedance monitoring (from Scarpignato [35])

patients do not respond to PPI therapy at standard doses [37]. To ascertain whether they are "truly" PPI-resistant, compliance and adherence to treatment should be checked. Indeed, PPIs are often taken inappropriately, with only 27% of GERD patients dosing their PPI correctly and only 12% dosing it optimally in a USA survey [38]. Although a standard PPI dose can occasionally control symptoms, nocturnal intragastric acidity often remains elevated (with Nocturnal Acid Breakthrough, NAB) in these patients. A split regimen (either standard or double dose) of PPIs b.i.d. (before breakfast and before evening meal) provides superior acid control. In patients with persistent nocturnal symptoms, the addition of an $H_2RA$ at bedtime may be indicated to control NAB and associated esophageal acidification [35, 39–41], despite the likely development of tolerance to $H_2RA$ [42]. The majority of patients, however, reported persistent improvement in GERD symptoms from nighttime $H_2RA$ use [40]. To reduce the development of tolerance, on demand or cyclic dosing may be preferable, but this approach has not been specifically studied.

## PPIs for Maintenance of GERD

GERD and NERD are chronic, relapsing diseases. Six months after cessation of treatment, symptomatic relapse is rapid and frequent (i.e. in 90% of endoscopy-positive and 75% of endoscopy-negative patients [6]). PPIs, both at a full and half dose, are able to maintain patients in remission, with a superior efficacy of the full dose (NNT = 9.1) [43]. Esomeprazole 20 mg is the only step-down dose PPI able to maintain in symptomatic remission a significantly higher proportion of GERD patients compared to lansoprazole 15 mg [23, 44] or pantoprazole 20 mg [23].

Since PPIs do not correct the underlying pathophysiological motor abnormalities responsible for GERD, a continuous treatment is required to maintain all patients in remission. In the LOTUS trial [45], comparing long-term esomeprazole therapy with anti-reflux surgery (ARS), the estimated remission rate at 5 years was 92%, higher than that (57%) reported with omeprazole in the SOPRAN study [46]. However, while the PPI dose in the SOPRAN trial was fixed, in the LOTUS investigation, patients whose reflux symptoms were not adequately controlled by a standard maintenance regimen (i.e., esomeprazole, 20 mg/ddaily) were allowed to increase the dosage to 40 mg once daily and then to 20 mg twice daily. This dose titration may have contributed to the improved remission rate and suggests that long-term maintenance therapy should be individualized. Indeed, the number and severity of relapses are highly variable amongst patients. Infrequent reflux symptoms are less likely to be chronic and may respond to different management strategies. There are basically three different long-term approaches for GERD treatment with PPIs (Fig. 23.4): continuous (i.e. every day), intermittent (i.e. cycles of daily PPI administration) or *on-demand* (i.e. symptom-driven) therapy, each selected on the basis of patients' clinical characteristics [47].

One third of patients, submitted for fundoplication, are reported to take acid-lowering compounds (mostly PPIs) after anti-reflux surgery, but only few studies have specified whether drug use was on a regular or occasional basis [48]. A

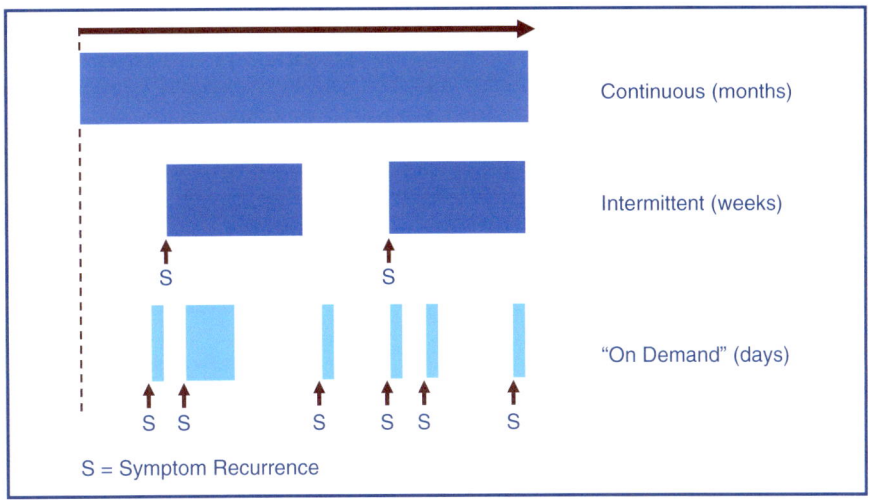

**Fig. 23.4** Long-term management strategies in GERD (from Bruley des Varannes et al. [47])

meta-analysis of RCTs [49] found that—after anti-reflux surgery—14% of patients still require antisecretory drugs. This figure increases with the duration of follow-up and up to one third of patients required antisecretory drugs after 10 years. The data from non-randomized studies [50], which are higher than the estimation provided by randomized studies (i.e. 20% of patients under acid suppression), are probably more representative of the current clinical practice.

Although medication use is often considered as an outcome measure for successful antireflux surgery, some studies have shown that antisecretory drug use does not correlate with true recurrent reflux in most patients [48], and does not necessarily indicate a failure of the procedure. A significant proportion of patients taking medications after operation are using them to relieve *non-reflux symptoms* and only one third of patients displays an abnormal esophageal exposure to acid after surgery [48]. Therefore, many patients take PPIs despite the lack of objective evidence of GERD on esophageal testing. The causes of persistent symptoms after surgery remain unclear. Non-GERD symptoms might be due to increased esophageal sensitivity while other symptoms (like bloating, early satiety and nausea) may be unmasked when reflux symptoms improve [51–53]. A careful selection of patients and thorough follow-up is needed to avoid unnecessary acid suppression in post-surgical patients.

Before embarking on long-term treatment, an attempt to stop acid suppression must always be considered. Of the various interventions (patient's education, lifestyle modifications, abrupt withdrawal and tapering), tapering is the more effective discontinuation strategy [54]. Abrupt withdrawal might be followed by rebound acid hypersecretion and exacerbation of symptoms [55], a finding observed however in healthy subjects but not in GERD patents [55]. Weight loss appears to be another strategy in obese/overweight patients (Fig. 23.5). Indeed, in one study, up to

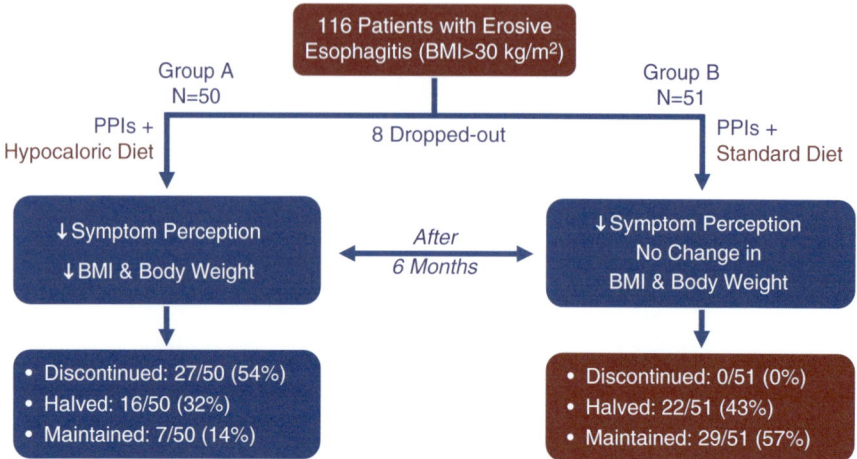

**Fig. 23.5** Reduction of symptoms as well as of PPI use and dose by weight loss in obese patients with GERD (drawn from data in de Bortoli et al. [56])

54% of subjects compliant to a hypocaloric diet were able to stop PPI therapy, with an additional 32% being able to halve the dose [56]. All the above attempts should be considered also in patients who are already on long-term acid suppression.

Continuous maintenance therapy is indicated in patients with Barrett's esophagus of any mucosal length, owing to the potential chemopreventive activity of PPIs against neoplastic transformation, a property advocated by the ACG [57] and AGA [58] but denied by the BSG guidelines [59]. Indeed, a recent meta-analysis of observational studies showed that PPI use is associated with a 71% reduction in risk of esophageal adenocarcinoma and/or high-grade dysplasia in this patient population (adjusted OR 0.29) [60]. Despite a contrary opinion of the AGA [58], current evidence suggests that standard PPI therapy is unable to normalize esophageal exposure to acid in the vast majority of patients with Barrett's esophagus. Profound and individually tailored maximal acid suppression is needed not only to control GER, but also in the hope to achieve a better chemopreventive effect [61].

In all those patients with GERD, requiring long-term PPI therapy, *H. pylori* should be sought and—if present—eradicated, particularly in young patients. This approach, recommended by international guidelines [62, 63], is needed to prevent the development of atrophic gastritis or worsening of any preexisting one, with potential for neoplastic transformation [64]. However, in accordance with the Food and Drug Administration (FDA), ACG guidelines [65] do not recommend *routine* screening for or treatment of *H. pylori* infection in GERD patients (strong recommendation, low level of evidence).

## PPIs for Extra-Digestive GERD

Typical GERD symptoms include heartburn and acid regurgitation. However, extra-esophageal manifestations of GERD, such as cough, laryngitis, asthma and even dental erosions also occur. Over the last 2 decades, these conditions, often called extra-esophageal, or better, extra-digestive manifestations of GERD, have gained increasing attention. In the ProGERD study, involving 6215 patients with heartburn, the prevalence of extra-esophageal symptom was 32.8%. Chest pain was the most frequent complaint (14.5%), followed by chronic cough (13%), laryngeal disorders (10.4%) and asthma (4.8%) [66]. It is worth mentioning that the costs of managing patients with suspected extra-digestive GERD has been estimated to be over 5 times that of patients with typical GERD symptoms [67].

During the Montreal meeting [3], four key principles regarding the extra-esophageal syndromes with established associations were emphasized:

1. An association between GERD and the manifestations of these syndromes exists;
2. These syndromes rarely occur in isolation without concomitant manifestations of the typical esophageal syndrome;
3. These syndromes are usually multifactorial, with GERD as one of several potential aggravating factors;
4. Data supporting a significant benefit of anti-reflux therapy for these syndromes are weak.

Although some symptoms may well be related to extra-digestive GERD, there is currently an *overdiagnosis* of GERD as the major contributing factor to the extra-esophageal syndromes. Patients with suspected extra-digestive GERD are usually referred to gastroenterologists - often without other manifestations of GERD—from ENT physicians, respirologists, cardiologists and primary care physicians.

The diagnosis of extra-digestive GERD is difficult due to the lack of gold standard diagnostic criteria for extra-digestive symptoms. Functional investigations and upper GI endoscopy are not always adequate diagnostic tools to definitively establish a causal link between reflux patterns and patients' chronic symptoms [68–70]. For this reason, empirical PPI therapy is recommended as an initial approach to diagnose and treat the potential underlying cause of these extra-esophageal symptoms. Diagnostic testing with naso-laryngoscopy, esophago-gastro-duodenoscopy and 24-h esophageal pH-impedance monitoring is usually reserved for those who continue to be symptomatic despite initial empiric trial of PPI therapy.

Conversely from typical symptoms, the efficacy of PPIs on extra-esophageal manifestations of GERD is uncertain. This uncertainty could result, at least in part, from the available studies, which are not homogenous, with differences in patient selection, end-point considered, drug used and regimen adopted. In addition, since extra-digestive symptoms may need higher PPI dose and clinical improvement may take a longer time to occur, only properly designed trials would be able to unravel a clinical response. Unfortunately, however, this has not always been the case.

The efficacy of PPIs in non-cardiac chest pain (NCCP) and extra-digestive GERD is disappointing. In these clinical conditions, PPIs are usually given twice daily and for extended periods (i.e. 3 or more months). However, evidence is often lacking and, where available, not strong enough to allow clear recommendations to be made.

GERD being the most common and best-studied cause of NCCP, acid suppression is the initial pharmacological approach in this patient population. A systematic review showed that patients with endoscopic or pH-monitoring evidence of GERD tend to improve, but not resolve, with PPI therapy, whereas GERD-negative patients display little or no response [32], a result confirmed by a more recent meta-analysis [71]. PPIs might also improve symptoms related to atrial fibrillation and other supra-ventricular arrhythmias, especially after meal, in patients with proven GERD [72].

Despite the negative conclusions of a Cochrane meta-analysis [73], a recent review [74] suggests that a therapeutic benefit for acid-suppressive therapy in patients with chronic cough cannot be dismissed, advocating a rigorous patient selection that could allow the identification of patient subgroups likely to be responsive. On the contrary, no systematic reviews and meta-analyses [75–80] found any significant clinical benefit of PPI therapy over placebo in reflux laryngitis.

Asthma and GERD can often coexist, with reflux disease being reported in 40–80% of patients with asthma. While asthma medications can trigger GERD [81, 82], PPIs might on the contrary improve asthma control. Here again, an early Cochrane review [83] showed no benefit of PPI therapy on nocturnal symptom score and lung function, but a recent meta-analysis [73]—by selecting the morning peak expiratory flow (PEF) rate as primary outcome—disclosed a benefit of PPIs over placebo, which was greater in patients with proven GERD.

Despite the widespread use of PPIs in dental practice to manage the oral manifestations of GERD [84], treatment of dental erosions represents the only *objectively* documented clinical use [85].

## Management of Extra-Digestive GERD: The Way Forward

A careful analysis of the available literature clearly shows that the efficacy of PPIs in extra-digestive GERD is less consistent than that observed in patients with typical symptoms. A synopsis of effectiveness and failure of PPIs in extra-esophageal manifestation of GERD is presented in Fig. 23.6.

In extra-digestive GERD, the complexity of patient presentation is matched only by the challenge in making an appropriate diagnosis of reflux as the cause for the patients' complaints. Upper GI endoscopy and pH-impedance monitoring suffer from poor sensitivity while laryngoscopy suffers from poor specificity in diagnosing reflux in this group of patients [68]. An empiric trial of PPIs could be the initial approach to diagnose and treat the potential underlying cause of these extra-digestive

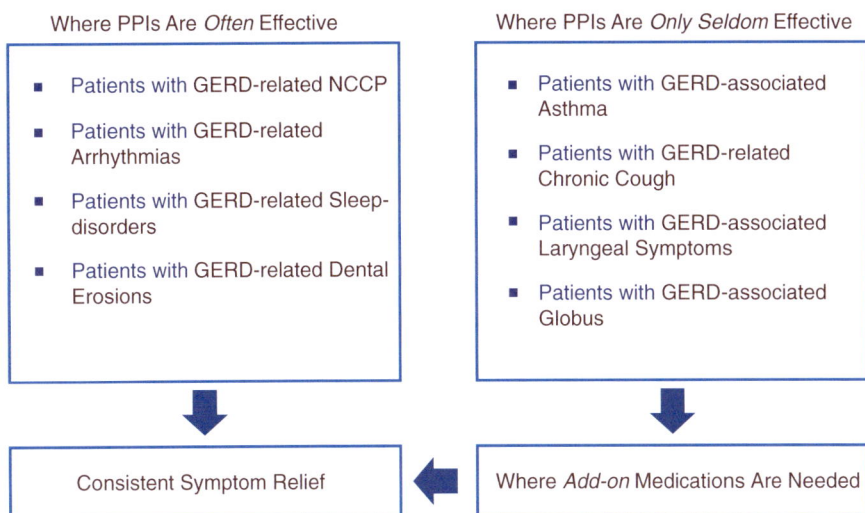

**Fig. 23.6** Effectiveness and failure of acid suppression in extra-digestive GERD

symptoms. Symptom resolution usually needs higher PPI dose and longer treatment time than those adopted in patients with typical GERD [86]. However, it is important to highlight that PPI therapy in extra-digestive GERD and twice daily dosing are both unapproved indications for these agents but one that is recommended by both GI [65, 87] and other specialty guidelines [88–90].

For patients, who improve with PPIs, GERD is presumed to be the most important etiological factor, but for those who do not respond, diagnostic testing with pH-impedance monitoring are reasonable to typically exclude continued acid or weakly acidic reflux. If this is the case, etiologies other than GERD should be pursued. However, there is increasing evidence suggesting that—in patients with proven GERD—PPIs alone may not suffice and the use of *add-on* medications can achieve a higher success rate (Table 23.2). Even with higher PPI doses and a longer duration of therapy, the response of patients with extra-digestive symptoms can be substantially less than that of patients with typical GERD symptoms. This may be due to the inclusion in the study cohorts of non-GERD patients or related to the exquisite sensitivity of the supra-esophageal structures to damage from even a small amount of acid. As outlined by Hunt [91], the currently adopted criteria for mucosal acid exposure are too insensitive with respect to symptoms. The Johnson–De Meester criteria (% time of pH <4 for >4.2% of the time) give equal weight to solutions of pH 4 and pH 1, despite a 1000-fold difference in $H^+$ concentration. In addition, at the cut-off of pH 4, the $H^+$ concentration can still be sufficient to damage supra-esophageal tissues while being less harmful for the distal esophageal mucosa. Last but not least, the pathogenesis of extra-digestive GERD is multifactorial and hence *isolated* acid suppression may not be effective, relegating the underlying cause(s) as being non-GERD related.

**Table 23.2** *Add-on* medications for the treatment of laryngo-pharyngeal reflux

| Authors, Year | Ref. | Compound | Symptoms and signs |
|---|---|---|---|
| Ezzat et al., 2011 | [93] | Itopride | Better improvement with combined therapy |
| Chun and Lee, 2013 | [94] | Itopride | Better improvement with combined therapy |
| Dabirmoghaddam et al., 2013 | [96] | N-acetylcysteine | Better improvement with combined therapy |
| Lieder and Issing, 2011 | [98] | Gaviscon® advance | Better improvement with combined therapy |
| Strugala and Dettmar, 2010 | [99] | Gaviscon® advance | Better improvement with combined therapy |

Although a recent systematic review does not recommend prokinetics as a treatment option for laryngo-pharyngeal reflux (LPR) [92], some studies found a better symptomatic improvement in patients with LPR [93, 94] or in those with GERD-related chronic cough [95] when a prokinetic was added to PPI therapy.

A randomized, placebo-controlled, double–blinded study [96] evaluated the effect of N-acetylcysteine (NAC, 600 mg daily), a mucolytic agent, combined with omeprazole (20 mg twice daily) in patients with LPR. After 3-month treatment, combined treatment achieved a significantly better improvement of objective (laryngoscopic findings) and subjective (both reflux symptom index, RSI, and reflux symptom score, RSS) findings.

In patients with LPR, alginate-containing formulations (e.g. Gaviscon® Advance) are able to achieve a significant improvement in symptom scores and clinical findings either alone [97] or in combination with PPIs [98]. Compared to acid suppression alone, the combination of esomeprazole and Gaviscon® Advance attained a significantly better reduction of the reflux symptom index (RSI) [99]. The efficacy of alginates in extra-esophageal manifestations of GERD are likely due to its barrier effect, which translates into a reduction of the proximal migration of the refluxed gastric contents [100] and binding and inactivation of pepsin [101]. The concentration and mucosal damaging activity of pepsin are potentially very high in the (acidic or nonacidic) refluxate that can reach the upper airways [102]. A mucosal protection from pepsin (and acid as well) is exerted also by Esoxx™ One (a mixture of hyaluronic acid and chondroitin sulfate in a bioadhesive carrier) [103]. This class 3 medical device proved to be effective in patients with refractory GERD symptoms either alone [104] or in combination with PPIs [105]. A trial in patients with extra-esophageal manifestations of GERD is ongoing and results are eagerly awaited.

A suggested algorithm for the management of extra-digestive GERD is presented in Fig. 23.7, where anti-reflux surgery is also considered. Fundoplication, which is able to address almost all the underlying pathophysiology of GERD (Table 23.3) [106], could be a reasonable choice in patients with moderate-to-severe reflux (both gastro-esophageal and duodeno-gastro-esophageal) and large hiatal hernia as well as regurgitation despite PPI therapy, in whom volume reflux may be the cause for patients' continued symptoms.

**Fig. 23.7** Suggested flow-chart for the management of extra-digestive GERD

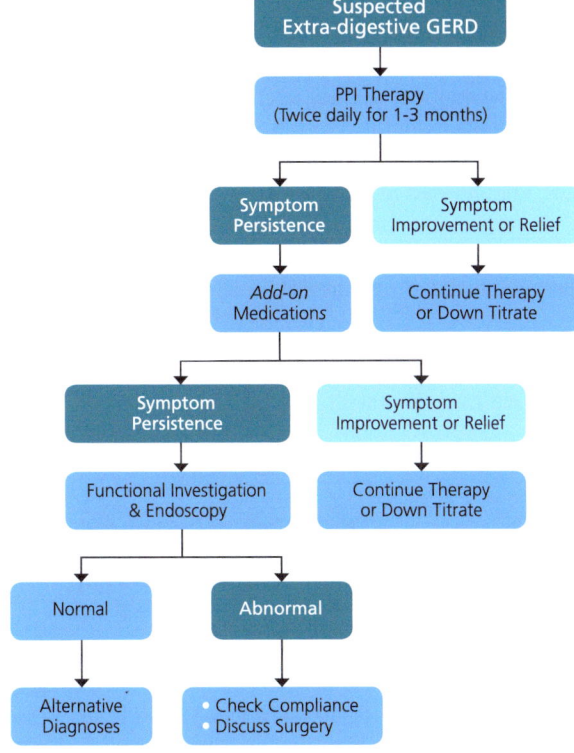

**Table 23.3** Management of GERD: comparative effects of medical and surgical therapies on the underlying pathophysiology (*modified from* Contini and Scarpignato [106])

|  | Antisecretory drugs | Prokinetic drugs | Anti-reflux surgery |
| --- | --- | --- | --- |
| Defective LES | 0 | ++ | +++ |
| Transient LESRs | 0 | + | +++ |
| Hiatal hernia | 0 | 0 | +++ |
| Impaired clearance | 0 | + | + (?) |
| Mucosal resistance | 0 | 0 | 0 |
| Acid-pepsin injury | +++ | + | +++ |
| DGE reflux | + | + (?) | +++ |
| Gastric emptying | 0 (−) | ++ | +++ |

*LES* lower esophageal sphincter, *DGE* duodeno-gastro-esophageal

## Safety Concerns with PPI Therapy

Although overuse and misuse may challenge the safety profile, the tolerability of PPIs has been remarkably good. Adverse events generally occur at a rate of 1–3%, without any significant differences among PPIs. Untoward effects most commonly include headaches, nausea, abdominal pain, constipation, flatulence, diarrhea, rash, and dizziness. Long-term studies indicate a tolerability profile similar to that found in short-term trials [107–110].

PPI-related adverse events involve the GI tract as well as other organs and systems. The majority of these events have been summarized in comprehensive reviews, to which the reader is referred [111–119]. The potential risks of long-term PPI therapy, along with the evidence summary and the recommendations for clinical practice, are outlined in Table 23.4.

Gastric pH is relevant for the absorption of several drugs and its modification by antisecretory therapy may significantly modify their pharmacokinetics [120]. PPIs also influence drug absorption and metabolism by interacting with adenosine

**Table 23.4** Summary of potential adverse effects of PPs and clinical recommendations (from Sheen and Triadafilopoulos [113])

| Theoretical risk | Evidence summary | Recommendations for clinical practice |
|---|---|---|
| *Nutritional deficiencies* | | |
| $B_{12}$ deficiency | Most patients consuming normal diet will not experience clinically significant $B_{12}$ deficiency. Elderly and malnourished patients at higher risk | Evidence does not justify routine screening |
| | | Screening may be reasonable for elderly or malnourished patients |
| Iron deficiency | Little data that long-term PPI use results in clinically significant iron deficiency | Evidence does not justify routine screening |
| | | Long-term PPI use does not result in clinically significant iron deficiency under normal clinical circumstances |
| | | Reduced iron absorption secondary to long-term PPI use may only be clinically significant in hemochromatosis and other iron overload states |
| Hypomagnesemia | <30 case reports published in peer-reviewed literature | Remain vigilant for unexplained hypomagnesemia, hypokalemia, or hypocalcemia in PPI users |
| Fracture risk | Inconsistent study results | Evidence does not justify routine pharmacologic prophylaxis or bone mineral density screening |
| | Possible that long-term PPI use in patients with risk factors for fracture may increase risk for certain fractures | Consider risks and benefits of long-term PPI therapy in patients with risk factors such as osteoporosis and steroid use |
| *Infections* | | |
| Community acquired pneumonia | No substantial increase in risk of community-acquired pneumonia after controlling for potential confounders | PPIs should not be withheld from patients with pulmonary disease if they have indications for treatment |

**Table 23.4** (continued)

| Theoretical risk | Evidence summary | Recommendations for clinical practice |
|---|---|---|
| | | Patients who are immunocompromised, elderly, smokers, and those with COPD or other risk factors for CAP should receive annual influenza vaccination |
| Enteric infections | Growing evidence that acid suppression increases risk of enteric infections by *C. difficile* and a variety of pathogens | Benefits and risks of long-term PPI therapy for inpatients who are immunocompromised or chronically ill should be weighed |
| | | PPI discontinuation should be considered in patients with life-threatening enteric infections without urgent indication for acid suppression |
| *Hypergastrinemia and malignancy* | | |
| Gastric polyps | Long-term PPI use is likely associated with increased frequency of fundic gland polyps (FGPs) in *H. pylori*-negative patients without familial adenomatous polyposis (FAP) | Majority of FGPs are benign, routine endoscopic surveillance or removal not indicated |
| | | FAP patients with FGPs may benefit from closer monitoring |
| Gastric cancer | No controlled human data supporting increased risk of gastric cancer from long-term PPI use | Maastricht consensus panel recommends *H. pylori* eradication before prolonged PPI use, while American College of Gastroenterology currently does not |
| | Acid suppression alters pattern of gastritis in *H. pylori*; unclear whether this increases gastric cancer risk | |
| Gastric carcinoids | No formal studies in humans, no studies showing increased risk of carcinoid development in any non-rat species | Risk does not justify altering current PPI prescribing practices or routine screening |
| Colon cancer | Clinical studies have not supported relationship between hypergastrinemia and increased risk of CRC | Risk does not justify altering current PPI prescribing or CRC screening practices |
| *Drug interactions* | | |
| Cytochrome $P_{450}$ interactions | Rare and usually clinically insignificant | Take note of established drug interactions and polypharmacy, monitor individual responses |
| Interactions with clopidogrel | Inconsistent study results | Consider risks and benefits of PPI therapy on an individual basis |
| Safety during pregnancy | Most studies have involved omeprazole; no significant association between omeprazole use and birth defects | Based on existing data, omeprazole appears to be safe during the first trimester of pregnancy |

triphosphate-dependent P-glycoprotein (e.g. inhibiting digoxin efflux) or with the cytochrome $P_{450}$ (CYP) enzyme system (e.g. decreasing simvastatin metabolism), thereby affecting both intestinal first-pass metabolism and hepatic clearance. A number of studies have shown that omeprazole (and, to a lesser extent, lansoprazole) carries a considerable potential for DDIs, since it has a high affinity for CYP2C19 and a somewhat lower affinity for CYP3A4. In contrast, pantoprazole and rabeprazole display a lower potential for drug-to-drug interactions (DDIs) [121, 122]. DDIs therefore represent a molecule-related effect rather than a class-effect [123].

These interactions are clinically relevant mostly for drugs with a narrow therapeutic index (e.g. diazepam, warfarin, antipsychotics, etc.) [121, 124]. In addition, PPIs metabolism is very rapid in most Caucasian subjects (extensive metabolizers), so that their half-life ranges from only 0.5 to 2.1 h [124]. Indeed, the prevalence of poor metabolizers, potentially at increased risk of drug interactions, is as low as 1.2–3.8% in Europe as compared to 23% in Asia [125]. This could explain why only few of the reported DDIs involving PPIs have been shown to be of clinical significance.

Recent studies have raised concerns about a possible adverse interaction between clopidogrel and PPIs (currently prescribed to patients, who are receiving dual antiplatelet therapy to prevent upper GI bleeding) that could reduce the antithrombotic effect of the former and, therefore, lessen protection against cardiovascular (CV) events in high-risk patients. However, current evidence shows that—while concomitant use of *some* PPIs with clopidogrel does attenuate the antiplatelet effect of clopidogrel—this effect is likely to be not clinically relevant [126–129]. Conversely, denying PPIs to patients at GI risk would result in increased life-threatening GI bleeding [130–132].

PPIs are among the most widely used prescription drugs. Although alarms have been raised about their long-term safety, the preponderance of the evidence does not strongly support the concerns, publicized over the last few years and the benefit to harm ratio remains favorable. Some adverse effects are plausible and predictable. Others are idiosyncratic, unpredictable, and rare.

The best available information on long-term safety of PPIs derives from the SOPRAN [46] and LOTUS [45] trials, comparing anti-reflux surgery with omeprazole or esomeprazole, respectively. Safety data were collected from patients during the 12-year period of the SOPRAN study (n = 298) and the 5-year period of the LOTUS study (n = 514). Serious adverse events and changes in laboratory parameters were analyzed. Across both studies, serious adverse events were reported at a similar frequency in the PPI and ARS treatment groups. Laboratory results, including routine hematology and tests for liver enzymes, electrolytes, vitamin D, vitamin $B_{12}$, folate and homocysteine, showed no clinically relevant changes over time. The only expected difference concerned gastrin and chromogranin A levels, which were elevated in the PPI group, with the greatest increases observed in the first year [133]. Despite a continued proliferative drive on enterochromaffin-like cells (ECL) during esomeprazole treatment, no dysplastic or neoplastic lesions were found [134].

Based on the quality of the overall evidence, the benefits of PPI treatment outweigh the potential risks in most patients, especially if PPI use is based on a relevant and appropriate indication [19, 135, 136]. On the contrary, patients treated without an appropriate therapeutic indication are *only* exposed to potential risks. Because PPIs are *overprescribed* in many patients, in particular for continued long-term use, the clinical effects should always be reviewed and justified attempts should be made to stop any therapy that may not be needed [115].

## References

1. Kahrilas PJ. GERD pathogenesis, pathophysiology, and clinical manifestations. Cleve Clin J Med. 2003;70(Suppl 5):S4–19.
2. Dent J, Brun J, Fendrick AM, et al. An evidence-based appraisal of reflux disease management—the Genval Workshop Report. Gut. 1999;44(Suppl 2):S1–16.
3. Vakil N, van Zanten SV, Kahrilas P, Dent J, Jones R, Global Consensus Group. The Montreal definition and classification of gastroesophageal reflux disease: a global evidence-based consensus. Am J Gastroenterol. 2006;101:1900–20; quiz 43.
4. El-Serag HB, Sweet S, Winchester CC, Dent J. Update on the epidemiology of gastro-oesophageal reflux disease: a systematic review. Gut. 2014;63:871–80.
5. Modlin IM, Hunt RH, Malfertheiner P, et al. Diagnosis and management of non-erosive reflux disease—the Vevey NERD Consensus Group. Digestion. 2009;80:74–88.
6. Carlsson R, Dent J, Watts R, et al. Gastro-oesophageal reflux disease in primary care: an international study of different treatment strategies with omeprazole. International GORD Study Group. Eur J Gastroenterol Hepatol. 1998;10:119–24.
7. Galmiche JP, Letessier E, Scarpignato C. Treatment of gastro-oesophageal reflux disease in adults. BMJ. 1998;316:1720–3.
8. Wang C, Hunt RH. Medical management of gastroesophageal reflux disease. Gastroenterol Clin N Am. 2008;37:879–99, ix.
9. Savarino V, Scarpignato C. Novità in tema di fisiopatologia della malattia da reflusso gastroesofageo—quale ruolo degli alginati nell'era degli inibitori della pompa protonica? Ther Perspect. 2011;14:1–37.
10. Boeckxstaens GE, Rohof WO. Pathophysiology of gastroesophageal reflux disease. Gastroenterol Clin N Am. 2014;43:15–25.
11. Kahrilas PJ, McColl K, Fox M, et al. The acid pocket: a target for treatment in reflux disease? Am J Gastroenterol. 2013;108:1058–64.
12. Anand G, Katz PO. Gastroesophageal reflux disease and obesity. Gastroenterol Clin N Am. 2010;39:39–46.
13. Chang P, Friedenberg F. Obesity and GERD. Gastroenterol Clin N Am. 2014;43:161–73.
14. Kahrilas PJ, Boeckxstaens G. Failure of reflux inhibitors in clinical trials: bad drugs or wrong patients? Gut. 2012;61:1501–9.
15. Looijer-van Langen M, Veldhuyzen van Zanten S. Does the evidence show that prokinetic agents are effective in healing esophagitis and improving symptoms of GERD? Open Med. 2007;1:e181–3.
16. Weijenborg PW, de Schepper HS, Smout AJ, Bredenoord AJ. Effects of antidepressants in patients with functional esophageal disorders or gastroesophageal reflux disease: a systematic review. Clin Gastroenterol Hepatol. 2015;13:251–59.e1.
17. Ford AC, Quigley EM, Lacy BE, et al. Effect of antidepressants and psychological therapies, including hypnotherapy, in irritable bowel syndrome: systematic review and meta-analysis. Am J Gastroenterol. 2014;109:1350–65; quiz 66.

18. Scarpignato C, Pelosini I, Di Mario F. Acid suppression therapy: where do we go from here? Dig Dis. 2006;24:11–46.
19. Savarino V, Di Mario F, Scarpignato C. Proton pump inhibitors in GORD. An overview of their pharmacology, efficacy and safety. Pharmacol Res. 2009;59:135–53.
20. Moayyedi P, Santana J, Khan M, Preston C, Donnellan C. Medical treatments in the short term management of reflux oesophagitis. Cochrane Database Syst Rev. 2007:CD003244.
21. Edwards SJ, Lind T, Lundell L. Systematic review: proton pump inhibitors (PPIs) for the healing of reflux oesophagitis—a comparison of esomeprazole with other PPIs. Aliment Pharmacol Ther. 2006;24:743–50.
22. Gralnek IM, Dulai GS, Fennerty MB, Spiegel BM. Esomeprazole versus other proton pump inhibitors in erosive esophagitis: a meta-analysis of randomized clinical trials. Clin Gastroenterol Hepatol. 2006;4:1452–8.
23. Labenz J, Armstrong D, Leodolter A, Baldycheva I. Management of reflux esophagitis: does the choice of proton pump inhibitor matter? Int J Clin Pract. 2015;69:796–801.
24. Armstrong D, Bennett JR, Blum AL, et al. The endoscopic assessment of esophagitis: a progress report on observer agreement. Gastroenterology. 1996;111:85–92.
25. Lundell LR, Dent J, Bennett JR, et al. Endoscopic assessment of oesophagitis: clinical and functional correlates and further validation of the Los Angeles classification. Gut. 1999;45:172–80.
26. Hunt RH, Scarpignato C. Potassium-competitive acid blockers (P-CABs): are they finally ready for prime time in acid-related disease? Clin Transl Gastroenterol. 2015;6:e119.
27. Iwakiri K, Umegaki E, Hiramatsu N, et al. A phase 3, randomized, double-blind, multi-center study to evaluate the efficacy and safety of TAK-438 (20 mg once-daily) compared to lansoprazole (30 mg once-daily) in patients with erosive esophagitis. Gastroenterology. 2014;146:S-741.
28. Umegaki E, Iwakiri K, Hiramatsu N, et al. A phase 3, randomized, double-blind, multicenter study to evaluate the efficacy and safety of TAK-438 (10 mg or 20 mg once-daily) compared to lansoprazole (15 mg once-daily) in a 24-week maintenance treatment for healed erosive esophagitis. Gastroenterology. 2014;146:S-738.
29. Goldstein JL, Miner PB Jr, Schlesinger PK, Liu S, Silberg DG. Intragastric acid control in non-steroidal anti-inflammatory drug users: comparison of esomeprazole, lansoprazole and pantoprazole. Aliment Pharmacol Ther. 2006;23:1189–96.
30. Kirchheiner J, Glatt S, Fuhr U, et al. Relative potency of proton-pump inhibitors-comparison of effects on intragastric pH. Eur J Clin Pharmacol. 2009;65:19–31.
31. Sigterman KE, van Pinxteren B, Bonis PA, Lau J, Numans ME. Short-term treatment with proton pump inhibitors, H2-receptor antagonists and prokinetics for gastro-oesophageal reflux disease-like symptoms and endoscopy negative reflux disease. Cochrane Database Syst Rev. 2013:CD002095.
32. Kahrilas PJ, Howden CW, Hughes N. Response of regurgitation to proton pump inhibitor therapy in clinical trials of gastroesophageal reflux disease. Am J Gastroenterol. 2011;106:1419–25.
33. Weijenborg PW, Cremonini F, Smout AJ, Bredenoord AJ. PPI therapy is equally effective in well-defined non-erosive reflux disease and in reflux esophagitis: a meta-analysis. Neurogastroenterol Motil. 2012;24:747–57.
34. Savarino E, Zentilin P, Savarino V. NERD: an umbrella term including heterogeneous subpopulations. Nat Rev Gastroenterol Hepatol. 2013;10:371–80.
35. Scarpignato C. Poor effectiveness of proton pump inhibitors in non-erosive reflux disease: the truth in the end! Neurogastroenterol Motil. 2012;24:697–704.
36. Aziz Q, Fass R, Gyawali CP, Miwa H, Pandolfino JE, Zerbib F. Esophageal disorders. Gastroenterology. 2016;150:1368–79.
37. Bytzer P, van Zanten SV, Mattsson H, Wernersson B. Partial symptom-response to proton pump inhibitors in patients with non-erosive reflux disease or reflux oesophagitis—a post hoc analysis of 5796 patients. Aliment Pharmacol Ther. 2012;36:635–43.

38. Gunaratnam NT, Jessup TP, Inadomi J, Lascewski DP. Sub-optimal proton pump inhibitor dosing is prevalent in patients with poorly controlled gastro-oesophageal reflux disease. Aliment Pharmacol Ther. 2006;23:1473–7.
39. Scarpignato C, Pelosini I. Review article: the opportunities and benefits of extended acid suppression. Aliment Pharmacol Ther. 2006;23(Suppl 2):23–34.
40. Rackoff A, Agrawal A, Hila A, Mainie I, Tutuian R, Castell DO. Histamine-2 receptor antagonists at night improve gastroesophageal reflux disease symptoms for patients on proton pump inhibitor therapy. Dis Esophagus. 2005;18:370–3.
41. Wang Y, Pan T, Wang Q, Guo Z. Additional bedtime H2-receptor antagonist for the control of nocturnal gastric acid breakthrough. Cochrane Database Syst Rev. 2009:CD004275.
42. Scarpignato C. Antisecretory drugs, helicobacter pylori infection and symptom relief in GORD: still an unexplored triangle. Dig Liver Dis. 2005;37:468–74.
43. Donnellan C, Sharma N, Preston C, Moayyedi P. Medical treatments for the maintenance therapy of reflux oesophagitis and endoscopic negative reflux disease. Cochrane Database Syst Rev. 2005:CD003245.
44. Edwards SJ, Lind T, Lundell L. Systematic review of proton pump inhibitors for the maintenance of healed reflux oesophagitis. J Outcomes Res. 2002;6:1–14.
45. Galmiche JP, Hatlebakk J, Attwood S, et al. Laparoscopic antireflux surgery vs esomeprazole treatment for chronic GERD: the LOTUS randomized clinical trial. JAMA. 2011;305:1969–77.
46. Lundell L, Miettinen P, Myrvold HE, et al. Comparison of outcomes twelve years after antireflux surgery or omeprazole maintenance therapy for reflux esophagitis. Clin Gastroenterol Hepatol. 2009;7:1292–8.
47. Bruley des Varannes S, Coron E, Galmiche JP. Short and long-term PPI treatment for GERD. Do we need more-potent anti-secretory drugs? Best Pract Res Clin Gastroenterol. 2010;24:905–21.
48. Contini S, Scarpignato C. Evaluation of clinical outcome after laparoscopic antireflux surgery in clinical practice: still a controversial issue. Minim Invasive Surg. 2011;2011:725472.
49. Yuan Y, Dattani ND, Scarpignato C, Hunt RH. Use of antisecretory medication after antireflux surgery for patients with gastroesophageal reflux disease (GERD): a systematic review of randomized control trials (RCTs). Am J Gastroenterol. 2009;104(Suppl 3):S25.
50. Yuan Y, Dattani ND, Scarpignato C, Hunt RH. Use of antisecretory medication (ARM) after antireflux surgery (ARS) for patients with gastroesophageal reflux disease (GERD): a systematic review of non-randomized studies. Gut. 2010;59(Suppl 1):A116–A17.
51. Rohof WO, Bisschops R, Tack J, Boeckxstaens GE. Postoperative problems 2011: fundoplication and obesity surgery. Gastroenterol Clin N Am. 2011;40:809–21.
52. Richter JE. Gastroesophageal reflux disease treatment: side effects and complications of fundoplication. Clin Gastroenterol Hepatol. 2013;11:465–71.
53. Lin DC, Chun CL, Triadafilopoulos G. Evaluation and management of patients with symptoms after anti-reflux surgery. Dis Esophagus. 2015;28:1–10.
54. Haastrup P, Paulsen MS, Begtrup LM, Hansen JM, Jarbol DE. Strategies for discontinuation of proton pump inhibitors: a systematic review. Fam Pract. 2014;31:625–30.
55. Lodrup AB, Reimer C, Bytzer P. Systematic review: symptoms of rebound acid hypersecretion following proton pump inhibitor treatment. Scand J Gastroenterol. 2013;48:515–22.
56. de Bortoli N, Guidi G, Martinucci I, et al. Voluntary and controlled weight loss can reduce symptoms and proton pump inhibitor use and dosage in patients with gastroesophageal reflux disease: a comparative study. Dis Esophagus. 2016;29:197–204.
57. Shaheen NJ, Falk GW, Iyer PG, Gerson LB, American College of Gastroenterology. ACG clinical guideline: diagnosis and management of Barrett's esophagus. Am J Gastroenterol. 2016;111:30–50.
58. Spechler SJ, Sharma P, Souza RF, Inadomi JM, Shaheen NJ. American Gastroenterological Association medical position statement on the management of Barrett's esophagus. Gastroenterology. 2011;140:1084–91.

59. Fitzgerald RC, di Pietro M, Ragunath K, et al. British Society of Gastroenterology guidelines on the diagnosis and management of Barrett's oesophagus. Gut. 2014;63:7–42.
60. Singh S, Garg SK, Singh PP, Iyer PG, El-Serag HB. Acid-suppressive medications and risk of oesophageal adenocarcinoma in patients with Barrett's oesophagus: a systematic review and meta-analysis. Gut. 2014;63:1229–37.
61. Akiyama J, Bertele A, Brock C, et al. Benign and precursor lesions in the esophagus. Ann N Y Acad Sci. 2014;1325:226–41.
62. Malfertheiner P, Megraud F, O'Morain CA, et al. Management of Helicobacter pylori infection-the Maastricht V/Florence Consensus Report. Gut. 2017;66:6.
63. World Gastroenterology Organisation Global Guidelines. GERD: Global Perspective on Gastroesophageal Reflux Disease. 2015. http://www.worldgastroenterology.org/guidelines/globalguidelines/gastroesophageal-reflux-disease/gastroesophageal-reflux-disease-english.
64. Lundell L, Vieth M, Gibson F, Nagy P, Kahrilas PJ. Systematic review: the effects of long-term proton pump inhibitor use on serum gastrin levels and gastric histology. Aliment Pharmacol Ther. 2015;42:649–63.
65. Katz PO, Gerson LB, Vela MF. Guidelines for the diagnosis and management of gastroesophageal reflux disease. Am J Gastroenterol. 2013;108:308–28.
66. Jaspersen D, Kulig M, Labenz J, et al. Prevalence of extra-oesophageal manifestations in gastro-oesophageal reflux disease: an analysis based on the ProGERD study. Aliment Pharmacol Ther. 2003;17:1515–20.
67. Francis DO, Rymer JA, Slaughter JC, et al. High economic burden of caring for patients with suspected extraesophageal reflux. Am J Gastroenterol. 2013;108:905–11.
68. Vaezi MF. Benefit of acid-suppressive therapy in chronic laryngitis: the devil is in the details. Clin Gastroenterol Hepatol. 2010;8:741–2.
69. de Bortoli N, Nacci A, Savarino E, et al. How many cases of laryngopharyngeal reflux suspected by laryngoscopy are gastroesophageal reflux disease-related? World J Gastroenterol. 2012;18:4363–70.
70. Mazzoleni G, Vailati C, Lisma DG, Testoni PA, Passaretti S. Correlation between oropharyngeal pH-monitoring and esophageal pH-impedance monitoring in patients with suspected GERD-related extra-esophageal symptoms. Neurogastroenterol Motil. 2014;26:1557–64.
71. Burgstaller JM, Jenni BF, Steurer J, Held U, Wertli MM. Treatment efficacy for non-cardiovascular chest pain: a systematic review and meta-analysis. PLoS One. 2014;9:e104722.
72. Roman C, Bruley des Varannes S, Muresan L, Picos A, Dumitrascu DL. Atrial fibrillation in patients with gastroesophageal reflux disease: a comprehensive review. World J Gastroenterol. 2014;20:9592–9.
73. Chang AB, Lasserson TJ, Gaffney J, Connor FL, Garske LA. Gastro-oesophageal reflux treatment for prolonged non-specific cough in children and adults. Cochrane Database Syst Rev. 2011:CD004823.
74. Kahrilas PJ, Howden CW, Hughes N, Molloy-Bland M. Response of chronic cough to acid-suppressive therapy in patients with gastroesophageal reflux disease. Chest. 2013;143:605–12.
75. Sen P, Georgalas C, Bhattacharyya AK. A systematic review of the role of proton pump inhibitors for symptoms of laryngopharyngeal reflux. Clin Otolaryngol. 2006;31:20–4.
76. Qadeer MA, Colabianchi N, Strome M, Vaezi MF. Gastroesophageal reflux and laryngeal cancer: causation or association? A critical review. Am J Otolaryngol. 2006;27:119–28.
77. Gatta L, Vaira D, Sorrenti G, Zucchini S, Sama C, Vakil N. Meta-analysis: the efficacy of proton pump inhibitors for laryngeal symptoms attributed to gastro-oesophageal reflux disease. Aliment Pharmacol Ther. 2007;25:385–92.
78. Guo H, Ma H, Wang J. Proton pump inhibitor therapy for the treatment of laryngopharyngeal reflux: a meta-analysis of randomized controlled trials. J Clin Gastroenterol. 2016;50:295–300.
79. Wei C. A meta-analysis for the role of proton pump inhibitor therapy in patients with laryngopharyngeal reflux. Eur Arch Otorhinolaryngol. 2016;273:3795.

80. Liu C, Wang H, Liu K. Meta-analysis of the efficacy of proton pump inhibitors for the symptoms of laryngopharyngeal reflux. Braz J Med Biol Res. 2016;49:S0100-879X2016000700704.
81. Harding SM. Gastroesophageal reflux, asthma, and mechanisms of interaction. Am J Med. 2001;111(Suppl 8A):8S–12S.
82. Scarpignato C. Pharmacological bases of the medical treatment of gastroesophageal reflux disease. Dig Dis. 1988;6:117–48.
83. Gibson PG, Henry RL, Coughlan JL. Gastro-oesophageal reflux treatment for asthma in adults and children. Cochrane Database Syst Rev. 2003:CD001496.
84. Ranjitkar S, Smales RJ, Kaidonis JA. Oral manifestations of gastroesophageal reflux disease. J Gastroenterol Hepatol. 2012;27:21–7.
85. Wilder-Smith CH, Wilder-Smith P, Kawakami-Wong H, Voronets J, Osann K, Lussi A. Quantification of dental erosions in patients with GERD using optical coherence tomography before and after double-blind, randomized treatment with esomeprazole or placebo. Am J Gastroenterol. 2009;104:2788–95.
86. Khalil HS. The diagnosis and management of globus: a perspective from the United Kingdom. Curr Opin Otolaryngol Head Neck Surg. 2008;16:516–20.
87. Kahrilas PJ, Shaheen NJ, Vaezi MF, American Gastroenterological Association Institute, Clinical Practice and Quality Management Committee. American Gastroenterological Association Institute technical review on the management of gastroesophageal reflux disease. Gastroenterology. 2008;135:1392–413.
88. Koufman JA, Aviv JE, Casiano RR, Shaw GY. Laryngopharyngeal reflux: position statement of the committee on speech, voice, and swallowing disorders of the American Academy of Otolaryngology-Head and Neck Surgery. Otolaryngol Head Neck Surg. 2002;127:32–5.
89. Irwin RS. Chronic cough due to gastroesophageal reflux disease: ACCP evidence-based clinical practice guidelines. Chest. 2006;129:80s–94s.
90. Altman KW, Prufer N, Vaezi MF. A review of clinical practice guidelines for reflux disease: toward creating a clinical protocol for the otolaryngologist. Laryngoscope. 2011;121:717–23.
91. Hunt R. Acid suppression for reflux disease: "off-the-peg" or a tailored approach? Clin Gastroenterol Hepatol. 2012;10:210–3.
92. Glicksman JT, Mick PT, Fung K, Carroll TL. Prokinetic agents and laryngopharyngeal reflux disease: prokinetic agents and laryngopharyngeal reflux disease: a systematic review. Laryngoscope. 2014;124:2375–9.
93. Ezzat WF, Fawaz SA, Fathey H, El Demerdash A. Virtue of adding prokinetics to proton pump inhibitors in the treatment of laryngopharyngeal reflux disease: prospective study. J Otolaryngol Head Neck Surg. 2011;40:350–6.
94. Chun BJ, Lee DS. The effect of itopride combined with lansoprazole in patients with laryngopharyngeal reflux disease. Eur Arch Otorhinolaryngol. 2013;270:1385–90.
95. Poe RH, Kallay MC. Chronic cough and gastroesophageal reflux disease: experience with specific therapy for diagnosis and treatment. Chest. 2003;123:679–84.
96. Dabirmoghaddam P, Amali A, Motiee Langroudi M, Samavati Fard MR, Hejazi M, Sharifian Razavi M. The effect of N-acetyl cysteine on laryngopharyngeal reflux. Acta Med Iran. 2013;51:757–64.
97. McGlashan JA, Johnstone LM, Sykes J, Strugala V, Dettmar PW. The value of a liquid alginate suspension (Gaviscon Advance) in the management of laryngopharyngeal reflux. Eur Arch Otorhinolaryngol. 2009;266:243–51.
98. Lieder A, Issing W. Treatment for resilient cough owing to laryngopharyngeal reflux with a combination of proton pump inhibitor and Gaviscon(R) Advance: how we do it. Clin Otolaryngol. 2011;36:583–7.
99. Strugala V, Dettmar PW. Alginate in the treatment of extra-oesophageal reflux. In: Johnson N, Toohill RJ, editors. Effects, diagnosis and management of extra-esophageal reflux. New York: Nova Science; 2010. p. 145–68.

100. Zentilin P, Dulbecco P, Savarino E, et al. An evaluation of the antireflux properties of sodium alginate by means of combined multichannel intraluminal impedance and pH-metry. Aliment Pharmacol Ther. 2005;21:29–34.
101. Strugala V, Avis J, Jolliffe IG, Johnstone LM, Dettmar PW. The role of an alginate suspension on pepsin and bile acids—key aggressors in the gastric refluxate. Does this have implications for the treatment of gastro-oesophageal reflux disease? J Pharm Pharmacol. 2009;61:1021–8.
102. Bardhan KD, Strugala V, Dettmar PW. Reflux revisited: advancing the role of pepsin. Int J Otolaryngol. 2012;2012:646901.
103. Di Simone MP, Baldi F, Vasina V, et al. Barrier effect of Esoxx((R)) on esophageal mucosal damage: experimental study on ex-vivo swine model. Clin Exp Gastroenterol. 2012;5:103–7.
104. Palmieri B, Merighi A, Corbascio D, Rottigni V, Fistetto G, Esposito A. Fixed combination of hyaluronic acid and chondroitin-sulphate oral formulation in a randomized double blind, placebo controlled study for the treatment of symptoms in patients with non-erosive gastro-esophageal reflux. Eur Rev Med Pharmacol Sci. 2013;17:3272–8.
105. Savarino V, Pace F, Scarpignato C. Randomized clinical trial: mucosal protection combined with acid suppression in the treatment of nor erosive reflux disease—efficacy of Esoxx, a hyaluronic acid-chondroitin sulphate based bioadhesive formulation. Aliment Pharmacol Ther. 2017;45:631–42.
106. Contini S, Scarpignato C. Endoscopic treatment of gastro-oesophageal reflux disease (GORD): a systematic review. Dig Liver Dis. 2003;35:818–38.
107. Blandizzi C, Scarpignato C. Gastrointestinal drugs. In: Aronson JK, editor. Side effects of drugs annual, Chap. 36. Amsterdam: Elsevier; 2011. p. 741–67.
108. Blandizzi C, Scarpignato C. Gastrointestinal drugs. In: Aronson JK, editor. Side effects of drugs annual, Chap. 36. Amsterdam: Elsevier; 2012. p. 555–78.
109. Blandizzi C, Scarpignato C. Gastrointestinal drugs. In: Aronson JK, editor. Side effects of drugs annual, Chap. 36. Amsterdam: Elsevier; 2014. p. 633–58.
110. Blandizzi C, Scarpignato C. Gastrointestinal drugs. In: Sidhartha DR, editor. Side effects of drugs annual, Chap. 36. Amsterdam: Elsevier; 2014. p. 539–60.
111. Ito T, Jensen RT. Association of long-term proton pump inhibitor therapy with bone fractures and effects on absorption of calcium, vitamin B12, iron, and magnesium. Curr Gastroenterol Rep. 2010;12:448–57.
112. Thomson AB, Sauve MD, Kassam N, Kamitakahara H. Safety of the long-term use of proton pump inhibitors. World J Gastroenterol. 2010;16:2323–30.
113. Sheen E, Triadafilopoulos G. Adverse effects of long-term proton pump inhibitor therapy. Dig Dis Sci. 2011;56:931–50.
114. Chen J, Yuan YC, Leontiadis GI, Howden CW. Recent safety concerns with proton pump inhibitors. J Clin Gastroenterol. 2012;46:93–114.
115. Johnson DA, Oldfield EC. Reported side effects and complications of long-term proton pump inhibitor use: dissecting the evidence. Clin Gastroenterol Hepatol. 2013;11:458–64.
116. de la Coba Ortiz C, Arguelles Arias F, Martin de Argila de Prados C, et al. Proton-pump inhibitors adverse effects: a review of the evidence and position statement by the Sociedad Espanola de Patologia Digestiva. Rev Esp Enferm Dig. 2016;108:207–24.
117. Mossner J. The indications, applications, and risks of proton pump inhibitors. Dtsch Arztebl Int. 2016;113:477–83.
118. Savarino V, Dulbecco P, Savarino E. Are proton pump inhibitors really so dangerous? Dig Liver Dis. 2016;48:851–9.
119. Vaezi MF, Yang YX, Howden CW. Complications of proton pump inhibitor therapy. Gastroenterology. 2017;153:35–48.
120. Lahner E, Annibale B, Delle Fave G. Systematic review: impaired drug absorption related to the co-administration of antisecretory therapy. Aliment Pharmacol Ther. 2009;29:1219–29.
121. Blume H, Donath F, Warnke A, Schug BS. Pharmacokinetic drug interaction profiles of proton pump inhibitors. Drug Saf. 2006;29:769–84.
122. Wedemeyer RS, Blume H. Pharmacokinetic drug interaction profiles of proton pump inhibitors: an update. Drug Saf. 2014;37:201–11.

123. Yucel E, Sancar M, Yucel A, Okuyan B. Adverse drug reactions due to drug-drug interactions with proton pump inhibitors: assessment of systematic reviews with AMSTAR method. Expert Opin Drug Saf. 2016;15:223–36.
124. Shi S, Klotz U. Proton pump inhibitors: an update of their clinical use and pharmacokinetics. Eur J Clin Pharmacol. 2008;64:935–51.
125. Desta Z, Zhao X, Shin JG, Flockhart DA. Clinical significance of the cytochrome P450 2C19 genetic polymorphism. Clin Pharmacokinet. 2002;41:913–58.
126. Agewall S, Cattaneo M, Collet JP, et al. Expert position paper on the use of proton pump inhibitors in patients with cardiovascular disease and antithrombotic therapy. Eur Heart J. 2013;34:1708–13.
127. Cardoso RN, Benjo AM, DiNicolantonio JJ, et al. Incidence of cardiovascular events and gastrointestinal bleeding in patients receiving clopidogrel with and without proton pump inhibitors: an updated meta-analysis. Open Heart. 2015;2:e000248.
128. Leontiadis GI, Yuan Y, Howden CW. The interaction between proton pump inhibitors and clopidogrel and upper gastrointestinal bleeding. Gastrointest Endosc Clin N Am. 2011;21:637–56.
129. Madanick RD. Proton pump inhibitor side effects and drug interactions: much ado about nothing? Cleve Clin J Med. 2011;78:39–49.
130. Vaduganathan M, Cannon CP, Cryer BL, et al. Efficacy and safety of proton-pump inhibitors in high-risk cardiovascular subsets of the COGENT trial. Am J Med. 2016;129:1002–5.
131. Bhatt DL, Cryer BL, Contant CF, et al. Clopidogrel with or without omeprazole in coronary artery disease. N Engl J Med. 2010;363:1909–17.
132. Vaduganathan M, Bhatt DL, Cryer BL, et al. Proton-pump inhibitors reduce gastrointestinal events regardless of aspirin dose in patients requiring dual antiplatelet therapy. J Am Coll Cardiol. 2016;67:1661–71.
133. Attwood SE, Ell C, Galmiche JP, et al. Long-term safety of proton pump inhibitor therapy assessed under controlled, randomised clinical trial conditions: data from the SOPRAN and LOTUS studies. Aliment Pharmacol Ther. 2015;41:1162–74.
134. Fiocca R, Mastracci L, Attwood SE, et al. Gastric exocrine and endocrine cell morphology under prolonged acid inhibition therapy: results of a 5-year follow-up in the LOTUS trial. Aliment Pharmacol Ther. 2012;36:959–71.
135. Vakil N. Prescribing proton pump inhibitors: is it time to pause and rethink? Drugs. 2012;72:437–45.
136. Scarpignato C, Gatta L, Zullo A, et al. Effective and safe proton pump inhibitor therapy in acid-related diseases—a position paper addressing benefits and potential harms of acid suppression. BMC Med. 2016;14:179.

# Reflux Inhibitors and Prokinetics

## 24

Woo-Jung Song

## Introduction

Gastro-oesophageal reflux disease (GORD) is a motility disorder that develops when reflux of stomach contents causes troublesome symptoms or complications [1]. This syndrome encompasses a broad range of pathological conditions in which reflux is the root cause of oesophageal or extra-oesophageal problems. Several factors are considered important in the pathophysiology of GORD, including the occurrence of reflux, refluxate constituents, clearance of refluxate, and oesophageal mucosal sensitivity [2]. The roles of each factor vary among individuals and respiratory conditions [3], and contribute to the heterogeneity of this syndrome.

Various airway disorders are frequently comorbid with GORD [4–7]. Reflux is increasingly recognised as a potential cause or modifier of airway diseases and symptoms [3, 6, 8–13]. Reflux is presumed to have clinical relevance in airway diseases refractory to conventional treatment. However, acid refluxate, a major cause of peptic reflux symptoms, appears to contribute very little to airway disorders [12]. A recent meta-analysis showed that proton pump inhibitor (PPI) therapy did not achieve real therapeutic gain in chronic cough patients with no pathological oesophageal acid exposure (vs. placebo; 0.0–8.6%). Although it improved cough outcomes in those with pathological acid exposure, the therapeutic gain was modest (12.5–35.8%) [14]. PPI therapy was also ineffective for managing patients with asthma comorbid with GERD or poorly controlled asthma [15–18]. Therefore, it may be reasonably hypothesised that 'reflux' itself (not confined to acid reflux) is relevant in unexplained or refractory airway diseases.

Several pharmacological agents have been developed to control reflux, by reducing reflux occurrence or promoting refluxate clearance. This chapter focuses on the

---

W.-J. Song
Department of Internal Medicine, Asan Medical Center, University of Ulsan College of Medicine, Seoul, South Korea

anti-reflux efficacy of two classes of agents—reflux inhibitors and prokinetics—and then estimates their therapeutic potential in reflux-related airway diseases.

## Reflux Inhibitors in GORD

Transient lower oesophageal sphincter relaxation (TLOSR) is the major event underlying the occurrence of gastro-oesophageal reflux, making it an attractive target for reflux inhibitor development. TLOSR is a vagally mediated reflex, and gastric distention is the major reflex trigger [19].

Among the neurotransmitters involved in the reflex pathway, γ-aminobutyric acid (GABA) has been one of the main therapeutic targets. GABA is a major inhibitory neurotransmitter within the central nervous system, and GABA type B ($GABA_B$) receptors are present in both the central and enteric nervous systems [20]. $GABA_B$ receptor stimulation mediates postsynaptic inhibition [21], and inhibits the mechano-sensitivity of the gastro-oesophageal vagal afferents [22].

Baclofen is a selective $GABA_B$ receptor agonist, which was originally used in the treatment of spasticity but also showed potential for treating reflux. Lidums et al. first demonstrated the effects of oral baclofen in modulating TLOSR in humans [23]. In studies of patients with GORD, baclofen significantly reduced the rate of TLOSR and reflux episodes and improved reflux symptoms [20, 24–26]. Notably, baclofen also effectively reduced reflux symptoms in 16 patients refractory to PPI therapy, demonstrating its potential to control non-acid reflux [27]. A meta-analysis of nine randomised trials involving 283 GORD patients also concluded that baclofen is potentially useful [28]. However, the use of baclofen is limited by safety concerns. Its frequent adverse events include neurological disturbances (such as dizziness, fatigue, somnolence, paraesthesia, and muscle weakness) and gastrointestinal discomfort (nausea, diarrhoea, and flatulence), which are related to its activity in the central nervous system [28, 29]. Although the meta-analysis of GORD patients identified its mild-to-moderate side effects [28], studies of patients with spasticity reported that adverse effects showed a prevalence of 26–73% in baclofen groups versus 4–27% in placebo groups [29].

Lesogaberan is a novel peripherally active $GABA_B$ receptor agonist, developed as a reflux inhibitor [30]. Early clinical trials using lesogaberan showed promising results in reducing TLOSR and improving reflux symptoms in GORD patients who remained symptomatic despite PPI therapy [31, 32]. However, in a large multicentre phase IIb trial involving 661 refractory GORD patients, lesogaberan failed to show clear benefits compared with placebo; the responder rate was only 26.2% in the high-dose (240 mg) lesogaberan group, which was not statistically different from the rate of 17.9% seen in the placebo group [33]. Therefore, despite its better safety profile [32, 33], development of lesogaberan as a reflux inhibitor was halted [34].

Arbaclofen placarbil is a baclofen prodrug designed to overcome the pharmacokinetic limitations of baclofen. Baclofen is mostly absorbed in the proximal small bowel, while arbaclofen is absorbed throughout the gastrointestinal tract by both passive and active mechanisms via the monocarboxylate type 1 transporter [35]. Therefore, sustained release of oral arbaclofen is possible, resulting in less fluctuation in plasma levels [36]. In a clinical trial using a single dose of arbaclofen placarbil (n = 50), it successfully decreased GORD episodes and related symptoms with good tolerability [37]. In two large multicentre phase II clinical trials (n = 156 and n = 460), however, arbaclofen placarbil did not show clear benefits over placebo in the primary analysis (frequency of heartburn), and only showed some potential in *post hoc* analyses confined to moderate to severe GORD cases [38, 39]. Currently, no clinical trials are examining arbaclofen placarbil as a treatment for GORD [40].

Recently, the metabotropic glutamate receptor 5 (mGluR5) has been identified as important in controlling TLOSR. [41] Several mGluR5 antagonists have been developed as reflux inhibitors. Raseglurant (ADX10059) was tested in patients with GERD, and a short course of therapy significantly reduced acid reflux and symptomatic reflux episodes [42]. In a 2-week trial of 103 patients with GORD responsive to PPI, raseglurant monotherapy improved GORD symptoms (heartburn and regurgitation) and reflux events [43]. However, raseglurant was discontinued because of the risk of hepatotoxicity, as observed in migraine patients with long-term use (https://clinicaltrials.gov/ct2/show/NCT00820105). Another mGluR5 inhibitor, mavoglurant, showed promising results in reducing postprandial reflux episodes in a trial of 36 patients with moderate to severe GORD [44].

## Reflux Inhibitors in Airway Diseases

No randomised controlled trial has examined the longterm use of these reflux inhibitors in a large group of patients with airway diseases (Table 24.1). In guinea pigs, baclofen and lesogaberan reduced citric acid-induced cough [49]. In a 4-week prospective open-label trial involving 7 patients with ACE inhibitor-induced cough, low dose baclofen showed potential anti-tussive effects [83]. In an 8-week open single-arm study of 16 patients with suspected reflux-cough refractory to PPI, add-on baclofen significantly improved cough scores, capsaicin cough sensitivity, and reflux scores. The responder rate was 56.3% (9/16) [45]. Meanwhile, in a 2-week randomized, double-blind, placebo-controlled, crossover study of six stable asthmatics, baclofen improved methacholine bronchial hyper-responsiveness [82].

## Prokinetics in GORD

Prokinetics are a diverse group of agents that can promote anterograde movement of the gastrointestinal tract via various mechanisms, such as increased lower oesophageal sphincter pressure, enhanced peristalsis, and gastric emptying (Table 24.1) [50].

The dopaminergic pathway is implicated in gastrointestinal motility, and the dopamine D2 receptor has been considered a target as its blockade had prokinetic effects [51]. Metoclopramide and domperidone are dopamine D2 receptor antagonists used as prokinetics, and domperidone has a better safety profile due to peripheral selectivity [52]. The use of metoclopramide is often limited by adverse central

**Table 24.1** Classification of reflux inhibitors and prokinetics and their clinical evidence in airway diseases

| Agent | Clinical evidence in airway diseases |
|---|---|
| *GABA$_B$ receptor agonist* | |
| Baclofen | 1. Population: patients with suspected reflux-cough refractory to PPI<br>Intervention: 8-week baclofen add-on to PPI<br>Comparison: none<br>Outcome: improvement in cough scores, capsaicin cough sensitivity and reflux scores [45]<br>2. Population: patients with ACE inhibitor-induced cough.<br>Intervention: 4-week baclofen.<br>Comparison: none<br>Outcome: improvement in cough [83].<br>3. Population: patients with stable asthma.<br>Intervention: 2-week baclofen.<br>Comparison: placebo.<br>Outcome: methacholine bronchial responsiveness [82]. |
| Lesogaberan | – |
| Arbaclofen placarbil | – |
| *Metabotropic glutamate receptor 5 antagonist* | |
| Raseglurant | – |
| Mavoglurant | – |
| *Dopamine D2 receptor antagonist* | |
| Metoclopramide | – |
| Domperidone | 1. Population: patients with laryngopharyngeal reflux (defined as reflux symptom index score 13 or more)<br>Intervention: 3-month domperidone add-on to omeprazole<br>Comparison: omeprazole monotherapy<br>Outcome: no significant difference in reflux symptom index score [46]<br>2. Population: children with difficult-to-treat asthma<br>Intervention: 12-week domperidone add-on to esomeprazole<br>Comparison: esomeprazole monotherapy<br>Outcome: improvement in endoscopic reflux score, asthma control test score and FEV1% [47] |
| *5-HT4 receptor agonist* | |
| Cisapride | – |
| Mosapride | – |
| Revexepride | – |
| Tegaserod | – |
| Prucalopride | – |
| *Dopamine D2 receptor antagonist with acetylcholine esterase inhibitor activity* | |
| Itopride | Population: patients with laryngopharyngeal reflux (defined as the presence of laryngeal and respiratory symptoms combined with laryngoscopic mucosal abnormality and reflux symptom index score >13)<br>Intervention: 12-week itopride add-on to lansoprazole<br>Comparison: lansoprazole monotherapy<br>Outcome: no improvement in reflux finding score but acceleration of relief of reflux symptoms [48] |

nervous system effects, such as drowsiness, agitation, depression, dystonic reactions, or tardive dyskinesia [53]. To date, there is no clear evidence to support the use of metoclopramide or domperidone in patients with GORD [54–59].

Cisapride, a non-selective 5-hydroxytryptamine receptor 4 (5-HTR$_4$) agonist, stimulates gastrointestinal motility by increasing the release of acetylcholine from the myenteric plexus [60]. It is more efficacious than metoclopramide for treating GORD [61, 62] and its use was approved for nocturnal heartburn. However, it was withdrawn from the market in 2000 because of severe cardiac toxicity, including QT prolongation and fatal arrhythmias [63]. The example of cisapride has led to the development of novel 5-HTR$_4$ agonists with better safety profiles, such as mosapride, revexepride, tegaserod, and prucalopride. Mosapride is a selective 5-HTR$_4$ agonist in the gastrointestinal tract [64], but randomised clinical trials with mosapride had conflicting results and it showed only modest efficacy at relieving GORD symptoms [65–67]. Revexepride, another selective 5-HTR$_4$ agonist, did not show clear benefits in reflux outcomes in two recent placebo-controlled trials [68, 69]. Tegaserod, a non-benzamide selective 5-HTR$_4$ agonist, did not influence the lower oesophageal sphincter pressure, but did show therapeutic potential in reflux patients, promoting oesophageal motility, reducing postprandial oesophageal acid exposure, or improving the mechanical sensitivity of the oesophagus [70–72]. However, the results of subsequent clinical trials of tegaserod in patients with refractory GORD have not been published [73]. Tegaserod is associated with an increased risk of cardiovascular events, such as ischemic colitis [63]. Prucalopride is a benzofurancarboxamide agonist with high affinity and selectivity for 5-HT$_4$ receptors in the gastrointestinal tract, showing promising prokinetic efficacy and good tolerability [74–79].

Itopride is a different type of prokinetic agent, acting as both a dopamine D2 receptor antagonist and an acetylcholine esterase inhibitor [79]. It inhibited meal-induced TLOSR in healthy volunteers [80], and effectively decreased pathological acid reflux in an open-label trial of 26 patients with mild GORD [81].

## Prokinetics in Airway Diseases

Only three randomised controlled trials have evaluated the efficacy of prokinetics (two with domperidone and one with itopride) in patients with airway disorders (Table 24.1). In a 3-month trial of 17 patients with laryngopharyngeal reflux (defined as a reflux symptom index score ≥13), domperidone in combination with omeprazole was not superior to omeprazole alone at improving symptom scores [46]. Itopride as an add-on to lansoprazole did not show benefits over lansoprazole monotherapy in terms of reflux scores, and was helpful only for accelerating the relief of reflux symptoms in 64 patients with laryngopharyngeal reflux [48]. In a randomised trial of 89 children with difficult-to-treat asthma, the combination of domperidone and esomeprazole was more effective at improving endoscopic reflux scores and asthma control test results than esomeprazole alone; however, the data have still been reported only in abstract form [47].

## Summary

Despite some promising results in early studies, most reflux inhibitors and prokinetic agents have not met expectations in large clinical trials of GORD patients. It is even more difficult to evaluate their efficacy in patients with reflux-related airway disease. However, the failures in GORD trials may need to be interpreted cautiously and should not hinder further trials in different clinical settings. The pathophysiology of GORD is multi-factorial, and impaired physiological barriers against reflux may vary by individual and comorbid airway condition. Considering emerging evidence for non-acid reflux in airway diseases, any pharmacological intervention targeting "reflux" itself should be evaluated on its own (population and outcome). Careful patient selection based on objective characterisation of reflux and airway diseases is the key to testing the true efficacy of these drugs in the intended population.

## References

1. Vakil N, Van Zanten SV, Kahrilas P, Dent J, Jones R. The Montreal definition and classification of gastroesophageal reflux disease: a global evidence-based consensus. Am J Gastroenterol. 2006;101:1900–20.
2. Kahrilas PJ, Boeckxstaens G. Failure of reflux inhibitors in clinical trials: bad drugs or wrong patients? Gut. 2012;61:1501–9.
3. Houghton LA, Lee AS, Badri H, DeVault KR, Smith JA. Respiratory disease and the oesophagus: reflux, reflexes and microaspiration. Nat Rev Gastroenterol Hepatol. 2016;13:445.
4. Cazzola M, Segreti A, Calzetta L, Rogliani P. Comorbidities of asthma: current knowledge and future research needs. Curr Opin Pulm Med. 2013;19:36–41.
5. Brown JP, Martinez CH. Chronic obstructive pulmonary disease comorbidities. Curr Opin Pulm Med. 2016;22:113–8.
6. Fahim A, Crooks M, Hart SP. Gastroesophageal reflux and idiopathic pulmonary fibrosis: a review. Pulm Med. 2011;2011:1.
7. Morice A. The diagnosis and management of chronic cough. Eur Respir J. 2004;24:481–92.
8. Morice AH. Airway reflux as a cause of respiratory disease. Breathe. 2013;9:256–66.
9. Johnston N, Ondrey F, Rosen R, Hurley BP, Gould J, Allen J, DelGaudio J, Altman KW. Airway reflux. Ann N Y Acad Sci. 2016;1381:5–13.
10. Komatsu Y, Hoppo T, Jobe BA. Proximal reflux as a cause of adult-onset asthma: the case for hypopharyngeal impedance testing to improve the sensitivity of diagnosis. JAMA Surg. 2013;148:50–8.
11. Lee AL, Goldstein RS. Gastroesophageal reflux disease in COPD: links and risks. Int J Chron Obstruct Pulmon Dis. 2015;10:1935–49.
12. Boeckxstaens G, El-Serag HB, Smout AJ, Kahrilas PJ. Symptomatic reflux disease: the present, the past and the future. Gut. 2014;63:1185–93.
13. Herregods TV, Pauwels A, Jafari J, Sifrim D, Bredenoord AJ, Tack J, Smout AJ. Determinants of reflux-induced chronic cough. Gut. 2017;66:2057.
14. Kahrilas PJ, Howden CW, Hughes N, Molloy-Bland M. Response of chronic cough to acid-suppressive therapy in patients with gastroesophageal reflux disease. Chest. 2013;143:605–12.
15. Holbrook JT, Wise RA, Gold BD, Blake K, Brown ED, Castro M, Dozor AJ, Lima JJ, Mastronarde JG, Sockrider MM. Lansoprazole for children with poorly controlled asthma: a randomized controlled trial. JAMA. 2012;307:373–81.

16. Kiljander TO, Junghard O, Beckman O, Lind T. Effect of esomeprazole 40 mg once or twice daily on asthma: a randomized, placebo-controlled study. Am J Respir Crit Care Med. 2010;181:1042–8.
17. Chan WW, Chiou E, Obstein KL, Tignor AS, Whitlock TL. The efficacy of proton pump inhibitors for the treatment of asthma in adults: a meta-analysis. Arch Intern Med. 2011;171: 620–9.
18. American Lung Association Asthma Clinical Research Centers. Efficacy of esomeprazole for treatment of poorly controlled asthma. N Engl J Med. 2009;360:1487–99.
19. Holloway RH, Hongo M, Berger K, McCallum RW. Gastric distention: a mechanism for postprandial gastroesophageal reflux. Gastroenterology. 1985;89:779–84.
20. Zhang Q, Lehmann A, Rigda R, Dent J, Holloway RH. Control of transient lower oesophageal sphincter relaxations and reflux by the GABAB agonist baclofen in patients with gastrooesophageal reflux disease. Gut. 2002;50:19–24.
21. Brooks P, Glaum S, Miller R, Spyer K. The actions of baclofen on neurones and synaptic transmission in the nucleus tractus solitarii of the rat in vitro. J Physiol. 1992;457:115.
22. Page AJ, Blackshaw LA. GABAB receptors inhibit mechanosensitivity of primary afferent endings. J Neurosci. 1999;19:8597–602.
23. Lidums I, Lehmann A, Checklin H, Dent J, Holloway RH. Control of transient lower esophageal sphincter relaxations and reflux by the GABA(B) agonist baclofen in normal subjects. Gastroenterology. 2000;118:7–13.
24. Cange L, Johnsson E, Rydholm H, Lehmann A, Finizia C, Lundell L, Ruth M. Baclofen-mediated gastro-oesophageal acid reflux control in patients with established reflux disease. Aliment Pharmacol Ther. 2002;16:869–73.
25. Van Herwaarden MA, Samsom M, Rydholm H, Smout AJPM. The effect of baclofen on gastro-oesophageal reflux, lower oesophageal sphincter function and reflux symptoms in patients with reflux disease. Aliment Pharmacol Ther. 2002;16:1655–62.
26. Ciccaglione AF, Marzio L. Effect of acute and chronic administration of the GABAB agonist baclofen on 24 hour pH metry and symptoms in control subjects and in patients with gastrooesophageal reflux disease. Gut. 2003;52:464–70.
27. Koek GH, Sifrim D, Lerut T, Janssens J, Tack J. Effect of the GABA(B) agonist baclofen in patients with symptoms and duodeno-gastro-oesophageal reflux refractory to proton pump inhibitors. Gut. 2003;52:1397–402.
28. Li S, Shi S, Chen F, Lin J. The effects of baclofen for the treatment of gastroesophageal reflux disease: a meta-analysis of randomized controlled trials. Gastroenterol Res Pract. 2014;2014:1.
29. Ertzgaard P, Campo C, Calabrese A. Efficacy and safety of oral baclofen in the management of spasticity: a rationale for intrathecal baclofen. J Rehabil Med. 2017;49:193–203.
30. Lehmann A, Antonsson M, Holmberg AA, Blackshaw LA, Brändén L, Bräuner-Osborne H, Christiansen B, Dent J, Elebring T, Jacobson B-M. (R)-(3-amino-2-fluoropropyl) phosphinic acid (AZD3355), a novel GABAB receptor agonist, inhibits transient lower esophageal sphincter relaxation through a peripheral mode of action. J Pharmacol Exp Ther. 2009;331:504–12.
31. Boeckxstaens G, Beaumont H, Mertens V, Denison H, Ruth M, Adler J, Silberg D, Sifrim D. Effects of lesogaberan on reflux and lower esophageal sphincter function in patients with gastroesophageal reflux disease. Gastroenterology. 2010;139:409–17.
32. Boeckxstaens GE, Beaumont H, Hatlebakk JG, Silberg DG, Björck K, Karlsson M, Denison H. A novel reflux inhibitor lesogaberan (AZD3355) as add-on treatment in patients with GORD with persistent reflux symptoms despite proton pump inhibitor therapy: a randomised placebo-controlled trial. Gut. 2011;60:1182–8.
33. Shaheen NJ, Denison H, Björck K, Karlsson M, Silberg DG. Efficacy and safety of lesogaberan in gastro-oesophageal reflux disease: a randomised controlled trial. Gut. 2013;62:1248–55.
34. Rydholm H, von Corswant C, Denison H, Jensen JM, Lehmann A, Ruth M, Soderlind E, Aurell-Holmberg A. Reducing adverse effects during drug development: the example of lesogaberan and paresthesia. Clin Ther. 2016;38:946–60.
35. Lal R, Sukbuntherng J, Tai EH, Upadhyay S, Yao F, Warren MS, Luo W, Bu L, Nguyen S, Zamora J. Arbaclofen placarbil, a novel R-baclofen prodrug: improved absorption, distribu-

36. Lal R, Zomorodi K, Huff FJ, Luo W, Tovera J, Blumenthal R, Bian A, Cundy KC. Clinical pharmacokinetics and pharmacodynamics of arbaclofen placarbil, a novel reflux inhibitor, in subjects with GERD. Neurogastroenterol Motil. 2010;22:48.
37. Gerson LB, Huff FJ, Hila A, Hirota WK, Reilley S, Agrawal A, Lal R, Luo W, Castell D. Arbaclofen placarbil decreases postprandial reflux in patients with gastroesophageal reflux disease. Am J Gastroenterol. 2010;105:1266–75.
38. Vakil NB, Huff FJ, Bian A, Jones DS, Stamler D. Arbaclofen placarbil in GERD: a randomized, double-blind, placebo-controlled study. Am J Gastroenterol. 2011;106:1427–38.
39. Vakil NB, Huff FJ, Cundy KC. Randomised clinical trial: arbaclofen placarbil in gastro-oesophageal reflux disease—insights into study design for transient lower sphincter relaxation inhibitors. Aliment Pharmacol Ther. 2013;38:107–17.
40. ClinicalTrials.gov. http://clinicaltrials.gov.
41. Frisby CL, Mattsson JP, Jensen JM, Lehmann A, Dent J, Blackshaw LA. Inhibition of transient lower esophageal sphincter relaxation and gastroesophageal reflux by metabotropic glutamate receptor ligands. Gastroenterology. 2005;129:995–1004.
42. Keywood C, Wakefield M, Tack J. A proof-of-concept study evaluating the effect of ADX10059, a metabotropic glutamate receptor-5 negative allosteric modulator, on acid exposure and symptoms in gastro-oesophageal reflux disease. Gut. 2009;58:1192–9.
43. Zerbib F, Bruley des Varannes S, Roman S, Tutuian R, Galmiche JP, Mion F, Tack J, Malfertheiner P, Keywood C. Randomised clinical trial: effects of monotherapy with ADX10059, a mGluR5 inhibitor, on symptoms and reflux events in patients with gastro-oesophageal reflux disease. Aliment Pharmacol Ther. 2011;33:911–21.
44. Rouzade-Dominguez ML, Pezous N, David OJ, Tutuian R, Bruley des Varannes S, Tack J, Malfertheiner P, Allescher HD, Ufer M, Ruhl A. The selective metabotropic glutamate receptor 5 antagonist mavoglurant (AFQ056) reduces the incidence of reflux episodes in dogs and patients with moderate to severe gastroesophageal reflux disease. Neurogastroenterol Motil. 2017;29(8). https://doi.org/10.1111/nmo.13058 Epub 2017 Mar 23.
45. Xu XH, Yang ZM, Chen Q, Yu L, Liang SW, Lv HJ, Qiu ZM. Therapeutic efficacy of baclofen in refractory gastroesophageal reflux-induced chronic cough. World J Gastroenterol. 2013;19:4386–92.
46. Hunchaisri N. Treatment of laryngopharyngeal reflux: a comparison between domperidone plus omeprazole and omeprazole alone. J Med Assoc Thail. 2012;95:73–80.
47. Al-Biltagi M, Bediwy AS, Deraz S, Amer HG, Saeed NK. Esomeprazole, versus esomeprazole and domperidone in treatment of gastroesophageal reflux in children with difficult-to-treat asthma. Eur Respir J. 2013;42:P1138.
48. Chun BJ, Lee DS. The effect of itopride combined with lansoprazole in patients with laryngopharyngeal reflux disease. Eur Arch Otorhinolaryngol. 2013;270:1385–90.
49. Canning BJ, Mori N, Lehmann A. Antitussive effects of the peripherally restricted GABA B receptor agonist lesogaberan in guinea pigs: comparison to baclofen and other GABA B receptor-selective agonists. Cough. 2012;8:7.
50. Tack J. Prokinetics and fundic relaxants in upper functional GI disorders. Curr Opin Pharmacol. 2008;8:690–6.
51. Tonini M, Cipollina L, Poluzzi E, Crema F, Corazza G, De Ponti F. Clinical implications of enteric and central D2 receptor blockade by antidopaminergic gastrointestinal prokinetics. Aliment Pharmacol Ther. 2004;19:379–90.
52. Barone JA. Domperidone: a peripherally acting dopamine2-receptor antagonist. Ann Pharmacother. 1999;33:429–40.
53. Rao A, Camilleri M. Review article: metoclopramide and tardive dyskinesia. Aliment Pharmacol Ther. 2010;31:11–9.
54. Richter JE, Sabesin SM, Kogut DG, Kerr RM, Wruble LD, Collen MJ. Omeprazole versus ranitidine or ranitidine/metoclopramide in poorly responsive symptomatic gastroesophageal reflux disease. Am J Gastroenterol. 1996;91:1766.

55. Maddern GJ, Kiroff GK, Leppard PI, Jamieson GG. Domperidone, metoclopramide, and placebo. All give symptomatic improvement in gastroesophageal reflux. J Clin Gastroenterol. 1986;8:135–40.
56. Bellissant E, Duhamel JF, Guillot M, Pariente-Khayat A, Olive G, Pons G. The triangular test to assess the efficacy of metoclopramide in gastroesophageal reflux. Clin Pharmacol Ther. 1997;61:377–84.
57. Hibbs AM, Lorch SA. Metoclopramide for the treatment of gastroesophageal reflux disease in infants: a systematic review. Pediatrics. 2006;118:746–52.
58. Bines JE, Quinlan JE, Treves S, Kleinman RE, Winter HS. Efficacy of domperidone in infants and children with gastroesophageal reflux. J Pediatr Gastroenterol Nutr. 1992;14:400–5.
59. Pritchard DS, Baber N, Stephenson T. Should domperidone be used for the treatment of gastro-oesophageal reflux in children? Systematic review of randomized controlled trials in children aged 1 month to 11 years old. Br J Clin Pharmacol. 2005;59:725–9.
60. Van Nueten J, Van Daele P, Reyntjens A, Janssen P, Schuurkes J. Gastrointestinal motility stimulating properties of cisapride, a non-antidopaminergic non-cholinergic compound. In: Gastrointestinal motility. Dordrecht: Springer; 1984. p. 513–20.
61. Arabehety JT, Leitao OR, Fassler S, Olarte M, Serrano C. Cisapride and metoclopramide in the treatment of gastroesophageal reflux disease. Clin Ther. 1988;10:421–8.
62. Bravo Matus CA, Flores RM. Comparative study of cisapride and methoclopramide in newborns with gastroesophageal reflex. Invest Med Int. 1995;22:3–7.
63. Tack J, Camilleri M, Chang L, Chey W, Galligan J, Lacy B, Müller-Lissner S, Quigley E, Schuurkes J, Maeyer J. Systematic review: cardiovascular safety profile of 5-HT4 agonists developed for gastrointestinal disorders. Aliment Pharmacol Ther. 2012;35:745–67.
64. Yoshida N, Ito T. Mosapride citrate (AS-4370), a new gastroprolinetic agent, is a partial 5-HT4 receptor agonist in the gut. Neurogastroenterol Motil. 1994;6:197–204.
65. Ruth M, Finizia C, Cange L, Lundell L. The effect of mosapride on oesophageal motor function and acid reflux in patients with gastro-oesophageal reflux disease. Eur J Gastroenterol Hepatol. 2003;15:1115–21.
66. Miwa H, Inoue K, Ashida K, Kogawa T, Nagahara A, Yoshida S, Tano N, Yamazaki Y, Wada T, Asaoka D, Fujita T, Tanaka J, Shimatani T, Manabe N, Oshima T, Haruma K, Azuma T, Yokoyama T. Randomised clinical trial: efficacy of the addition of a prokinetic, mosapride citrate, to omeprazole in the treatment of patients with non-erosive reflux disease—a double-blind, placebo-controlled study. Aliment Pharmacol Ther. 2011;33:323–32.
67. Hsu YC, Yang TH, Hsu WL, Wu HT, Cheng YC, Chiang MF, Wang CS, Lin HJ. Mosapride as an adjunct to lansoprazole for symptom relief of reflux oesophagitis. Br J Clin Pharmacol. 2010;70:171–9.
68. Shaheen NJ, Adler J, Dedrie S, Johnson D, Malfertheiner P, Miner P, Meulemans A, Poole L, Tack J, Thielemans L, Troy S, Vakil N, Zerbib F, Ruth M. Randomised clinical trial: the 5-HT4 agonist revexepride in patients with gastro-oesophageal reflux disease who have persistent symptoms despite PPI therapy. Aliment Pharmacol Ther. 2015;41:649–61.
69. Tack J, Zerbib F, Blondeau K, Varannes S, Piessevaux H, Borovicka J, Mion F, Fox M, Bredenoord A, Louis H, Dedrie S, Hoppenbrouwers M, Meulemans A, Rykx A, Thielemans L, Ruth M. Randomized clinical trial: effect of the 5-HT4 receptor agonist revexepride on reflux parameters in patients with persistent reflux symptoms despite PPI treatment. Neurogastroenterol Motil. 2015;27:258–68.
70. Kahrilas PJ, Quigley EMM, Castell DO, Spechler SJ. The effects of tegaserod (HTF 919) on oesophageal acid exposure in gastro-oesophageal reflux disease. Aliment Pharmacol Ther. 2000;14:1503–9.
71. Fox M, Menne D, Stutz B, Fried M, Schwizer W. The effects of tegaserod on oesophageal function and bolus transport in healthy volunteers: studies using concurrent high-resolution manometry and videofluoroscopy. Aliment Pharmacol Ther. 2006;24:1017–27.
72. Rodriguez-Stanley S, Zubaidi S, Proskin H, Kralstein J, Shetzline M, Miner P. Effect of tegaserod on esophageal pain threshold, regurgitation, and symptom relief in patients with functional heartburn and mechanical sensitivity. Clin Gastroenterol Hepatol. 2006;4:442–50.

73. Scarpellini E, Ang D, Pauwels A, De Santis A, Vanuytsel T, Tack J. Management of refractory typical GERD symptoms. Nat Rev Gastroenterol Hepatol. 2016;13:281.
74. Kessing BF, Smout AJPM, Bennink RJ, Kraaijpoel N, Oors JM, Bredenoord AJ. Prucalopride decreases esophageal acid exposure and accelerates gastric emptying in healthy subjects. Neurogastroenterol Motil. 2014;26:1079–86.
75. Nennstiel S, Bajbouj M, Schmid RM, Becker V. Prucalopride reduces the number of reflux episodes and improves subjective symptoms in gastroesophageal reflux disease: a case series. J Med Case Rep. 2014;8:34.
76. Pitocco A, Grossi L, Di Berardino M, Ciccaglione AF, Marzio L. Prucalopride increases basal LES tone in patients with esophageal motility disorders. United European Gastroenterol J. 2015;3:A477.
77. Carbone F, Rotondo A, Andrews CN, Holvoet L, Van Oudenhove L, Vanuytsel T, Bisschops R, Caenepeel P, Arts J, Papathanasopoulos A, Tack J. Prucalopride improves symptoms and quality of life in a controlled cross-over trial in gastroparesis. Neurogastroenterol Motil. 2016;28:80.
78. Vigone B, Caronni M, Severino A, Bellocchi C, Baldassarri AR, Montanelli G, Santaniello A, Beretta L. Efficacy of prucalopride in the treatment of systemic sclerosis-related intestinal involvement: results from an open label cross-over study. Arthritis Rheumatol. 2016;68:1128–9.
79. Holtmann G, Talley NJ, Liebregts T, Adam B, Parow C. A placebo-controlled trial of itopride in functional dyspepsia. N Engl J Med. 2006;354:832–40.
80. Scarpellini E, Vos R, Blondeau K, Boecxstaens V, Farré R, Gasbarrini A, Tack J. The effects of itopride on oesophageal motility and lower oesophageal sphincter function in man. Aliment Pharmacol Ther. 2011;33:99–105.
81. Kim YS, Kim TH, Choi CS, Shon YW, Kim SW, Seo GS, Nah YH, Choi MG, Choi SC. Effect of itopride, a new prokinetic, in patients with mild GERD: a pilot study. World J Gastroenterol. 2005;11:4210–4.
82. Dicpinigaitis PV. Effect of the GABA-agonist Baclofen on Bronchial Responsiveness in Asthmatics. Pulm Pharmacol Ther. 1999;12(4):257–60.
83. Dicpinigaitis PV. Use of baclofen to suppress cough induced by angiotensin-converting enzyme inhibitors. Ann Pharmacother. 1996;30(11):1242–5.

# Macrolides, Reflux and Respiratory Disease

## 25

Michael G. Crooks and Tamsin Nash

## Introduction

Macrolides are a family of compounds that belong to the polyketides class. They are characterised by a large macrocyclic lactone ring that is produced by chain extension of propionates to which one or more sugars (usually cladinose and desosamine) attach. Macrolides are widely used in healthcare, primarily owing to their antimicrobial properties. The spectrum of antimicrobial activity and tissue penetration makes them particularly suitable for respiratory infections (Gram-positive and some Gram-negative organisms, Chlamydia, Legionella, Mycobacteria and Mycoplasma) [1]. However, macrolides are increasingly being used for their immunomodulatory and prokinetic effects with newer agents having no discernible antimicrobial activity (e.g. Tacrolimus, Sirolimus and Everolimus) [2].

A large number of macrolides exist and can be differentiated by the size of their macrocyclic lactone ring. The three macrolides most commonly used in the management of lung disease are erythromycin, clarithromycin and azithromycin that have 14, 14 and 15-membered rings respectively (Fig. 25.1). Erythromycin is the original macrolide antibiotic and has a similar antimicrobial spectrum to penicillin with additional cover of the 'atypical', intracellular organisms associated with community acquired pneumonia. Subsequent development of clarithromycin and azithromycin offers a broader spectrum of antimicrobial cover with favourable pharmacokinetics allowing lower dosing frequency and fewer adverse effects. These drugs form the cornerstone of antimicrobial therapy for respiratory infection, either as monotherapy or used in combination with penicillins or cephalosporins. However,

M. G. Crooks (✉)
Hull York Medical School, University of Hull, Hull, UK
e-mail: m.g.crooks@hull.ac.uk

T. Nash
Hull and East Yorkshire Hospitals NHS Trust, Hull, UK
e-mail: tamsin.nash@hey.nhs.uk

© Springer International Publishing AG, part of Springer Nature 2018
A. H. Morice, P. W. Dettmar (eds.), *Reflux Aspiration and Lung Disease*,
https://doi.org/10.1007/978-3-319-90525-9_25

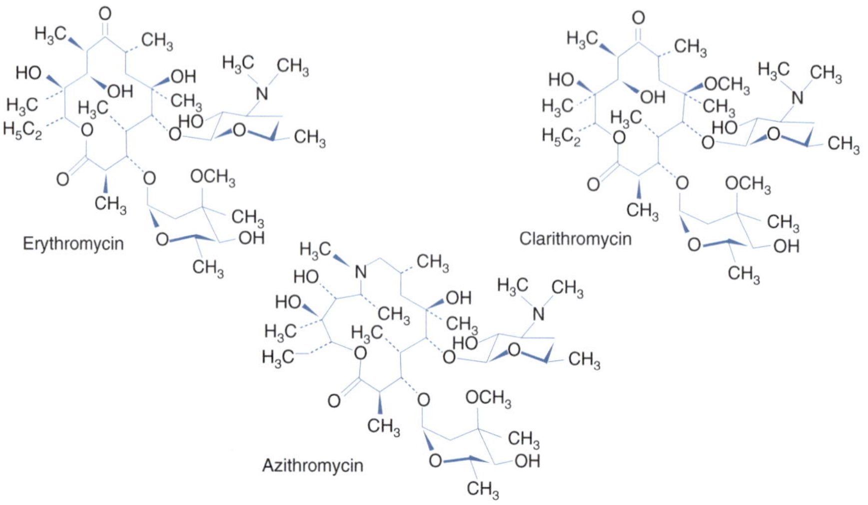

**Fig. 25.1** Structure of macrolides commonly used in the management of respiratory disease

macrolides have also become established treatments for patients with a range of other chronic lung diseases including cystic fibrosis (CF) [3–5]; non-CF bronchiectasis [6, 7], diffuse panbronchiolitis [8, 9], bronchiolitis obliterans syndrome, asthma and chronic obstructive pulmonary disease (COPD) [10, 11] in which they are credited with improving lung function and/or reducing exacerbation frequency. The mechanism of these beneficial effects remains subject to debate with the full spectrum of macrolide effects being proposed.

This chapter will focus on the three most commonly used macrolide antibiotics used to treat lung disease: erythromycin, clarithromycin and azithromycin. A brief history of macrolides and their respective structures will be discussed before focussing on their anti-reflux effects and their benefits in treating a selection of lung diseases.

## History of Macrolide Antibiotics and Their Structure

Erythromycin was the first macrolide to be discovered when it was isolated from Streptomyces erythraeus (later reclassified as Saccharopolyspora erythraea) in 1952. Erythromycin A was subsequently manufactured and launched by Eli Lilly as a broad spectrum antimicrobial providing an alternative for patients sensitive to penicillin [12]. However, erythromycin A's instability in an acidic environment resulted in its degradation to inactive metabolites within the stomach limiting its oral bioavailability [13]. Efforts to increase stability in an acidic environment and therefore improve oral bioavailability led to the production of the first semisynthetic macrolides: erythromycin estolate (Ilosone, Eli Lilly) and erythromycin acistrate (Erasis, Orion Pharma). Subsequently roxithromycin and dirithromycin were produced through modification of the 9-keto group of erythromycin A. However, it was 6-*O*-methylation that led to the production of what would become the market leader, clarithromycin [13].

Clarithromycin (6-*O*-methylerythromycin A) is a semisynthetic macrolide antibiotic created by Taisho Pharmaceutical Co by the addition of a 6-*O*-Methyl group to erythromycin A. 6-*O*-methylation resulted in greater stability in acidic conditions giving it better biological properties and antibacterial activity than erythromycin [14]. Erythromycin A remained the most important base substance for the development of semisynthetic macrolides. Through a series of reactions, including the addition of a nitrogen atom to the lactone ring to form a 15-membered ring, a new class of macrolides called the 'azalides' was created. Azithromycin was the first in this class [13].

Azithromycin (9-dihydro-9-deoxo-9a-methyl-9a-aza-9a-homoerythromycin A) was developed in 1980 and patented in 1981 by PLIVA, a Croatian pharmaceutical company [13]. Azithromycin was subsequently licenced for sale in Western Europe and America by Pfizer, becoming the most prescribed out-patient antibiotic in America in 2010 [15].

## Macrolides in Lung Disease: Protective Properties

### Prokinetic Effect

It has been proposed that the beneficial effects of macrolides in chronic lung diseases may relate to their prokinetic properties, reducing the deleterious consequences of reflux and aspiration events [16].

Since the introduction of erythromycin it has been associated with a series of gastrointestinal side effects. Originally it was suggested that these related to its antibacterial activity leading to alterations in the normal intestinal flora. However, the prominence of gastrointestinal side effects during intravenous administration led to investigation of the effect of macrolides directly on the gut of dogs [17]. It was discovered that intravenous and oral administration of erythromycin and other macrolides induced a dose-dependent strong and sustained contractile response within the stomach and small bowel. It was observed that the effects with erythromycin were similar to those following administration of motilin and therefore it was proposed that the gastrointestinal effects of erythromycin resulted from increased endogenous motilin release [18]. The observation that exposure of muscle strips from dogs to erythromycin does not result in contraction supports the hypothesis that the prokinetic effect in dogs is not due to the direct action of erythromycin on smooth muscle but a secondary phenomenon requiring motilin synthesis and release [18].

Studies in rabbits demonstrated that the prokinetic activity of macrolides varies between species. In contrast to dogs, muscle strips from rabbits do contract in response to erythromycin [19]. This suggests that erythromycin acts directly on the smooth muscle without the need for endogenous motilin production. Indeed, macrolides inhibit the binding of iodinated motilin to rabbit duodenal and colonic muscle in a dose dependent fashion while mimicking the action of motilin. This suggests that erythromycin and other macrolides act as motilin receptor agonists in rabbits [19, 20]. This is supported by the lack of an additive effect of administering motilin and erythromycin in combination.

Similar effects have been observed in humans. Erythromycin has been shown to potentiate gastric and small bowel motility [21], increase lower oesophageal sphincter pressure [22, 23] and effect colonic transit and gall bladder function [18]. However, no increase in motilin concentration occurs following erythromycin infusion in humans [21]. This suggests that it is not endogenous motilin secretion that is responsible for these effects in humans, rather erythromycin is acting as a motilin receptor agonist as seen in rabbits.

The prokinetic effects of erythromycin led to its therapeutic use in conditions with reduced gastric motility including diabetic gastroparesis [24], anorexia nervosa [25], colonic pseudo-obstruction, postoperative ileus [26] and in critical care patients [27].

The prokinetic effects of the other commonly used macrolides have been studied less. Clarithromycin has been shown to increase gastroduodenal motility compared to amoxicillin in patient with *H. pylori* gastritis and functional dyspepsia [28]. Likewise a study of gallbladder emptying following administration of clarithromycin, erythromycin or no drug demonstrated similarly improved gall bladder emptying with both macrolides although the duration of the effect appeared shorter with clarithromycin than erythromycin [29].

Azithromycin also acts as a motilin receptor agonist [30] and has been demonstrated to increase gastric motility in healthy subjects [31]. In patients with impaired gastrointestinal motility, azithromycin has shown comparable positive effects on gastric and duodenal motility to erythromycin [32, 33]. Interestingly, azithromycin has been investigated in 19 patients with GOR disease and using concurrent high resolution manometry and PH-impedance monitoring was found to reduce the number of acid reflux events and the total oesophageal acid exposure [34]. In patients with a hiatus hernia, azithromycin treatment was associated with a reduction in hiatus hernia size.

GOR is common in patients with chronic respiratory disease and in many cases appears to be associated with disease severity. Although it is difficult to identify the chronology of this relationship there is clear scientific and clinical plausibility for the argument that reflux with or without aspiration of gastric contents can have deleterious effects on the airways and result in lung injury. It is therefore conceivable that the beneficial effects of macrolide antibiotics relate to their effects on lower oesophageal sphincter tone and gastroduodenal motility.

## Antibacterial Effects

Bacterial infections are a common reason for presentation with respiratory symptoms in patients with and without underlying lung disease. Indeed, infections can be critical in the pathogenesis of some lung diseases (e.g. cystic fibrosis and bronchiectasis) and have a detrimental effect on the clinical course of others through precipitating acute exacerbations (e.g. COPD).

Macrolides exert their antibacterial effects primarily through binding to the bacterial 50s ribosomal subunits and thereby preventing bacterial protein synthesis. Although they are considered to be primarily bacteriostatic, at higher doses they can be bactericidal. The antimicrobial properties of macrolides are not the primary focus of this chapter and have previously been reviewed elsewhere [35].

## Immunomodulatory Effects

Macrolides have been demonstrated to have a number of protective effects across a wide range of cells including bronchial epithelium, eosinophils, lymphocytes, alveolar macrophages, monocytes, and neutrophils. The majority of immunomodulatory effects are common to the discussed 14 and 15-member compounds however there is a degree of variability [36]. Potentially beneficial effects include: down-regulation of pro-inflammatory cytokine production (IL-5, IL-6, IL-8, IL-10, IL-1β, tumour necrosis factor (TNF)-α and granulocyte-monocyte-colony stimulating factor) [37], inhibition of NF-κB activation, impaired neutrophil superoxide production [38], down regulation of adhesion molecule expression (e.g. ICAM-1) with reduced inflammatory cell influx into the lung [39], and attenuation of extracellular matrix and vascular remodelling [40, 41]. Azithromycin has also been shown to increase the ability of alveolar macrophages to phagocytose apoptotic cells and clear bacteria and cellular debris, reducing local and systemic inflammation [42, 43].

Macrolides have additional beneficial effects in patients colonised with Pseudomonas aeruginosa despite this organism's inherent macrolide resistance. Through destruction of the pseudomonal biofilm, macrolides potentiate killing by anti-pseudomonal antibiotics. Quorum sensing is a system of intercommunication between bacteria that controls biofilm formation and virulence factors. Macrolides interfere with his process by inhibiting the transcription of several genes involved in this process [37]. Additionally, macrolides inhibit bacterial flagellin synthesis, impeding bacterial motility and impairing biofilm formation [44].

The effect of macrolides on inflammation is frequently discussed in clinical trials of their use in individual respiratory diseases.

## Macrolides in Respiratory Diseases

### Asthma

Asthma is a heterogeneous condition characterised by variable airflow obstruction and airways inflammation. The evolution of asthma therapies is seeing the development of treatments that target specific phenotypes, for example omalizumab in atopic asthma and mepolizumab for patients with eosinophilia. However, it is important that available therapies reflect the diversity of the disease and allow targeting of the different facets of an individual patient's airways disease [45].

The association of GORD with asthma is well-known (see Chap. 12). Havemann et al. [46] performed a systematic review in 2007 and identified 28 studies that reported the incidence or prevalence of GORD in asthmatics and vice versa. The average prevalence of GORD symptoms was 59.2% in asthma patients compared to 38.1% in controls. Furthermore, a pooled analysis of three studies that evaluated the severity of asthma related to GORD symptoms revealed that reflux symptoms were more prevalent in patients with increasing asthma severity. However, the temporal relationship between reflux and asthma remains unclear and there remains debate about causality.

The mechanisms underlying the deleterious effects of reflux in asthma are incompletely understood but a number of processes have been described including: micro and macro aspiration of gastric contents; bronchoconstriction mediated by vagal reflexes [47] and neurogenic inflammation in the lung [48]. Although direct airway injury related to aspiration of gastric contents may be important in asthma, reflux of gastric contents into the oesophagus that do not reach the airways can also have deleterious effects.

The prokinetic effect of macrolides has the potential to benefit patients with asthma. Macrolides have been studied in a number of randomised controlled trials across a range of asthma phenotypes. The heterogeneity of trial design and quality and inconsistent outcomes makes it difficult to draw firm conclusions regarding the role of macrolides in the management of asthma. Despite the potential therapeutic effect of macrolides on GOR in asthma patients, no randomised controlled trials have studied this association or stratified patients according to reflux status. In contrast, studies have focussed on assessing the potential immunomodulatory and antimicrobial effects through pre-specified patient stratification and sub-group analyses. The key features of the available randomised trials of macrolides in adult asthma are presented in Table 25.1. Macrolides in childhood asthma is addressed in Chap. 21.

## Bronchiolitis Obliterans

Bronchiolitis obliterans is a progressive condition marked by dyspnoea, wheeze, dry cough and an irreversible obstructive pattern on pulmonary function testing, with an absence of parenchymal abnormality on radiographic studies. It is associated with environmental exposure to occupational fumes and rheumatoid arthritis. Bronchiolitis Obliterans Syndrome (BOS) refers to presentation of the syndrome in transplant recipients: it affects up to 50% of patients in the first 5 years following lung transplantation and is the most common cause of death after 1 year. The disease is characterised by small airway injury, dysregulation of inflammatory pathways, fibroblast proliferation and fibrosis resulting in progressive bronchiolar narrowing and airway obstruction.

GORD is known to cause chronic non-immune airway injury and neutrophilic inflammation, and has been extensively described as a strong predictive risk factor for BOS. A causal relationship between the two conditions is supported by several investigations showing pepsin and bile acids in BAL aspirate from lung allograft recipients. The highest levels were detected in those who developed BOS. Those

**Table 25.1** Summary of randomised controlled trials of macrolides in adult asthma

| Author | Year | Population | Intervention | Summary of main findings |
|---|---|---|---|---|
| Johnston et al. [49] | 2016 | 199 adult patients with a history of asthma experiencing an acute exacerbation requiring corticosteroids | A randomised, double-blind, placebo-controlled trial of azithromycin 500 mg once daily or placebo for 3 days | • No significant difference was observed in terms of symptoms or quality of life with azithromycin<br>• Study limited by high screen failure rate |
| Cameron et al. [50] | 2013 | 77 adult asthmatic current smokers | Randomised, double blind, placebo-controlled trial of azithromycin 250 mg once daily for 12 weeks | • No difference was observed in lung function, quality of life or markers of airway inflammation with azithromycin |
| Brusselle et al. [51] | 2013 | 109 subjects with exacerbation-prone severe asthma | Double blind randomised placebo-controlled trial of low dose azithromycin (250 mg once daily for 5 days followed by 3 times weekly) or placebo for 26 weeks Predefined sub-group analysis was performed in patients with non-eosinophilic asthma | • There was no change in rate of severe exacerbations or LRTI requiring treatment<br>• Azithromycin was associated with a lower rate of severe exacerbations and LRTI requiring treatment in patients with non-eosinophilic asthma |
| Hahn et al. [52] | 2012 | 97 adults with persistent asthma | Randomised, double-blind, placebo-controlled trial of azithromycin 600 mg daily for 3 days followed by 11 once weekly doses. An open label azithromycin group was included for those that declined randomisation Outcome data was evaluated over 12 months | • No difference observed in terms of asthma symptoms, QoL or asthma control in participants randomised to azithromycin compared to placebo<br>• Participants in the open label azithromycin group experienced improvements in symptoms, quality of life and asthma control |

(continued)

**Table 25.1** (continued)

| Author | Year | Population | Intervention | Summary of main findings |
|---|---|---|---|---|
| Sutherland et al. [53] | 2010 | 92 patients with poorly controlled mild—moderate persistent asthma | Randomised placebo controlled trial of clarithromycin 500 mg twice daily or placebo for 16 weeks. Participants were stratified according to PCR evidence of mycoplasma or chlamydia pneumoniae on bronchial biopsy | • Clarithromycin did not lead to improvement in symptom/QoL scores or lung function regardless of PCR status |
| Simpson et al. [54] | 2008 | 45 subjects with severe refractory asthma | Randomised to receive clarithromycin 500 mg twice daily (n = 23) or placebo (n = 22) for 8 weeks | • Significant reduction in IL-8 levels, IL-8 gene expression, neutrophil numbers and neutrophil activation following clarithromycin<br>• Significant improvements in quality of life following clarithromycin<br>• Significant reduction in proportion of participants reporting wheeze in the clarithromycin group<br>• No change in FEV1% predicted, dose-response slope to hypertonic saline, or asthma control score<br>• Positive effects of clarithromycin most prominent in non-eosinophilic asthma |
| Hahn et al. [55] | 2006 | 45 adults with stable persistent asthma | Pilot, randomised, double-blind, placebo-controlled trial of azithromycin 600 mg daily for 3 days followed by once weekly for a further 5 weeks | • Feasibility confirmed for future trial<br>• Improvements seen in terms of symptoms in patients on azithromycin<br>• No significant difference in QoL between groups |

**Table 25.1** (continued)

| Author | Year | Population | Intervention | Summary of main findings |
|---|---|---|---|---|
| Kostadima et al. [56] | 2004 | 63 adult asthma patients | Randomised, double-blind, placebo controlled trial of clarithromycin 250 mg two or three times daily compared to placebo for 8 weeks | • Both doses of clarithromycin were associated with improvement in bronchial hyper-responsiveness with compared to placebo |
| Kraft et al. [57] | 2002 | 55 patients with chronic stable asthma | Randomised double blind placebo controlled trial of clarithromycin 500 mg twice daily or placebo for 6 weeks. Analysis was performed with reference to evidence of mycoplasma or chlamydia pneumoniae on PCR (31/55 patients were PCR positive) | • Improvements in FEV-1 and markers of airway inflammation were observed following clarithromycin in patients with evidence of mycoplasma or chlamydia pneumoniae on PCR<br>• No improvements were observed in PCR negative patients |
| Amayasu et al. [58] | 2000 | 17 adults with stable mild or moderate asthma | Clarithromycin 200 mg or placebo twice daily for 8 weeks. Double blind, randomised cross over trial. Airway responsiveness assessed using methacholine provocation testing | • Airway responsiveness improved in all patients after clarithromycin<br>• Reduced markers of airway inflammation occurred following clarithromycin<br>• Patients had significant decrease in symptoms following clarithromycin |
| Shoji et al. [59] | 1999 | 14 adults with mild—moderate aspirin-intolerant asthma | Randomised, double-blind, placebo controlled cross-over trial of Roxithromycin 150 mg twice daily or placebo for 8 weeks | • No change was observed in airway responsiveness following roxithromycin<br>• Roxithromycin resulted in improvements in symptoms, blood eosinophils and sputum eosinophilic cationic protein |

*FEV-1* forced expiratory volume in 1 s, *IL-8* interleukin 8, *LRTI* lower respiratory tract infection, *PCR* polymerase chain reaction, *QoL* quality of life with raised BAL bile acid concentration demonstrated a greater degree of neutrophilia and higher concentrations of IL-8, suggesting that non-acid reflux disease was the trigger of neutrophilic inflammation in these patients [60–62]. Furthermore, several studies have shown that surgical control of GORD by Nissen fundoplication is associated with improved lung function in transplant recipients [63].

Macrolides have the potential to benefit patients with obliterative bronchiolitis through their immunomodulatory and prokinetic properties. Beneficial effects of azithromycin have been described in a number of observational and randomised controlled trials in BOS. A summary of the randomised controlled trials and larger observational studies is provided in Table 25.2. Despite the limited available evidence, azithromycin does appear to have a role in the management of BOS with the greatest benefits described in the earlier stages of the condition and in patients with evidence of

**Table 25.2** Summary of the randomised controlled trials and larger observational studies of macrolides in bronchiolitis obliterans syndrome

| Author | Year | Study population | Study design and intervention | Summary of main findings |
|---|---|---|---|---|
| Corris et al. [65] | 2015 | 48 patients with BOS post lung transplant (25 azithromycin and 23 placebo) | Randomised, placebo-controlled trial of azithromycin 250 mg on alternate days vs placebo for 12 weeks | • No difference in FEV-1 at 12 weeks in ITT analysis (5 patients in placebo group withdrew and received open-label azithromycin)<br>• Significant improvement in FEV-1 at 12 weeks with azithromycin in study completers |
| Vos et al. [66] | 2011 | 83 patients following lung transplant (40 azithromycin and 43 placebo) | Randomised, double-blind, placebo-controlled trial of azithromycin 250 mg or placebo three times weekly for 2 years. Patients that developed BOS were treated with open-label azithromycin | • BOS occurred less in patients receiving azithromycin (12.5% vs 44%; p = 0.002)<br>• Those receiving azithromycin demonstrated better FEV1 (p = 0.028) and lower airway neutrophilia (p = 0.015) and CRP (p = 0.05)<br>• FEV1 improved in 52.2% of patients receiving open-label azithromycin for BOS<br>• No difference in GOR reflux prevalence following azithromycin |

**Table 25.2** (continued)

| Author | Year | Study population | Study design and intervention | Summary of main findings |
|---|---|---|---|---|
| Federica et al. [67] | 2011 | 62 lung transplant recipients; 25 with potential BOS and 37 with BOS grade 1–3 | Retrospective cohort study Participants received azithromycin for 12 months (250 mg daily for 5 days, then three times weekly) | • 13 (21%) demonstrated ≥10% FEV1 increase; 35 had graft function stabilisation; 14 deteriorated<br>• Higher response rate in potential BOS (44%) compared to BOS grade 1–3 (6%) |
| Lam et al. [68] | 2010 | 22 patients diagnosed with BOS following HSCT (10 azithromycin and 12 controls) | Randomised, double-blind, placebo-controlled trial of azithromycin 250 mg or placebo daily for 12 weeks | • No significant difference in lung functions test results at 1, 2, 3, or 4 months between treatment and control groups<br>• No significant difference in respiratory symptom, impact or activities scores between groups |
| Vos et al. [69] | 2010 | 107 patients with BOS post-transplant treated with azithromycin | Retrospective cohort study | • FEV1 increased by ≥10% in 40% (responders)<br>• Pre-treatment neutrophilia in 29.2% of responders compared to 11.5% non-responders<br>• Responders demonstrated improved survival compared to non-responders |
| Jain et al. [70] | 2010 | 179 consecutive patients who developed BOS following lung transplant | Retrospective cohort study between 1999 and 2007 84 patients were treated with azithromycin (6 excluded as received azithromycin for other indications) and 95 did not receive macrolides | • Lower risk of death in those started on azithromycin prior to development of stage 2 disease (HR 0.29, CI 0.11–0.82, p = 0.02)<br>• No difference in risk of death for those started on azithromycin after BOS stage 2 |

(continued)

**Table 25.2** (continued)

| Author | Year | Study population | Study design and intervention | Summary of main findings |
|---|---|---|---|---|
| Gottlieb et al. [71] | 2008 | 81 patients diagnosed with BOS following lung transplant | Single centre observational study of azithromycin 250 mg three times weekly for 6 months | • 30% showed improvement in FEV1 at 3 months<br>• Responders at 6 months had higher pre-treatment BAL neutrophils<br>• Pre-treatment BAL showing <20% neutrophils had negative predictive value of 0.91 for response to treatment<br>• Concomitant PPI use was a negative predictor for disease progression |

*FEV-1* forced expiratory volume in 1 s, *ITT* intention to treat, *HSCT* haematopoietic stem-cell transplant

pre-treatment neutrophilia. Azithromycin has been shown to reduce the number of reflux events in patients following lung transplantation and reduce bile acid concentration in bronchoalveolar lavage samples suggesting it also reduces microaspiration [64].

## Non-CF Bronchiectasis

Bronchiectasis is characterised by chronic bronchial inflammation, bronchial wall thickening and dilatation. Excessive sputum production and failure of the mucociliary escalator is associated with infection and a vicious cycle of progressive airway inflammation and fibrosis. Patients experience chronic cough, wheeze and breathlessness, and frequently experience infective exacerbations. The lungs become colonised with multiple pathogens, for example, Haemophilus influenza and Pseudomonas aeruginosa. The inflammatory response to infection in bronchiectasis is predominantly neutrophilic with elevated levels of associated proinflammatory cytokines [72].

The remodelling that occurs in bronchiectasis can be secondary to a number of infectious and inflammatory conditions. GORD has been considered as a factor contributing to lung injury and chronic inflammation via a process of chronic aspiration. Indeed, a study of 27 bronchiectasis patients revealed the presence of GOR in 40% using 24 h oesophageal pH monitoring, frequently in the absence of typical symptoms and therefore termed clinically silent [73]. In a case series of seven patients, Hu et al. reviewed the role of GORD and its treatment in bronchiectasis. Five patients underwent laparoscopic fundoplication, and two underwent repair of hiatus hernias; all demonstrated resolution of their reflux symptoms and to a variable degree, wheeze, cough, sputum production and haemoptysis [74].

Macrolides have the potential to benefit patients with bronchiectasis through their antimicrobial properties, immunomodulatory effects and prokinetic activity. As such, a number of studies have investigated the efficacy of long term macrolide therapy in non-CF bronchiectasis. A summary of randomised-controlled trials of azithromycin in adults with non-CF bronchiectasis is provided in Table 25.3. Although the available trials are methodologically varied in terms of the studied population, choice of macrolide, dosing regimen and duration of treatment; a

**Table 25.3** Summary of randomised controlled trials of azithromycin in adults with non-CF bronchiectasis

| Author | Year | Study population | Intervention (n) | Summary of main findings |
|---|---|---|---|---|
| Serisier et al. [76] | 2013 | 117 non-smoking adults with non-CF bronchiectasis and 2 or more infective exacerbations in the past year | Randomised, double-blind, placebo-controlled trial of erythromycin 400 mg twice daily (n = 59), or placebo (n = 58) for 48 weeks | Erythromycin had the following effects:<br>• Reduction in exacerbations (incidence rate ratio 0.57 $P = 0.003$)<br>• Reduced 24 h sputum production.<br>• Reduced lung function decline ($P = 0.04$)<br>• Increased proportion of macrolide resistant oropharyngeal streptococci |
| Diego et al. [77] | 2013 | 30 adults with stable non-CF bronchiectasis | Randomised, open-label study of azithromycin 250 mg three times weekly for 3 months (n = 16) versus controls (n = 14) | • Significant reduction in sputum volume with azithromycin ($-9.9$ vs $+2.1$ ml, $P < 0.05$)<br>• Significant reduction in exacerbation frequency with azithromycin (0.1 vs 1.2, $P < 0.05$)<br>• Significant reductions in dyspnoea and SGRQ scores with azithromycin ($P < 0.05$) |
| Altenburg et al. [6] | 2013 | 83 patients with non-CF bronchiectasis and ≥3 LRTIs in preceding year | Randomised, double-blind, placebo-controlled trial of azithromycin 250 mg daily (n = 43) compared to placebo (n = 40) for 12 months | • Reduced number of exacerbations with azithromycin (median 0 vs 2 in placebo group ($p < 0.001$)<br>• 32 placebo-treated patients vs 20 azithromycin treated patients had at least 1 exacerbation (HR 0.29 CI 0.15–0.51)<br>• FEV1 increase of 1.03% per 3 months treatment of azithromycin compared to decrease of 0.1% per 3 months in the placebo group ($P = 0.047$) |

(continued)

**Table 25.3** (continued)

| Author | Year | Study population | Intervention (n) | Summary of main findings |
|---|---|---|---|---|
| Wong et al. [7] | 2012 | 141 patients with bronchiectasis defined on HRCT and at least 1 exacerbation in the previous year | Randomised, double-blind, placebo-controlled trial of 500 mg azithromycin (n = 71) or placebo (n = 70) three times a week for 6 months | • Reduced exacerbation rate with azithromycin (rate ratio 0.38, CI 0.26–0.54; p < 0.0001)<br>• No change in pre-bronchodilator FEV1 from baseline or between groups<br>• No difference in SGRQ score between groups |
| Cymbala et al. [78] | 2005 | 11 patients with bronchiectasis confirmed on HRCT | Randomised, non-placebo controlled cross-over trial of oral azithromycin 500 mg twice weekly for 6 months in addition to usual care compared to usual care alone | • Significantly reduced incidence of exacerbations with azithromycin (5 vs 16 p = 0.019)<br>• No significant change in pulmonary function tests |
| Tsang et al. [79] | 1999 | 21 patients with steady state idiopathic bronchiectasis | Double-blind, placebo-controlled pilot study of erythromycin 500 mg twice daily (n = 11) or placebo (n = 10) for 8 weeks | • Significant improvement in FEV1 and FVC compared to baseline with erythromycin (P < 0.05)<br>• Reduced 24 h sputum volume compared to baseline with erythromycin (p < 0.05)<br>• No difference in respiratory pathogen density or markers of inflammation from baseline or between groups |

*FEV-1* forced expiratory volume in 1 s, *FVC* forced vital capacity, *SGRQ* St Georges respiratory questionnaire

consistent observation is a reduction in exacerbation frequency. When making a clinical decision regarding the use of macrolides in non-CF bronchiectasis it is important to balance this benefit with the potential risks of macrolide resistance and the potential association with atypical mycobacterial infection that has been observed in CF [75]. The impact of macrolide therapy on GOR in patients with non-CF bronchiectasis has not been studied and therefore the contribution of this effect to exacerbation reduction remains unknown.

## Chronic Obstructive Pulmonary Disease

The clinical course of COPD is characterised by chronic and progressive symptoms of shortness of breath and cough with episodes of acute worsening out-with normal day-to-day variability termed acute exacerbations. Exacerbations are a significant cause of morbidity and mortality in COPD and represent a challenge for health services, often resulting in contact with unscheduled care services [80, 81]. COPD exacerbations have been suggested to have a number of possible causes including infection (viral or bacterial) [82–85] environmental pollution [86] and aspiration of gastric contents [87].

Numerous studies have demonstrated that gastroesophageal reflux (GOR) is prevalent in COPD patients and correlates with an increased risk of exacerbation and health care utilisation [87–90]. See Chap. 13 for a more detailed analysis. Briefly, GOR is more common in females and is associated with a chronic bronchitis phenotype, a more significant symptom burden and poorer quality of life [91, 92]. A small study of stable COPD patients has demonstrated that an abnormal swallowing reflex is also more common among COPD patients than controls and is associated with GOR disease symptoms and an increased exacerbation frequency [93]. Interestingly, in this patient cohort bacteria were isolated more frequently in the induced sputum of patients with an abnormal swallowing reflex identifying aspiration as a potential route for bacterial colonisation of the respiratory tract. The association between GOR and COPD is not surprising when one considers their pathophysiology.

Pathological GOR results from the failure of the bodies usual protective mechanisms. In health, GOR is prevented by the action of the oesophageal musculature, most importantly the lower oesophageal sphincter that maintains a normal tone and frequency of transient relaxations. In addition, the diaphragmatic crura applies an extrinsic pressure on the lower oesophagus providing additional protection against reflux of gastric contents [94]. Disruption of these mechanisms results in GOR.

Cigarette smoking is recognised to cause relaxation of the lower oesophageal sphincter with the potential to precipitate reflux events [95]. Likewise, it is possible that alterations in the pressure gradient between the abdomen and thorax related to the altered respiratory dynamics in COPD may precipitate reflux. Reflux of gastric contents into the upper airways with subsequent aspiration may contribute to the inflammatory response and bacterial colonisation observed in the lungs of patients with COPD [96]. The respiratory complications of aspiration of gastric contents are frequently encountered by practicing clinicians and encompass a spectrum of presentations. It is not surprising that patients with COPD, who have a high prevalence of GOR will experience related complications that manifest as acute deterioration in their clinical state, i.e. acute exacerbations.

Conventionally, studies exploring the effect of GOR treatment on respiratory outcomes have adopted a strategy of acid suppression. This approach has provided conflicting results. A study of COPD patients included in the Copenhagen City Heart Study identified an increased risk of exacerbations in COPD patients with comorbid GOR who were not using acid suppression but not in patients using acid suppressing therapy regularly [92]. This was not observed in a recent large observational study of the ECLIPSE cohort with increased exacerbation rates observed in patients with GOR irrespective of acid suppression [97]. However, a randomised trial of acid suppression using a proton pump inhibitor (PPI) demonstrated a significant reduction in COPD exacerbation frequency [98]. This trial was small and single-blind with no placebo administered to the control group and therefore further investigation in a large, double-blind, placebo-controlled, randomised trial is required to investigate this further. However, acid suppression alone fails to address the deleterious effects of non-acid elements of refluxate. The prokinetic properties of macrolides have potential advantages in this regard. Indeed, their described immunomodulatory and antimicrobial properties broadens their therapeutic potential in COPD.

A number of clinical studies have investigated the role of macrolide antibiotics in preventing COPD exacerbations. These studies are summarised below:

## Erythromycin

Suzuki et al. [99] conducted an open label, randomised-controlled trial of erythromycin at a dose of 200–400 mg per day for 1 year in COPD patients. One hundred and nine patients were randomised and observed for symptoms of a common cold and COPD exacerbation. There was a significant reduction in the number of patients experiencing symptoms of a common cold and suffering COPD exacerbations in patients receiving erythromycin compared with controls. The relative risk of experiencing an exacerbation in the control group was 4.71 (95% CI 1.53–14.5. P = 0.007).

Seemungal et al. [100] undertook a randomised, double-blind, placebo-controlled trial of erythromycin 250 mg twice per day for 1 year in COPD patients. This study used co-primary outcome measures of exacerbation frequency and airway inflammation. The latter was measured by sputum IL-6, IL-8 and myeloperoxidase (MPO) and serum IL-6 and C-reactive protein. One hundred and fifteen patients were recruited with 109 undergoing randomisation. Daily erythromycin was associated with a significant reduction in exacerbation rate (rate ratio 0.648 (95% CI 0.489–0.859, P = 0.003) and prolonged time to first exacerbation (median 271 days versus 89 days in the placebo arm. P = 0.02). Exacerbations occurring in patients receiving erythromycin were on average of shorter duration than those in the placebo group. There was no difference between markers of airway or systemic inflammation between the groups.

He et al. [101] investigated the role of erythromycin at a dose of 125 mg three times a day for 6 months in a double-blind, placebo-controlled, randomised trial. Thirty one patients completed this study and patients taking erythromycin experienced a prolonged time to first exacerbation and reduced exacerbation rate compared with controls. It was also noted that sputum neutrophil counts were lower in the erythromycin treated group suggesting reduced airways inflammation.

The 3 studies of long term erythromycin in COPD patients are all small and are of variable quality. However, the consistent demonstration of a reduction in the rate of COPD exacerbations associated with daily erythromycin is promising and supports a role for macrolides in COPD exacerbation prevention. However, erythromycin requires more frequent dosing and has a higher propensity to cause gastrointestinal side effects than other macrolide antibiotics and therefore is a less attractive option for long term treatment regimens.

## Clarithromycin

Banerjee et al. [102] investigated the role of clarithromycin in a randomised, double-blind, placebo-controlled trial of patients with moderate-severe COPD. Sixty-seven patients were randomised to receive oral clarithromycin at a dose of 500 mg once per day (n = 31) or placebo (n = 36) for 3 months. The primary outcome in this study was health status measured using the St Georges Respiratory Questionnaire (SGRQ) and short form 36-item questionnaire (SF-36) with secondary outcome measures including sputum bacterial load, infective exacerbation rate, exercise capacity measured by shuttle walk test, and serum C-reactive protein. It is noteworthy that there was a significant difference in measures of health status at baseline with higher SGRQ and SF-36 scores observed in those randomised to receive clarithromycin. However, there was no significant change in health status between the groups at 3 months. Few exacerbations occurred during the study (5 in the clarithromycin group and 2 in the placebo group) with no significant difference between the groups. No difference was observed in sputum microbiology or any of the other secondary outcome measures.

The negative outcome of this study is somewhat disappointing given the positive results seen with erythromycin. However, the short duration of this study and low number of exacerbations limits its power. It remains possible that clarithromycin may offer the same benefits as its fellow macrolides but there have not been trials of sufficient size or duration to evaluate this. Therefore, a larger trial of sufficient duration is required to assess the role for daily clarithromycin in COPD.

## Azithromycin

In 2010, Blasi et al. [103] published a randomised trial of azithromycin 500 mg three times per week versus standard care for 6 months in 22 patients with severe COPD and tracheostomy. This was an open label pilot study aiming to evaluate the safety and efficacy of this treatment regimen. Patients were monitored for a total of 1 year (6 months treatment followed by 6 months observation) and the primary outcome measure was the number of exacerbations and hospitalisations during the study period. Secondary outcome measures included the time to first exacerbation and hospitalisation, airways inflammation measured by inflammatory cytokine levels in exhaled breath condensate, mortality, quality of life and safety. Despite the small number of patients in this study a significantly lower number of exacerbations and hospitalisations were observed in the Azithromycin group compared to standard care during the treatment period. It is noteworthy that there were significantly fewer exacerbations during the treatment period compared to the subsequent 6 month follow-up period in those randomised to receive Azithromycin suggesting that the benefit is limited to the time that the patient is receiving the drug. Although there was a trend towards reduced mortality in the Azithromycin group (27% versus 46% with standard care) this did not reach statistical significance. Exhaled breath condensate was only measured in 3 patients receiving Azithromycin and 2 patients receiving standard care. Levels of IL-6 and TNF-α decreased during Azithromycin treatment, returning to baseline following discontinuation of treatment. There was a small rise in IL-6 and TNF-α in the standard care group. Azithromycin was also associated with improvement in quality of life measured by MRF26 score, no change was observed in the standard care group. Few adverse events were described in the Azithromycin group with 4 patients describing mild gastrointestinal side effects.

The findings of Blasi et al. [103] were promising and consistent with the earlier erythromycin studies. The finding during the 6 month observation period following Azithromycin discontinuation suggests that the beneficial effects are limited to the treatment period. However, the limited sample size and open-label nature of the study made it impossible to draw firm, generalisable conclusions.

Albert et al. [10] addressed any uncertainty regarding the beneficial effects of azithromycin when they published their large, randomised, placebo-controlled trial of Azithromycin in COPD patients with a prior history of exacerbations. A total of 1142 patients were randomised to receive Azithromycin 250 mg once per day or placebo for 1 year. The primary outcome was the time to first exacerbation and secondary outcomes included quality of life, nasopharyngeal colonisation with respiratory pathogens, and study medication adherence. Patients randomised to receive azithromycin experienced a prolonged time to first exacerbation (median 266 days versus 174 days with placebo) and a reduction in exacerbation frequency by 0.35 exacerbations per patient-year. Patients in the azithromycin group also experienced an improvement in quality of life measured by the St Georges Respiratory Questionnaire. No difference in mortality was observed between the groups and most importantly the cardiovascular mortality was the same (0.2%) in both groups. The main adverse event observed in the Azithromycin group was an increased frequency of audiogram confirmed hearing decrement compared with the placebo group (25% and 20% respectively). With regard to nasopharyngeal bacteriology, patients in the azithromycin group were less likely to become colonized during the study period however the rate of macrolide resistance was higher in the azithromycin group (81% and 41% respectively).

The publication of this large clinical trial has led to azithromycin becoming the macrolide of choice in COPD patients. A series of further randomised trials have been undertaken since 2011 and have confirmed the associated reduction in exacerbation frequency [104]. A summary of clinical trials of azithromycin in COPD are presented in Table 25.4.

Interestingly, Berkhof et al. [105] undertook a randomised, double-blind, placebo-controlled trial to assess the effect of azithromycin 250 mg three times a week for 3 months on cough-specific health status in COPD patients. This study is worthy of individual mention because it investigates a different facet of COPD symptomatology with cough often a prominent symptom in patients with reflux and microaspiration. In this study, 84 patients were randomised and cough-specific health status assessed using the Leicester Cough Questionnaire (LCQ). Patients randomised to receive Azithromycin had a significant improvement in LCQ score

**Table 25.4** Summary of randomised controlled trials of azithromycin in COPD

| Author | Year | Intervention (n) | Summary of main findings |
|---|---|---|---|
| Blasi et al. [103] | 2010 | Azithromycin 500 mg 3 × per week (n = 11) Standard care (n = 11) | • Reduction in exacerbations and hospitalisations with azithromycin<br>• Improved quality of life with azithromycin |
| Albert et al. [10] | 2011 | Azithromycin 250 mg od (n = 570) Placebo (n = 572) | • Reduced exacerbation frequency with azithromycin<br>• Prolonged time to first exacerbation with azithromycin<br>• Improved quality of life with azithromycin<br>• Reduced nasopharyngeal colonisation during study with azithromycin but increased macrolide resistance |
| Berkhof et al. [105] | 2013 | Azithromycin 250 mg 3 × per week (n = 42) Placebo (n = 42) | • Improved cough-specific health status with azithromycin<br>• Improved quality of life with azithromycin<br>• Trend towards reduced exacerbations with azithromycin |
| Uzun et al. [104] | 2014 | Azithromycin 500 mg 3 × per week (n = 47) Placebo (n = 45) | • Reduced exacerbation rate with azithromycin<br>• Prolonged time to first exacerbation in azithromycin group<br>• Increased diarrhoea reported with azithromycin |
| Simpson et al. [106] | 2014 | Azithromycin 250 mg od (n = 15) Placebo (n = 15) | • Nonsignificant reduction in sputum neutrophils, CXCL8 and bacterial load with azithromycin<br>• Trend towards reduction in exacerbations with azithromycin |

compared with placebo with benefits mainly observed in patients with lower scores at baseline (i.e. those with worse cough-specific health status at baseline). Consistent with the findings of Blasi et al. [103] the beneficial effects of Azithromycin were limited to during treatment with LCQ scores falling following cessation of the drug. Azithromycin also resulted in significant improvements in SGRQ and SF-36 scores and although there was a trend towards fewer exacerbations and prolonged time to first exacerbation in the Azithromycin group this failed to reach statistical significance. No differences were observed between the groups in terms of spirometry measures.

Macrolides have repeatedly been shown to reduce exacerbation frequency in patients with COPD. Azithromycin has become the favoured macrolide for this indication, partly due to its favourable pharmacokinetics meaning it can be administered less frequently, but predominantly due to the larger body of evidence supporting it. However, there remains uncertainty regarding the optimum dosing regimen with a range of doses and frequencies used in clinical trials resulting in heterogeneous prescribing in practice. Another area of debate relates to which macrolide effect is responsible for their benefit.

## Cystic Fibrosis (CF)

Cystic fibrosis is the most commonly inherited genetic disease in Caucasian populations effecting approximately 1 in 2500 newborns [107]. It is an autosomal recessive multisystem disorder caused by mutations in the cystic fibrosis transmembrane conductance regulator (CFTR) gene. Although over 1600 different mutations have been described, approximately 70% of patients have the $\Delta$F508 mutation (deletion of phenylalanine at codon 508). Lung disease is usually the most prominent feature in older children and adults with cystic fibrosis and is the most common cause of death [107]. Recurrent and often chronic suppurative lower respiratory infections are a hallmark feature of CF with colonisation and infection with pathogenic organisms associated with different stages of disease progression including Haemophilus influenza, *Staphylococcus aureus*, Pseudomonas aeruginosa and Burkholderia cepacia complex. In recent years additional organisms including methicillin resistant *Staphylococcus aureus* (MRSA), non-tuberculous mycobacteria (NTM) and Stenotrophomonas maltophilia are emerging as important pathogens [108]. As such, treatment of CF related lung disease focuses on the prevention and early treatment of pulmonary infections using a range of non-pharmacological and pharmacological strategies.

GOR is prevalent in patients with cystic fibrosis and appears to be associated with more severe lung disease and more frequent exacerbations [109]. Mechanisms predisposing to GOR in CF include reduced lower oesophageal sphincter tone with frequent transient relaxations, delayed gastric emptying and lower intrathoracic pressures during inspiration altering the thoracoabdominal pressure gradient in favour of reflux [109, 110]. Interventions targeting the GOR in CF have been trialled. A retrospective review of 48 CF patients and uncontrolled GOR who underwent Nissen fundoplication demonstrated a significant improvement in FEV-1, pulmonary exacerbation rate and weight over the 2 years following surgery [111]. Similarly, a smaller case-series of 6 patients with intractable cough, GOR and CF that underwent Nissen fundoplication experienced reduction in cough, improved spirometry and reduced exacerbation frequency [112]. Although these studies are small and not randomised or controlled, they suggest that selected CF patients with GOR benefit from anti-reflux treatment in terms of symptoms and lung function.

Data on acid suppression in CF is of poor quality. Retrospective data of lansoprazole use in children with CF suggested potential benefits in terms of weight gain and respiratory dynamics [113]. However, a small randomised trial of PPI treatment did not reveal any benefit in frequently exacerbating CF patients without reflux symptoms despite 62% having evidence of acid reflux on PH-monitoring [114]. Therefore, there is limited evidence to support the routine use of PPI's to treat GOR in CF.

There have been a number of clinical trials evaluating the effects of long term azithromycin in CF and it is the subject of a Cochrane review [5]. A summary of the key randomised, double-blind, placebo-controlled azithromycin trials are presented in Table 25.5. Other macrolides have been studied in CF but with limited effect [115].

**Table 25.5** Summary of the key randomised, double-blind, placebo-controlled trials of azithromycin in CF

| Author | Year | Study population | Intervention (n) | Summary of main findings |
|---|---|---|---|---|
| Saiman et al. [116] | 2010 | CF patients aged 6–18 years without pseudomonas | Azithromycin 250–500 mg 3 times a week (n = 131) Placebo (n = 129) | • No difference in FEV1 between groups<br>• 50% reduction in exacerbations with azithromycin<br>• Reduced cough in azithromycin group<br>Weight gain with azithromycin |
| Kabra et al. [117] | 2010 | Children (aged 5–18) with CF | Azithromycin 5 mg/kg od (n = 28) Azithromycin 15 mg/kg od (n = 28) | • No difference between groups in terms of clinical scores, FEV1 or exacerbations<br>• Significant increase in exacerbations following stopping azithromycin |
| Steinkamp et al. [118] | 2008 | CF patients aged ≥8 years with Pseudomonas | Azithromycin 500-1250 mg once per week (n = 21) Placebo (n = 17) | • No difference in FEV1 between groups<br>• Reduced markers of inflammation with azithromycin (CRP, IL-8, LBP)<br>• Improved symptoms and quality of life with azithromycin |
| McCormack et al. [119] | 2007 | CF patients aged 6–58 years | Azithromycin 250 mg od (n = 103) Azithromycin 1200 mg once weekly (n = 105) | • No difference between groups in terms of lung function, hospital admission and inflammatory markers.<br>• Increased GI side effects with once weekly therapy |
| Clement et al. [4] | 2006 | CF patients aged ≥6 years | Azithromycin 250–500 mg 3 times per week (n = 40) Placebo (n = 42) | • No difference in change in FEV1 between the groups<br>• Reduction in exacerbations and prolonged time to first exacerbation with azithromycin |
| Saiman et al. [3] | 2003 | CF patients aged ≥6 years with Pseudomonas | Azithromycin 250–500 mg 3 times a week (n = 87) Placebo (n = 98) | • Improved FEV1 with azithromycin<br>• Reduced exacerbation risk with azithromycin<br>• Increased weight with azithromycin<br>• Increased GI side effects with azithromycin |

(continued)

**Table 25.5** (continued)

| Author | Year | Study population | Intervention (n) | Summary of main findings |
|---|---|---|---|---|
| Equi et al. [120] | 2002 | CF patients aged 8–18 years | Azithromycin 250–500 mg od or placebo (n = 41) cross-over trial design | • Increased FEV1 with azithromycin<br>• Fewer additional oral antibiotic courses with azithromycin<br>• No difference in exacerbations or IV antibiotic use |
| Wolter et al. [121] | 2002 | Adult CF patients | Azithromycin 250 mg od (n = 30) Placebo (n = 30) | • FEV1 and FVC maintained with azithromycin, declined with placebo<br>• Fewer IV antibiotic courses with azithromycin<br>• Reduced CRP with azithromycin<br>• Improved quality of life with azithromycin |

*CRP* C-reactive protein, *FEV-1* forced expiratory volume in 1 s, *FVC* forced vital capacity, *GI* gastrointestinal, *IL-8* interleukin 8, *IV* intravenous, *LBP* lipopolysaccharide binding protein

## Conclusions

Macrolides have played a central role in the management of respiratory infections for over 50 years. However, their role in the treatment across a broad range of respiratory diseases is only now being realised. The effect of macrolides on the gastrointestinal tract is well established. It is increasingly understood that abnormal gastrointestinal tract function in the form of GOR is associated with adverse outcomes in patients with respiratory disease. Despite this, the effect of macrolides on GOR is rarely addressed or acknowledged in randomised trials evaluating their efficacy in these patients. Rather, investigators appear to favour exploration of their antimicrobial and/or immunomodulatory effects. As a result, the mechanism underlying macrolides beneficial effects in respiratory disease remains incompletely understood. However, it is both scientifically and clinically plausible that macrolides effect on the GI tract, reducing GOR, contributes to their protective properties.

Despite the discussed benefits of macrolide therapy, there are concerns about potential harms. It is essential that these are considered in the context of the burden of the disease that macrolides are being used to treat. Therefore, clinicians and patients should make an informed decision about the appropriateness of macrolide therapy based on balancing risks and benefits on a case by case basis.

## References

1. Baldwin DR, Wise R, Andrews JM, Ashby JP, Honeybourne D. Azithromycin concentrations at the sites of pulmonary infection. Eur Respir J. 1990;3(8):886–90.
2. Kwiatkowska B, Maslinska M. Macrolide therapy in chronic inflammatory diseases. Mediat Inflamm. 2012;2012:636157.
3. Saiman L, Marshall BC, Mayer-Hamblett N, Burns JL, Quittner AL, Cibene DA, et al. Azithromycin in patients with cystic fibrosis chronically infected with Pseudomonas aeruginosa: a randomized controlled trial. JAMA. 2003;290(13):1749–56.
4. Clement A, Tamalet A, Leroux E, Ravilly S, Fauroux B, Jais JP. Long term effects of azithromycin in patients with cystic fibrosis: a double blind, placebo controlled trial. Thorax. 2006;61(10):895–902.
5. Southern KW, Barker PM, Solis-Moya A, Patel L. Macrolide antibiotics for cystic fibrosis. Cochrane Database Syst Rev. 2012;11:Cd002203.
6. Altenburg J, de Graaff CS, Stienstra Y, Sloos JH, van Haren EH, Koppers RJ, et al. Effect of azithromycin maintenance treatment on infectious exacerbations among patients with non-cystic fibrosis bronchiectasis: the BAT randomized controlled trial. JAMA. 2013;309(12):1251–9.
7. Wong C, Jayaram L, Karalus N, Eaton T, Tong C, Hockey H, et al. Azithromycin for prevention of exacerbations in non-cystic fibrosis bronchiectasis (EMBRACE): a randomised, double-blind, placebo-controlled trial. Lancet. 2012;380(9842):660–7.
8. Hui D, Yan F, Chen RH. The effects of azithromycin on patients with diffuse panbronchiolitis: a retrospective study of 29 cases. J Thorac Dis. 2013;5(5):613–7.
9. Lin X, Lu J, Yang M, Dong BR, Wu HM. Macrolides for diffuse panbronchiolitis. Cochrane Database Syst Rev. 2015;(1):Cd007716.
10. Albert RK, Connett J, Bailey WC, Casaburi R, Cooper JA Jr, Criner GJ, et al. Azithromycin for prevention of exacerbations of COPD. N Engl J Med. 2011;365(8):689–98.
11. Ni W, Shao X, Cai X, Wei C, Cui J, Wang R, et al. Prophylactic use of macrolide antibiotics for the prevention of chronic obstructive pulmonary disease exacerbation: a meta-analysis. PLoS One. 2015;10(3):e0121257.
12. McGuire J, Bunch RL, Anderson RC, Boaz HE, Flynn EH, Powell HM, et al. Ilotycin, a new antibiotic. Antibiot Chemother. 1952;2(6):281–3.
13. Mutak S. Azalides from azithromycin to new azalide derivatives. J Antibiot. 2007;60(2):85–122.
14. Morimoto S, Takahashi Y, Watanabe Y, Omura S. Chemical modification of erythromycins. I. Synthesis and antibacterial activity of 6-O-methylerythromycins A. J Antibiot. 1984;37(2):187–9.
15. Hicks LA, Taylor TH Jr, Hunkler RJ. U.S. outpatient antibiotic prescribing, 2010. N Engl J Med. 2013;368(15):1461–2.
16. Crooks MG, Hart SP, Morice AH. Azithromycin for prevention of exacerbations of COPD. N Engl J Med. 2011;365(23):2234–5; author reply 6.
17. Itoh Z, Suzuki T, Nakaya M, Inoue M, Mitsuhashi S. Gastrointestinal motor-stimulating activity of macrolide antibiotics and analysis of their side effects on the canine gut. Antimicrob Agents Chemother. 1984;26(6):863–9.
18. Catnach SM, Fairclough PD. Erythromycin and the gut. Gut. 1992;33(3):397–401.
19. Hasler WL, Heldsinger A, Chung OY. Erythromycin contracts rabbit colon myocytes via occupation of motilin receptors. Am J Phys. 1992;262(1 Pt 1):G50–5.
20. Kondo Y, Torii K, Itoh Z, Omura S. Erythromycin and its derivatives with motilin-like biological activities inhibit the specific binding of 125I-motilin to duodenal muscle. Biochem Biophys Res Commun. 1988;150(2):877–82.

21. Tomomasa T, Kuroume T, Arai H, Wakabayashi K, Itoh Z. Erythromycin induces migrating motor complex in human gastrointestinal tract. Dig Dis Sci. 1986;31(2):157–61.
22. Tzovaras G, Xynos E, Chrysos E, Mantides A, Vassilakis JS. The effect of intravenous erythromycin on esophageal motility in healthy subjects. Am J Surg. 1996;171(3):316–9.
23. Pennathur A, Tran A, Cioppi M, Fayad J, Sieren GL, Little AG. Erythromycin strengthens the defective lower esophageal sphincter in patients with gastroesophageal reflux disease. Am J Surg. 1994;167(1):169–72; discussion 72-3.
24. Janssens J, Peeters TL, Vantrappen G, Tack J, Urbain JL, De Roo M, et al. Improvement of gastric emptying in diabetic gastroparesis by erythromycin. Preliminary studies. N Engl J Med. 1990;322(15):1028–31.
25. Stacher G, Peeters TL, Bergmann H, Wiesnagrotzki S, Schneider C, Granser-Vacariu GV, et al. Erythromycin effects on gastric emptying, antral motility and plasma motilin and pancreatic polypeptide concentrations in anorexia nervosa. Gut. 1993;34(2):166–72.
26. Longo WE, Vernava AM 3rd. Prokinetic agents for lower gastrointestinal motility disorders. Dis Colon Rectum. 1993;36(7):696–708.
27. Rohm KD, Boldt J, Piper SN. Motility disorders in the ICU: recent therapeutic options and clinical practice. Curr Opin Clin Nutr Metab Care. 2009;12(2):161–7.
28. Bortolotti M, Brunelli F, Sarti P, Mari C, Miglioli M. Effects of oral clarithromycin and amoxycillin on interdigestive gastrointestinal motility of patients with functional dyspepsia and Helicobacter pylori gastritis. Aliment Pharmacol Ther. 1998;12(10):1021–5.
29. Acalovschi M, Dumitrascu DL, Hagiu C. Oral clarithromycin enhances gallbladder emptying induced by a mixed meal in healthy subjects. Eur J Intern Med. 2002;13(2):104–7.
30. Broad J, Sanger GJ. The antibiotic azithromycin is a motilin receptor agonist in human stomach: comparison with erythromycin. Br J Pharmacol. 2013;168(8):1859–67.
31. Sifrim D, Matsuo H, Janssens J, Vantrappen G. Comparison of the effects of midecamycin acetate and azithromycin on gastrointestinal motility in man. Drugs Exp Clin Res. 1994;20(3):121–6.
32. Moshiree B, McDonald R, Hou W, Toskes PP. Comparison of the effect of azithromycin versus erythromycin on antroduodenal pressure profiles of patients with chronic functional gastrointestinal pain and gastroparesis. Dig Dis Sci. 2010;55(3):675–83.
33. Chini P, Toskes PP, Waseem S, Hou W, McDonald R, Moshiree B. Effect of azithromycin on small bowel motility in patients with gastrointestinal dysmotility. Scand J Gastroenterol. 2012;47(4):422–7.
34. Rohof WO, Bennink RJ, de Ruigh AA, Hirsch DP, Zwinderman AH, Boeckxstaens GE. Effect of azithromycin on acid reflux, hiatus hernia and proximal acid pocket in the postprandial period. Gut. 2012;61(12):1670–7.
35. Jelic D, Antolovic R. From erythromycin to azithromycin and new potential ribosome-binding antimicrobials. Antibiotics. 2016;5(3):29.
36. Martinez FJ, Curtis JL, Albert R. Role of macrolide therapy in chronic obstructive pulmonary disease. Int J Chron Obstruct Pulmon Dis. 2008;3(3):331–50.
37. Suresh Babu K, Kastelik J, Morjaria JB. Role of long term antibiotics in chronic respiratory diseases. Respir Med. 2013;107(6):800–15.
38. Villagrasa V, Berto L, Cortijo J, Perpina M, Sanz C, Morcillo EJ. Effects of erythromycin on chemoattractant-activated human polymorphonuclear leukocytes. Gen Pharmacol. 1997;29(4):605–9.
39. Zalewska-Kaszubska J, Gorska D. Anti-inflammatory capabilities of macrolides. Pharmacol Res. 2001;44(6):451–4.
40. Willems-Widyastuti A, Vanaudenaerde BM, Vos R, Dilisen E, Verleden SE, De Vleeschauwer SI, et al. Azithromycin attenuates fibroblast growth factors induced vascular endothelial growth factor via p38(MAPK) signaling in human airway smooth muscle cells. Cell Biochem Biophys. 2013;67(2):331–9.
41. Verleden SE, Vandooren J, Vos R, Willems S, Dupont LJ, Verleden GM, et al. Azithromycin decreases MMP-9 expression in the airways of lung transplant recipients. Transpl Immunol. 2011;25(2-3):159–62.

42. Hodge S, Hodge G, Jersmann H, Matthews G, Ahern J, Holmes M, et al. Azithromycin improves macrophage phagocytic function and expression of mannose receptor in chronic obstructive pulmonary disease. Am J Respir Crit Care Med. 2008;178(2):139–48.
43. Hodge S, Reynolds PN. Low-dose azithromycin improves phagocytosis of bacteria by both alveolar and monocyte-derived macrophages in chronic obstructive pulmonary disease subjects. Respirology. 2012;17(5):802–7.
44. Nalca Y, Jansch L, Bredenbruch F, Geffers R, Buer J, Haussler S. Quorum-sensing antagonistic activities of azithromycin in Pseudomonas aeruginosa PAO1: a global approach. Antimicrob Agents Chemother. 2006;50(5):1680–8.
45. Koczulla AR, Vogelmeier CF, Garn H, Renz H. New concepts in asthma: clinical phenotypes and pathophysiological mechanisms. Drug Discov Today. 2017;22(2):388–96.
46. Havemann BD, Henderson CA, El-Serag HB. The association between gastro-oesophageal reflux disease and asthma: a systematic review. Gut. 2007;56(12):1654–64.
47. Amarasiri DL, Pathmeswaran A, de Silva HJ, Ranasinha CD. Response of the airways and autonomic nervous system to acid perfusion of the esophagus in patients with asthma: a laboratory study. BMC Pulm Med. 2013;13:33.
48. Lazenby JP, Harding SM. Chronic cough, asthma, and gastroesophageal reflux. Curr Gastroenterol Rep. 2000;2(3):217–23.
49. Johnston SL, Szigeti M, Cross M, Brightling C, Chaudhuri R, Harrison T, et al. Efficacy and Mechanism Evaluation. A randomised, double-blind, placebo-controlled study to evaluate the efficacy of oral azithromycin as a supplement to standard care for adult patients with acute exacerbations of asthma (the AZALEA trial). Southampton: NIHR Journals Library. Copyright (c) Queen's Printer and Controller of HMSO 2016. This work was produced by Johnston et al. under the terms of a commissioning contract issued by the Secretary of State for Health. This issue may be freely reproduced for the purposes of private research and study and extracts (or indeed, the full report) may be included in professional journals provided that suitable acknowledgement is made and the reproduction is not associated with any form of advertising. Applications for commercial reproduction should be addressed to: NIHR Journals Library, National Institute for Health Research, Evaluation, Trials and Studies Coordinating Centre, Alpha House, University of Southampton Science Park, Southampton SO16 7NS, UK; 2016.
50. Cameron EJ, Chaudhuri R, Mair F, McSharry C, Greenlaw N, Weir CJ, et al. Randomised controlled trial of azithromycin in smokers with asthma. Eur Respir J. 2013;42(5):1412–5.
51. Brusselle GG, Vanderstichele C, Jordens P, Deman R, Slabbynck H, Ringoet V, et al. Azithromycin for prevention of exacerbations in severe asthma (AZISAST): a multicentre randomised double-blind placebo-controlled trial. Thorax. 2013;68(4):322–9.
52. Hahn DL, Grasmick M, Hetzel S, Yale S. Azithromycin for bronchial asthma in adults: an effectiveness trial. J Am Board Fam Med. 2012;25(4):442–59.
53. Sutherland ER, King TS, Icitovic N, Ameredes BT, Bleecker E, Boushey HA, et al. A trial of clarithromycin for the treatment of suboptimally controlled asthma. J Allergy Clin Immunol. 2010;126(4):747–53.
54. Simpson JL, Powell H, Boyle MJ, Scott RJ, Gibson PG. Clarithromycin targets neutrophilic airway inflammation in refractory asthma. Am J Respir Crit Care Med. 2008;177(2):148–55.
55. Hahn DL, Plane MB, Mahdi OS, Byrne GI. Secondary outcomes of a pilot randomized trial of azithromycin treatment for asthma. PLoS Clin Trials. 2006;1(2):e11.
56. Kostadima E, Tsiodras S, Alexopoulos EI, Kaditis AG, Mavrou I, Georgatou N, et al. Clarithromycin reduces the severity of bronchial hyperresponsiveness in patients with asthma. Eur Respir J. 2004;23(5):714–7.
57. Kraft M, Cassell GH, Pak J, Martin RJ. Mycoplasma pneumoniae and Chlamydia pneumoniae in asthma: effect of clarithromycin. Chest. 2002;121(6):1782–8.
58. Amayasu H, Yoshida S, Ebana S, Yamamoto Y, Nishikawa T, Shoji T, et al. Clarithromycin suppresses bronchial hyperresponsiveness associated with eosinophilic inflammation in patients with asthma. Ann Allergy Asthma Immunol. 2000;84(6):594–8.
59. Shoji T, Yoshida S, Sakamoto H, Hasegawa H, Nakagawa H, Amayasu H. Anti-inflammatory effect of roxithromycin in patients with aspirin-intolerant asthma. Clin Exp Allergy. 1999;29(7):950–6.

60. Cantu E 3rd, Appel JZ 3rd, Hartwig MG, Woreta H, Green C, Messier R, et al. J. Maxwell Chamberlain Memorial Paper. Early fundoplication prevents chronic allograft dysfunction in patients with gastroesophageal reflux disease. Ann Thorac Surg. 2004;78(4):1142–51; discussion 1142-51.
61. Hadjiliadis D, Duane Davis R, Steele MP, Messier RH, Lau CL, Eubanks SS, et al. Gastroesophageal reflux disease in lung transplant recipients. Clin Transpl. 2003;17(4):363–8.
62. Lau CL, Palmer SM, Howell DN, McMahon R, Hadjiliadis D, Gaca J, et al. Laparoscopic antireflux surgery in the lung transplant population. Surg Endosc. 2002;16(12):1674–8.
63. Hathorn KE, Chan WW, Lo WK. Role of gastroesophageal reflux disease in lung transplantation. World J Transplant. 2017;7(2):103–16.
64. Mertens V, Blondeau K, Pauwels A, Farre R, Vanaudenaerde B, Vos R, et al. Azithromycin reduces gastroesophageal reflux and aspiration in lung transplant recipients. Dig Dis Sci. 2009;54(5):972–9.
65. Corris PA, Ryan VA, Small T, Lordan J, Fisher AJ, Meachery G, et al. A randomised controlled trial of azithromycin therapy in bronchiolitis obliterans syndrome (BOS) post lung transplantation. Thorax. 2015;70(5):442–50.
66. Vos R, Vanaudenaerde BM, Verleden SE, De Vleeschauwer SI, Willems-Widyastuti A, Van Raemdonck DE, et al. A randomised controlled trial of azithromycin to prevent chronic rejection after lung transplantation. Eur Respir J. 2011;37(1):164–72.
67. Federica M, Nadia S, Monica M, Alessandro C, Tiberio O, Francesco B, et al. Clinical and immunological evaluation of 12-month azithromycin therapy in chronic lung allograft rejection. Clin Transpl. 2011;25(4):E381–9.
68. Lam DC, Lam B, Wong MK, Lu C, Au WY, Tse EW, et al. Effects of azithromycin in bronchiolitis obliterans syndrome after hematopoietic SCT—a randomized double-blinded placebo-controlled study. Bone Marrow Transplant. 2011;46(12):1551–6.
69. Vos R, Vanaudenaerde BM, Ottevaere A, Verleden SE, De Vleeschauwer SI, Willems-Widyastuti A, et al. Long-term azithromycin therapy for bronchiolitis obliterans syndrome: divide and conquer? J Heart Lung Transplant. 2010;29(12):1358–68.
70. Jain R, Hachem RR, Morrell MR, Trulock EP, Chakinala MM, Yusen RD, et al. Azithromycin is associated with increased survival in lung transplant recipients with bronchiolitis obliterans syndrome. J Heart Lung Transplant. 2010;29(5):531–7.
71. Gottlieb J, Szangolies J, Koehnlein T, Golpon H, Simon A, Welte T. Long-term azithromycin for bronchiolitis obliterans syndrome after lung transplantation. Transplantation. 2008;85(1):36–41.
72. Chalmers JD, Aliberti S, Blasi F. Management of bronchiectasis in adults. Eur Respir J. 2015;45(5):1446–62.
73. Lee AL, Button BM, Denehy L, Roberts SJ, Bamford TL, Ellis SJ, et al. Proximal and distal gastro-oesophageal reflux in chronic obstructive pulmonary disease and bronchiectasis. Respirology. 2014;19(2):211–7.
74. Hu ZW, Wang ZG, Zhang Y, Wu JM, Liu JJ, Lu FF, et al. Gastroesophageal reflux in bronchiectasis and the effect of anti-reflux treatment. BMC Pulm Med. 2013;13:34.
75. Renna M, Schaffner C, Brown K, Shang S, Tamayo MH, Hegyi K, et al. Azithromycin blocks autophagy and may predispose cystic fibrosis patients to mycobacterial infection. J Clin Invest. 2011;121(9):3554–63.
76. Serisier DJ, Martin ML, McGuckin MA, Lourie R, Chen AC, Brain B, et al. Effect of long-term, low-dose erythromycin on pulmonary exacerbations among patients with non-cystic fibrosis bronchiectasis: the BLESS randomized controlled trial. JAMA. 2013;309(12):1260–7.
77. Diego AD, Milara J, Martinez-Moragon E, Palop M, Leon M, Cortijo J. Effects of long-term azithromycin therapy on airway oxidative stress markers in non-cystic fibrosis bronchiectasis. Respirology. 2013;18(7):1056–62.
78. Cymbala AA, Edmonds LC, Bauer MA, Jederlinic PJ, May JJ, Victory JM, et al. The disease-modifying effects of twice-weekly oral azithromycin in patients with bronchiectasis. Treat Respir Med. 2005;4(2):117–22.

79. Tsang KW, Ho PI, Chan KN, Ip MS, Lam WK, Ho CS, et al. A pilot study of low-dose erythromycin in bronchiectasis. Eur Respir J. 1999;13(2):361–4.
80. Wedzicha JA, Seemungal TA. COPD exacerbations: defining their cause and prevention. Lancet. 2007;370(9589):786–96.
81. Seemungal TA, Donaldson GC, Paul EA, Bestall JC, Jeffries DJ, Wedzicha JA. Effect of exacerbation on quality of life in patients with chronic obstructive pulmonary disease. Am J Respir Crit Care Med. 1998;157(5 Pt 1):1418–22.
82. Seemungal T, Harper-Owen R, Bhowmik A, Moric I, Sanderson G, Message S, et al. Respiratory viruses, symptoms, and inflammatory markers in acute exacerbations and stable chronic obstructive pulmonary disease. Am J Respir Crit Care Med. 2001;164(9):1618–23.
83. Rohde G, Wiethege A, Borg I, Kauth M, Bauer TT, Gillissen A, et al. Respiratory viruses in exacerbations of chronic obstructive pulmonary disease requiring hospitalisation: a case-control study. Thorax. 2003;58(1):37–42.
84. Wilkinson TM, Hurst JR, Perera WR, Wilks M, Donaldson GC, Wedzicha JA. Effect of interactions between lower airway bacterial and rhinoviral infection in exacerbations of COPD. Chest. 2006;129(2):317–24.
85. Anthonisen NR, Manfreda J, Warren CP, Hershfield ES, Harding GK, Nelson NA. Antibiotic therapy in exacerbations of chronic obstructive pulmonary disease. Ann Intern Med. 1987;106(2):196–204.
86. Anderson HR, Spix C, Medina S, Schouten JP, Castellsague J, Rossi G, et al. Air pollution and daily admissions for chronic obstructive pulmonary disease in 6 European cities: results from the APHEA project. Eur Respir J. 1997;10(5):1064–71.
87. Sakae TM, Pizzichini MM, Teixeira PJ, Silva RM, Trevisol DJ, Pizzichini E. Exacerbations of COPD and symptoms of gastroesophageal reflux: a systematic review and meta-analysis. J Bras Pneumol. 2013;39(3):259–71.
88. Terada K, Muro S, Sato S, Ohara T, Haruna A, Marumo S, et al. Impact of gastro-oesophageal reflux disease symptoms on COPD exacerbation. Thorax. 2008;63(11):951–5.
89. Lin YH, Tsai CL, Chien LN, Chiou HY, Jeng C. Newly diagnosed gastroesophageal reflux disease increased the risk of acute exacerbation of chronic obstructive pulmonary disease during the first year following diagnosis—a nationwide population-based cohort study. Int J Clin Pract. 2015;69(3):350–7.
90. Kim J, Lee JH, Kim Y, Kim K, Oh YM, Yoo KH, et al. Association between chronic obstructive pulmonary disease and gastroesophageal reflux disease: a national cross-sectional cohort study. BMC Pulm Med. 2013;13:51.
91. Martinez CH, Okajima Y, Murray S, Washko GR, Martinez FJ, Silverman EK, et al. Impact of self-reported gastroesophageal reflux disease in subjects from COPDGene cohort. Respir Res. 2014;15:62.
92. Ingebrigtsen TS, Marott JL, Vestbo J, Nordestgaard BG, Hallas J, Lange P. Gastro-esophageal reflux disease and exacerbations in chronic obstructive pulmonary disease. Respirology. 2015;20(1):101–7.
93. Terada K, Muro S, Ohara T, Kudo M, Ogawa E, Hoshino Y, et al. Abnormal swallowing reflex and COPD exacerbations. Chest. 2010;137(2):326–32.
94. Fahim A, Crooks M, Hart SP. Gastroesophageal reflux and idiopathic pulmonary fibrosis: a review. Pulm Med. 2011;2011:634613.
95. Dennish GW, Castell DO. Inhibitory effect of smoking on the lower esophageal sphincter. N Engl J Med. 1971;284(20):1136–7.
96. Wedzicha JA, Brill SE, Allinson JP, Donaldson GC. Mechanisms and impact of the frequent exacerbator phenotype in chronic obstructive pulmonary disease. BMC Med. 2013;11:181.
97. Benson VS, Mullerova H, Vestbo J, Wedzicha JA, Patel A, Hurst JR. Associations between gastro-oesophageal reflux, its management and exacerbations of chronic obstructive pulmonary disease. Respir Med. 2015;109(9):1147–54.
98. Sasaki T, Nakayama K, Yasuda H, Yoshida M, Asamura T, Ohrui T, et al. A randomized, single-blind study of lansoprazole for the prevention of exacerbations of chronic obstructive pulmonary disease in older patients. J Am Geriatr Soc. 2009;57(8):1453–7.

99. Suzuki T, Yanai M, Yamaya M, Satoh-Nakagawa T, Sekizawa K, Ishida S, et al. Erythromycin and common cold in COPD. Chest. 2001;120(3):730–3.
100. Seemungal TA, Wilkinson TM, Hurst JR, Perera WR, Sapsford RJ, Wedzicha JA. Long-term erythromycin therapy is associated with decreased chronic obstructive pulmonary disease exacerbations. Am J Respir Crit Care Med. 2008;178(11):1139–47.
101. He ZY, Ou LM, Zhang JQ, Bai J, Liu GN, Li MH, et al. Effect of 6 months of erythromycin treatment on inflammatory cells in induced sputum and exacerbations in chronic obstructive pulmonary disease. Respiration. 2010;80(6):445–52.
102. Banerjee D, Khair OA, Honeybourne D. The effect of oral clarithromycin on health status and sputum bacteriology in stable COPD. Respir Med. 2005;99(2):208–15.
103. Blasi F, Bonardi D, Aliberti S, Tarsia P, Confalonieri M, Amir O, et al. Long-term azithromycin use in patients with chronic obstructive pulmonary disease and tracheostomy. Pulm Pharmacol Ther. 2010;23(3):200–7.
104. Uzun S, Djamin RS, Kluytmans JA, Mulder PG, van't Veer NE, Ermens AA, et al. Azithromycin maintenance treatment in patients with frequent exacerbations of chronic obstructive pulmonary disease (COLUMBUS): a randomised, double-blind, placebo-controlled trial. Lancet Respir Med. 2014;2(5):361–8.
105. Berkhof FF, Doornewaard-ten Hertog NE, Uil SM, Kerstjens HA, van den Berg JW. Azithromycin and cough-specific health status in patients with chronic obstructive pulmonary disease and chronic cough: a randomised controlled trial. Respir Res. 2013;14:125.
106. Simpson JL, Powell H, Baines KJ, Milne D, Coxson HO, Hansbro PM, et al. The effect of azithromycin in adults with stable neutrophilic COPD: a double blind randomised, placebo controlled trial. PLoS One. 2014;9(8):e105609.
107. Davies JC, Alton EW, Bush A. Cystic fibrosis. BMJ. 2007;335(7632):1255–9.
108. Parkins MD, Floto RA. Emerging bacterial pathogens and changing concepts of bacterial pathogenesis in cystic fibrosis. J Cyst Fibros. 2015;14(3):293–304.
109. Robinson NB, DiMango E. Prevalence of gastroesophageal reflux in cystic fibrosis and implications for lung disease. Ann Am Thorac Soc. 2014;11(6):964–8.
110. Pauwels A, Blondeau K, Dupont LJ, Sifrim D. Mechanisms of increased gastroesophageal reflux in patients with cystic fibrosis. Am J Gastroenterol. 2012;107(9):1346–53.
111. Sheikh SI, Ryan-Wenger NA, McCoy KS. Outcomes of surgical management of severe GERD in patients with cystic fibrosis. Pediatr Pulmonol. 2013;48(6):556–62.
112. Fathi H, Moon T, Donaldson J, Jackson W, Sedman P, Morice AH. Cough in adult cystic fibrosis: diagnosis and response to fundoplication. Cough. 2009;5:1.
113. Hendriks JJ, Kester AD, Donckerwolcke R, Forget PP, Wouters EF. Changes in pulmonary hyperinflation and bronchial hyperresponsiveness following treatment with lansoprazole in children with cystic fibrosis. Pediatr Pulmonol. 2001;31(1):59–66.
114. Dimango E, Walker P, Keating C, Berdella M, Robinson N, Langfelder-Schwind E, et al. Effect of esomeprazole versus placebo on pulmonary exacerbations in cystic fibrosis. BMC Pulm Med. 2014;14:21.
115. Robinson P, Schechter MS, Sly PD, Winfield K, Smith J, Brennan S, et al. Clarithromycin therapy for patients with cystic fibrosis: a randomized controlled trial. Pediatr Pulmonol. 2012;47(6):551–7.
116. Saiman L, Anstead M, Mayer-Hamblett N, Lands LC, Kloster M, Hocevar-Trnka J, et al. Effect of azithromycin on pulmonary function in patients with cystic fibrosis uninfected with Pseudomonas aeruginosa: a randomized controlled trial. JAMA. 2010;303(17):1707–15.
117. Kabra SK, Pawaiya R, Lodha R, Kapil A, Kabra M, Vani AS, et al. Long-term daily high and low doses of azithromycin in children with cystic fibrosis: a randomized controlled trial. J Cyst Fibros. 2010;9(1):17–23.
118. Steinkamp G, Schmitt-Grohe S, Doring G, Staab D, Pfrunder D, Beck G, et al. Once-weekly azithromycin in cystic fibrosis with chronic Pseudomonas aeruginosa infection. Respir Med. 2008;102(11):1643–53.
119. McCormack J, Bell S, Senini S, Walmsley K, Patel K, Wainwright C, et al. Daily versus weekly azithromycin in cystic fibrosis patients. Eur Respir J. 2007;30(3):487–95.

120. Equi A, Balfour-Lynn IM, Bush A, Rosenthal M. Long term azithromycin in children with cystic fibrosis: a randomised, placebo-controlled crossover trial. Lancet. 2002;360(9338):978–84.
121. Wolter J, Seeney S, Bell S, Bowler S, Masel P, McCormack J. Effect of long term treatment with azithromycin on disease parameters in cystic fibrosis: a randomised trial. Thorax. 2002;57(3):212–6.

# Inhaled, Nebulised and Oral Bronchodilators in Reflux Disease

**26**

K. Suresh Babu and Jaymin B. Morjaria

## Introduction

Gastro-oesophageal reflux disease (GORD) is associated with many chronic respiratory conditions including pulmonary fibrosis, asthma and chronic obstructive pulmonary disease (COPD) [1, 2]. Whether the association of these respiratory conditions with GORD are cause or effect is not known. The importance of GORD in respiratory conditions is that it may cause worsening symptoms of bronchospasm, wheeze, dyspnoea or coughing which may eventually result in an exacerbation of the underlying respiratory condition [3–6]. The prevalence of GORD in asthma varies from 36 to 55%, which is more common in difficult to control asthma and more severe asthma [7, 8] and as a matter of fact some older studies have reported prevalence of up to 82% [9, 10]. The prevalence of GORD in COPD is even more wide-ranging (between 19 to 57%) [2, 11, 12]. These disparities may be attributed to study demographics, GORD monitoring techniques and pH criteria [13, 14]. The mainstay pharmacological agents used in the treatment of airways diseases (asthma and COPD) include the use of inhaled (and nebulised) bronchodilators ($\beta_2$ agonists and anti-cholinergics), inhaled corticosteroids, leukotriene antagonists (LTRAs) and less commonly theophylline, cromlyn sodium, and oral steroids and $\beta_2$ agonists [15]. Evidence in the literature suggests that $\beta_2$ agonists and

K. Suresh Babu
Department of Respiratory Medicine, Queen Alexandra Hospital, Portsmouth, UK

J. B. Morjaria (✉)
Department of Respiratory Medicine, Castle Hill Hospital, Cottingham, UK

Department of Academic Respiratory Medicine, Hull York Medical School, University of Hull, Cottingham, UK

Department of Respiratory Medicine, Royal Brompton and Harefield NHS Trust, Harefield Hospital, Harefield, UK
e-mail: j.morjaria@rbht.nhs.uk

theophyllines may attenuate the lower oesophageal sphincter (LOS) and hence promote GORD, however there is some debate about the clinical importance of these observations. Also there is limited information in favour of a protective effect of anti-cholinergics. In this chapter we provide an overview and discuss the various studies of inhaled and oral bronchodilators that have been proposed in the promotion or attenuation of GOR.

## Drugs Implicated in Promoting GOR

### $\beta_2$ Agonists

The evidence for and against $\beta_2$ agonists in promoting GOR is reported in healthy individuals and patients with asthma.

Some of the initial work of the effect of $\beta_2$ agonists on the LOS was conducted a couple of decades ago [16]. Following an oral dose of carbuterol it was observed that there was a mean LOS pressure reduction of 7 mmHg, indicating the possibility of $\beta_2$ adrenergic receptors being involved in attenuating LOS tone. Moreover in patients with achalasia the reduction was more profound, suggesting a possible therapeutic benefit in this condition. In a subsequent study by a different group in healthy volunteers using pneumohydraulically perfused multi-lumen manometry tubes and 24-hour pH profiles, inhaled albuterol (salbutamol) had no effect on LOS pressure or oesophageal peristaltic amplitudes [17]. They reported similar GOR irrespective of patient position (recombinant and supine) with inhaled albuterol and placebo. Later, Crowell and colleagues reassessed the pharmacodynamics of albuterol on oesophageal function in nine healthy volunteers [18]. This study overcame some of the limitations of Schindlbeck and colleagues' study i.e. the total dose of nebulised albuterol was only 1.25 mg whereas most patients would receive at least 2.5 mg in a single dose, and secondly the pharmacodynamics of cumulative dosing of $\beta_2$ agonists may significantly vary from that of a single dose. The relevance of the latter is that self nebulisation, especially in emergencies, may result in increased $\beta_2$ agonist levels and hence impair oesophageal function. This may be clinically significant in an acute situation wherein $\beta_2$ agonists are administered back to back during exacerbations.

Crowell and colleagues' prospective, randomised, double-blind crossover study of nebulised albuterol (2.5–10 mg; increments of 2.5 mg every 20 min) or placebo in healthy volunteers a week apart used a 6 cm manometry assembly and a low-compliance pneumohydraulic pump. They assessed the proportion of LOS relaxations, number of transient LOS relaxations (TLOSRs) as well as the amplitude, duration and propagation velocity of the oesophageal contractions at 5 and 10 cm above the LOS. It was observed that albuterol treatment resulted in a significant attenuation of LOS basal tone in a dose-dependent manner compared to placebo. At 5 cm above the LOS, the amplitude of oesophageal contractions was significantly reduced compared to placebo in a dose proportional manner. These were noted in the cumulative dose of 5 mg and upwards. Although the occurrence of TLOSRs, contractile amplitudes at 10 cm, duration of primary oesophageal contractions and the propagation velocity decreased with albuterol use compared to placebo, there were no notable differences. Although there were no safety or tolerability issues, subjects in the albuterol group had significantly increased mean heart rates and systolic blood pressure at the 10 mg albuterol cumulative dose compared to placebo. These findings support the hypothesis that inhaled albuterol therapy attenuated LOS basal tone and contractile amplitudes in smooth-muscle oesophageal body in a dose-dependent manner. This would imply that when administered in higher doses or infrequent sequential doses $\beta_2$ agonists may increase the likelihood of GOR and thus may increase oesophageal acidification in susceptible patients. Importantly, it has been reported previously that acid infusion into the distal oesophagus causes reflux bronchoconstriction [19] and that intraoesophageal acid infusion results in a decline in peak inspiratory flow in the absence of micro-aspiration [20]. Thus increased inhaled $\beta_2$ agonist exposure accompanied by the ineffective oesophageal motility and reflux bronchoconstriction which is known in some respiratory conditions such as asthma [10] and persistent GORD [21] may result in worsening symptoms.

Sontag and colleagues assessed LOS pressures and 24-h GOR patterns in controls and adult asthmatics to assess their relationship between GOR and asthma [10]. Asthmatics had significantly attenuated LOS pressures, increased oesophageal acid exposure times, recurrent reflux episodes and prolonged clearance times irrespective of body position compared to placebo. Of note there were no differences in any of the measured parameters between asthmatics that needed inhaled bronchodilators compared to those who did not. In a smaller study Michoud and colleagues investigated the effect of $\beta_2$ agonists in GOR using oesophageal manometry before and every 30 min for a total of 210 min in healthy volunteers and asthmatic patients receiving 4 mg of oral salbutamol or placebo (on separate days) [22]. Akin to the findings of Sontag and colleagues, they observed that asthmatics had a lower resting oesophageal sphincter pressure compared to healthy subjects and that salbutamol had no effect on the LOS pressure gradient, peak oesophageal contraction pressure or the number and duration of reflux episodes in patients with asthma and normal individuals. Using a questionnaire based, cross-sectional analytical survey, Field and colleagues assessed reflux associated respiratory symptoms and $\beta_2$ agonist inhaler use in asthmatics [9]. They reported that in the week prior to completing the questionnaire over 40% of the asthmatics had reflux associated symptoms of cough, dyspnoea and wheeze and that more than a quarter used their inhalers while experiencing these GOR symptoms. Importantly, none of the asthma medications ($\beta_2$ agonists, ICS, theophyllines and oral corticosteroids) were associated with increased symptomatic GOR. Also, they noted weak associations of inhaler use with the severity of heartburn and regurgitation.

More recently in a prospective, randomised, placebo-controlled, double-blind, crossover trial oesophageal function in response to nebulised albuterol or placebo were evaluated over two sessions 1 week apart in asthmatic patients [23]. This was conducted by the same group (Crowell and colleagues) using the same oesophageal manometry assessment methodology and study design. As noted in the healthy controls, nebulised albuterol compared to control (nebulised saline) induced a dose-dependent attenuation in the LOS basal pressure with a threshold as low as 2.5 mg, and significantly low at higher cumulative doses and a greater than 50% reduction at the cumulative dose of 10 mg. However there were no differences between nebulised albuterol and normal saline control on the amplitude and duration of primary oesophageal contractions, as well as oesophageal propagation velocity. Given the results of this study and that of the same group in healthy volunteers easily helps to envision how inhaled albuterol may have an effect on attenuating LOS pressure in susceptible individuals and predisposing them to episodes of reflux. These may directly (GOR) or indirectly (through a reflex mechanism) precipitate an asthma exacerbation or worsen an ongoing one.

## Theophyllines

Theophyllines, which are bronchodilators medications, have been observed to increase gastric acid secretion as well as decrease LOS pressure [24, 25]. Theophyllines belong to a group of drugs that act by inhibiting phospho-di-esterases (PDE). There are different isoenzymes of PDE's. These are categorised based on their substrate specificity and response to specific inhibitors. There is functional evidence that three PDEs are present in the LOS, PDE types I, III and V [26, 27]. There is biochemical evidence that type IV PDE is also present, but its functional activity appears low. Park and colleagues have shown that theophylline, a non-selective PDE inhibitor decreases LOS tone and this is likely to be mediated by the nitric oxide/cyclic GMP pathway [28].

Hubert and colleagues conducted a randomised double-blind crossover study in 16 asthmatics comparing 1-week conventional slow-release theophylline to 1-week placebo treatment [29]. All the enrolled subjects were on inhaled $\beta_2$ agonists with seven on ICS, and none on oral or parenteral corticosteroids. At the end of each treatment period (theophyllines or placebo), subjects were interrogated for respiratory and digestive symptoms, forced expiratory flows and GOR were assessed using prolonged nocturnal intra-oesophageal pH monitoring. The expiratory flows were measured three times a day throughout the study. They observed no significant increase in GOR with theophylline use compared to placebo, however a significant improvement was noted in forced expiratory flows in favour of theophylline use. There were no associations between GOR, duration of asthma and forced expiratory flows. The observations would suggest that slow-release theophyllines improved lung function and had no adverse GOR effects in asthmatic patients. In interpreting the findings one should take into consideration that the subjects had no historical evidence of GOR or GOR-provoked asthma, small numbers (n = 14) and that all the GOR indices assessed were numerically but not significantly much higher.

Ekstrom and Tibbling investigated whether normal theophylline use increased GOR and if so whether this was detrimental to lung function in asthmatic subjects [30]. Twenty-five subjects with moderate-to-severe asthma and a history of asthma exacerbated by GOR underwent two consecutive 24-h oesophageal pH assessments i.e. one with and one without regular administration of oral slow-release theophylline. It was observed that theophylline use resulted in a significant increase in GOR time and symptoms but had no influence on asthma worsenings. In subjects with therapeutic theophylline levels there was a 24% increase in total oesophageal acid exposure and a 170% increase in reflux symptoms, and had no lung function improvement. However in subjects with sub-therapeutic theophylline levels there was not only a significant improvement in lung function but they had no significant increased reflux parameters assessed. The same group conducted a further study to assess whether bronchial challenge with histamine or saline in asthmatics with GORD and on theophylline had worsening GOR [31]. Bronchial provocation was similar irrespective of theophylline treatment or not, implying that mild bronchospasm is unlikely to provoke GOR.

In another small study (n = 9) the severity of GOR in patients with GORD and obstructive lung disease nebulised albuterol (0.5 mg qds) was compared to sustained-release oral theophylline (200 mg bd or for long term users with a theophylline level of 55–110 μmol/L) [32]. The drugs were administered on 2 separate days along with 24-h oesophageal monitoring. A 40% reduction in total time with a pH <4 was observed with albuterol than with theophylline treatment. Seven of the nine subjects had less GOR with albuterol administration. This would suggest that the use of inhaled $\beta_2$ agonists would result in an attenuated GOR in patients with obstructive lung disease and GORD than with sustained-release theophylline.

It seems the evidence from studies in patients with asthma and GOR that therapeutic levels of theophyllines can promote reflux symptoms the same is not true in subjects with sub therapeutic levels. This could also suggest that when studies were done with slow release formulations the subjects might not have achieved therapeutic levels to have reflux symptoms. On the other hand theophylline and $\beta_2$ agonists' ability to reduce the tonicity of the oesophageal musculature and LOS tone could provide a pharmacological option in hypercontractile conditions like achalasia. Theophyllines resulted in relaxation of esophageal smooth muscle and improved chest pain in those with non-cardiac chest pain [33].

## Drugs Implicated in Inhibiting GOR

### Anti-Cholinergics

Perfusion of hydrochloric acid into the distal oesophagus can result in bronchoconstriction and a reduction in forced expiratory flow at 50% of vital capacity in asthmatic subjects with GOR [34]. These changes may be considerably attenuated with atropine pre-treatment. In animal studies bilateral vagotomy or atropine pre-treatment not only improved the area resistance but also the microvascular leakage induced by oesophageal acid installation [35, 36]. Numerous studies in asthmatic patients implicating vagal/anti-cholinergic involvement have been reported [20, 37, 38]. More recently in a rodent study investigating lung inflammation and remodelling of chronic GORD using intra-oesophageal hydrochloric acid was conducted [39]. As would be expected there was a large inflammatory response, however this was considerably inhibited with pre-treatment of dexamethasone, intraperitoneal atropine or nebulised tiotropium. These observations confirm a possible role for acetylcholine in airway inflammation and remodelling in a GORD model which can be abrogated with anti-cholinergic treatment.

## Recombinant DNase

Nebulised recombinant human DNase (rhDNase) reduces sputum viscosity and improves lung function as well as acute respiratory exacerbations in suppurative lung diseases such as cystic fibrosis. In a case report of a teenager with Kartagener's syndrome with worsening lung function and severe GOR refractory to conventional treatment, the regular use of rhDNase not only improved respiratory symptoms and lung function parameters but also produced a marked reduction in gastrointestinal symptoms [40]. This could suggest that there may be a role for rhDNase in patients with suppurative lung disease both from a respiratory and a gastrointestinal perspective. These observations to be confirmed in randomised controlled trials.

### Conclusion

GORD is a common co-morbidity of respiratory conditions. While the exact cause of GORD is not clear, various factors that weaken or relax the LOS tone can make reflux worse. There is some evidence to suggest that the use of $\beta_2$ agonists can in some patients make reflux worse especially in the context of nebulised albuterol/salbutamol. The evidence for inhaled or nebulised anti-muscarinic agents are encouraging but need further investigation. PDE inhibitors, such as theophylline, can reduce the tone of the LOS and this could be attributable to the presence of PDE receptors on the LOS. Some of the evidence originates from studies conducted over two decades ago, in which time new and improved GORD assessment techniques have been developed and are being put to test [41, 42]. There is a dearth of data on oral or inhaled bronchodilator therapies easing GORD, but future studies may help to delineate as to whether some inhaled/oral bronchodilator therapies may contribute to and also see if others would aid in the attenuation of GORD.

**Conflict of Interest** None declared with regards to the chapter.

**Declarations** KSB has received honoraria for speaking and financial support to attend meetings from Wyeth, Chiesi, GSK, Teva, Novartis and AstraZeneca. JBM has received honoraria for speaking and financial support to attend meetings/advisory boards from Wyeth, Chiesi, Pfizer, MSD, Boehringer Ingelheim, Teva, Glaxo Smithkline/Allen & Hanburys, Napp, Almirall, AstraZeneca, Trudell Medical International and Novartis.

## References

1. Amarasiri LD, Pathmeswaran A, de Silva HJ, Ranasinha CD. Prevalence of gastro-oesophageal reflux disease symptoms and reflux-associated respiratory symptoms in asthma. BMC Pulm Med. 2010;10:49.
2. Kim J, Lee JH, Kim Y, Kim K, Oh YM, Yoo KH, Rhee CK, Yoon HK, Kim YS, Park YB, Lee SW, Lee SD. Association between chronic obstructive pulmonary disease and gastroesophageal reflux disease: a national cross-sectional cohort study. BMC Pulm Med. 2013;13:51.
3. Canning BJ, Mazzone SB. Reflex mechanisms in gastroesophageal reflux disease and asthma. Am J Med. 2003;115(Suppl 3A):45S–8S.
4. Hurst JR, Vestbo J, Anzueto A, Locantore N, Mullerova H, Tal-Singer R, Miller B, Lomas DA, Agusti A, Macnee W, Calverley P, Rennard S, Wouters EF, Wedzicha JA. Susceptibility to exacerbation in chronic obstructive pulmonary disease. N Engl J Med. 2010;363:1128–38.
5. Rascon-Aguilar IE, Pamer M, Wludyka P, Cury J, Coultas D, Lambiase LR, Nahman NS, Vega KJ. Role of gastroesophageal reflux symptoms in exacerbations of COPD. Chest. 2006;130:1096–101.
6. Terada K, Muro S, Sato S, Ohara T, Haruna A, Marumo S, Kinose D, Ogawa E, Hoshino Y, Niimi A, Terada T, Mishima M. Impact of gastro-oesophageal reflux disease symptoms on COPD exacerbation. Thorax. 2008;63:951–5.
7. Kiljander TO, Laitinen JO. The prevalence of gastroesophageal reflux disease in adult asthmatics. Chest. 2004;126:1490–4.
8. Leggett JJ, Johnston BT, Mills M, Gamble J, Heaney LG. Prevalence of gastroesophageal reflux in difficult asthma: relationship to asthma outcome. Chest. 2005;127:1227–31.
9. Field SK, Underwood M, Brant R, Cowie RL. Prevalence of gastroesophageal reflux symptoms in asthma. Chest. 1996;109:316–22.
10. Sontag SJ, O'Connell S, Khandelwal S, Miller T, Nemchausky B, Schnell TG, Serlovsky R. Most asthmatics have gastroesophageal reflux with or without bronchodilator therapy. Gastroenterology. 1990;99:613–20.
11. Dent J, El-Serag HB, Wallander MA, Johansson S. Epidemiology of gastro-oesophageal reflux disease: a systematic review. Gut. 2005;54:710–7.
12. Kempainen RR, Savik K, Whelan TP, Dunitz JM, Herrington CS, Billings JL. High prevalence of proximal and distal gastroesophageal reflux disease in advanced COPD. Chest. 2007;131:1666–71.
13. Casanova C, Baudet JS, del Valle Velasco M, Martin JM, Aguirre-Jaime A, de Torres JP, Celli BR. Increased gastro-oesophageal reflux disease in patients with severe COPD. Eur Respir J. 2004;23:841–5.
14. Delaney BC. Review article: prevalence and epidemiology of gastro-oesophageal reflux disease. Aliment Pharmacol Ther. 2004;20(Suppl 8):2–4.
15. Global Initiative for Asthma. Global strategy for asthma management and prevention [updated 2015]. 2015.
16. Dimarino AJ Jr, Cohen S. Effect of an oral beta2-adrenergic agonist on lower esophageal sphincter pressure in normals and in patients with achalasia. Dig Dis Sci. 1982;27:1063–6.
17. Schindlbeck NE, Heinrich C, Huber RM, Muller-Lissner SA. Effects of albuterol (salbutamol) on esophageal motility and gastroesophageal reflux in healthy volunteers. JAMA. 1988;260:3156–8.
18. Crowell MD, Zayat EN, Lacy BE, Schettler-Duncan A, Liu MC. The effects of an inhaled beta(2)-adrenergic agonist on lower esophageal function: a dose-response study. Chest. 2001;120:1184–9.
19. Mansfield LE, Stein MR. Gastroesophageal reflux and asthma: a possible reflex mechanism. Ann Allergy. 1978;41:224–6.
20. Schan CA, Harding SM, Haile JM, Bradley LA, Richter JE. Gastroesophageal reflux-induced bronchoconstriction. An intraesophageal acid infusion study using state-of-the-art technology. Chest. 1994;106:731–7.

21. Fouad YM, Katz PO, Hatlebakk JG, Castell DO. Ineffective esophageal motility: the most common motility abnormality in patients with GERD-associated respiratory symptoms. Am J Gastroenterol. 1999;94:1464–7.
22. Michoud MC, Leduc T, Proulx F, Perreault S, DU Souich P, Duranceau A, Amyot R. Effect of salbutamol on gastroesophageal reflux in healthy volunteers and patients with asthma. J Allergy Clin Immunol. 1991;87:762–7.
23. Lacy BE, Mathis C, DesBiens J, Liu MC. The effects of nebulized albuterol on esophageal function in asthmatic patients. Dig Dis Sci. 2008;53:2627–33.
24. Johannesson N, Andersson KE, Joelsson B, Persson CG. Relaxation of lower esophageal sphincter and stimulation of gastric secretion and diuresis by antiasthmatic xanthines. Role of adenosine antagonism. Am Rev Respir Dis. 1985;131:26–30.
25. Stein MR, Towner TG, Weber RW, Mansfield LE, Jacobson KW, McDonnell JT, Nelson HS. The effect of theophylline on the lower esophageal sphincter pressure. Ann Allergy. 1980;45:238–41.
26. Barnette MS, Barone FC, Fowler PJ, Grous M, Price WJ, Ormsbee HS. Human lower oesophageal sphincter relaxation is associated with raised cyclic nucleotide content. Gut. 1991;32:4–9.
27. Osinski MA, Bass P, Gaumnitz EA. Effects of selective phosphodiesterase inhibitors on the opossum lower esophageal sphincter. Gastroenterology. 1998;114:A816.
28. Park H, Clark E, Conklin JL. Effects of phosphodiesterase inhibitors on oesophageal neuromuscular functions. Neurogastroenterol Motil. 2003;15:625–33.
29. Hubert D, Gaudric M, Guerre J, Lockhart A, Marsac J. Effect of theophylline on gastroesophageal reflux in patients with asthma. J Allergy Clin Immunol. 1988;81:1168–74.
30. Ekstrom T, Tibbling L. Influence of theophylline on gastro-oesophageal reflux and asthma. Eur J Clin Pharmacol. 1988;35:353–6.
31. Ekstrom TK, Tibbling LI. Can mild bronchospasm reduce gastroesophageal reflux? Am Rev Respir Dis. 1989;139:52–5.
32. Ruzkowski CJ, Sanowski RA, Austin J, Rohwedder JJ, Waring JP. The effects of inhaled albuterol and oral theophylline on gastroesophageal reflux in patients with gastroesophageal reflux disease and obstructive lung disease. Arch Intern Med. 1992;152:783–5.
33. Rao SS, Mudipalli RS, Remes-Troche JM, Utech CL, Zimmerman B. Theophylline improves esophageal chest pain—a randomized, placebo-controlled study. Am J Gastroenterol. 2007;102:930–8.
34. Herve P, Denjean A, Jian R, Simonneau G, Duroux P. Intraesophageal perfusion of acid increases the bronchomotor response to methacholine and to isocapnic hyperventilation in asthmatic subjects. Am Rev Respir Dis. 1986;134:986–9.
35. Daoui S, D'Agostino B, Gallelli L, Alt XE, Rossi F, Advenier C. Tachykinins and airway microvascular leakage induced by HCl intra-oesophageal instillation. Eur Respir J. 2002;20:268–73.
36. Hamamoto J, Kohrogi H, Kawano O, Iwagoe H, Fujii K, Hirata N, Ando M. Esophageal stimulation by hydrochloric acid causes neurogenic inflammation in the airways in guinea pigs. J Appl Physiol. 1997;82:738–45.
37. Harding SM, Guzzo MR, Maples RV, Alexander RW, Richter JE. Gastroesophageal reflux induced bronchoconstriction: vagolytic doses of atropine diminish airway responses to esophageal acid infusion [Abstract]. Am J Respir Crit Care Med. 1995;151:A589.
38. Harding SM, Schan CA, Guzzo MR, Alexander RW, Bradley LA, Richter JE. Gastroesophageal reflux-induced bronchoconstriction. Is microaspiration a factor? Chest. 1995;108:1220–7.
39. Cui Y, Devillier P, Kuang X, Wang H, Zhu L, Xu Z, Xia Z, Zemoura L, Advenier C, Chen H. Tiotropium reduction of lung inflammation in a model of chronic gastro-oesophageal reflux. Eur Respir J. 2010;35:1370–6.
40. Desai M, Weller PH, Spencer DA. Clinical benefit from nebulized human recombinant DNase in Kartagener's syndrome. Pediatr Pulmonol. 1995;20:307–8.

41. Hayat JO, Gabieta-Somnez S, Yazaki E, Kang JY, Woodcock A, Dettmar P, Mabary J, Knowles CH, Sifrim D. Pepsin in saliva for the diagnosis of gastro-oesophageal reflux disease. Gut. 2015;64:373–80.
42. Timms C, Thomas PS, Yates DH. Detection of gastro-oesophageal reflux disease (GORD) in patients with obstructive lung disease using exhaled breath profiling. J Breath Res. 2012;6:016003.

# Speech Pathology: Reflux Aspiration and Lung Diseases

## Anne E. Vertigan

### Abstract

There are a range of conditions associated with reflux, aspiration and lung disease that are managed by speech-language pathologists (SLP). In many cases the SLP role is to treat the symptoms or consequences of the disease while management of the underlying disease is the role of the medical practitioner. Laryngeal conditions related to reflux, aspiration and lung disease can result in hypo or hyperlaryngeal function. They include oropharyngeal dysphagia, and laryngeal hyperresponsiveness syndromes such as chronic refractory cough, paradoxical vocal fold movement, muscle tension dysphonia and globus pharyngeus. This chapter outlines the speech pathology assessment and treatment of these conditions.

### Introduction

There are a range of conditions associated with reflux, aspiration and lung disease that are managed by speech-language pathologists (SLP). In many cases the SLP role is to treat the symptoms or consequences of the disease while management of the underlying disease is the role of the medical practitioner. It is therefore essential for the SLP to work in close collaboration with other members of the multidisciplinary team.

A. E. Vertigan
John Hunter Hospital, New Lambton Heights, NSW, Australia

Centre for Asthma and Respiratory Diseases, University of Newcastle, Callaghan, NSW, Australia

Hunter Medical Research Institute, New Lambton Heights, NSW, Australia
e-mail: anne.vertigan@hnehealth.nsw.gov.au

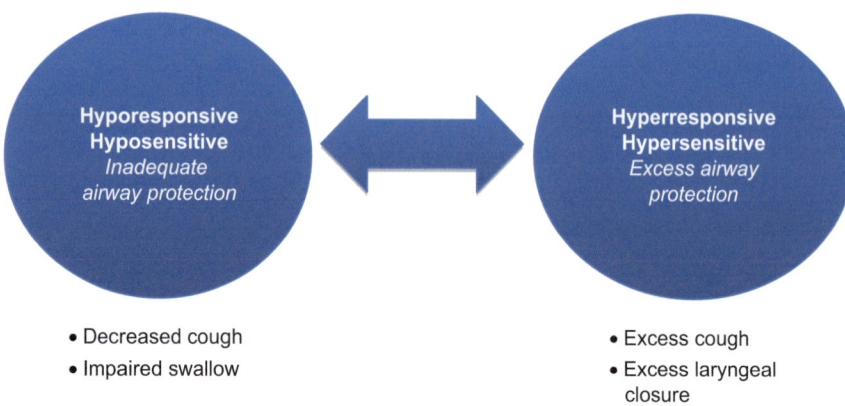

**Fig. 27.1** Comparison of laryngeal hypo- and hyper-responsiveness

Laryngeal conditions related to reflux, aspiration and lung disease can result in hypo or hyperlaryngeal function. They include oropharyngeal dysphagia, and laryngeal hyperresponsiveness syndromes such as chronic refractory cough, paradoxical vocal fold movement, muscle tension dysphonia and globus pharyngeus. Oropharyngeal dysphagia is typically associated with hyporesponsiveness and hyposensitivity resulting in decreased airway protection (Fig. 27.1). Swallowing is impaired and cough may be absent or ineffective in clearing airway penetration. The primary role of SLP intervention in oropharyngeal dysphagia is to prevent aspiration. In contrast, laryngeal hyperresponsiveness syndromes are associated with laryngeal hypersensitivity and excess airway protection in the form of excessive cough and laryngeal closure (Fig. 27.1). The role of SLP intervention for laryngeal hyperresponsiveness is to reduce sensitivity and consequent maladaptive laryngeal behaviour.

## Oropharyngeal Dysphagia

Swallowing is a complex behaviour involving numerous muscles and cranial nerves. Airway protection during swallowing relies on finely tuned coordination between the swallowing and respiratory systems to produce apnoea during the pharyngeal phase of the swallow and return of respiration in the expiratory phase to prevent aspiration [1]. Airway protection is achieved by superior and anterior hyolaryngeal elevation and epiglottic inversion during swallowing. Oropharyngeal dysphagia affects the oral preparatory, oral propulsive and pharyngeal phases of the swallow. It is a common cause of aspiration and can result from neurological impairment, respiratory disease, oesophageal disorders and head/neck cancer [2].

Dysphagia resulting from neurological disease such as stroke results from impaired cranial nerve and neuromuscular function. The oral and pharyngeal phases of the swallow can be impaired leading to difficulty with mastication, bolus control and preparation, triggering of the swallow and airway protection. Furthermore, both reflexive and voluntary cough are impaired even in the presence of preserved expiratory muscle strength. Cough reflex sensitivity is also reduced which can lead to silent aspiration [3–5].

Dysphagia resulting from respiratory disease is not typically due to neuromuscular weakness but due to the timing and coordination between respiration and swallowing. For example in chronic obstructive pulmonary disease dysphagia can occur due to dyspnoea and abnormal thoracoabdominal biomechanics [1]. Individuals may inhale before the pharyngeal phase of the swallow is completed and thus increasing aspiration risk [1]. Furthermore, aspiration can exacerbate the condition of chronic obstructive pulmonary disease.

The consequences of oropharyngeal dysphagia can be serious and life threatening. A study of 57 patients undergoing autopsy of aspiration related pulmonary disease identified risk factors for aspiration as reduced consciousness, dysphagia, GERD, vomiting and reduced airway protection due to vocal fold immobility, anatomical oropharyngeal abnormalities and endotracheal intubation [6]. Aspiration pneumonia was present in 46% of patients, aspiration pneumonitis in 44% and large airway obstruction in 11% [6]. The majority of patients with aspiration pneumonitis and large airway obstruction lead to death within 72 h. Aspiration may be clinically unsuspected. The authors [6] concluded that dysphagia due to neurologic disease is the commonest cause of death due to aspiration.

Aspiration pneumonia, an infection that develops from pathologic oropharyngeal microbes entering the lung [7], is a well-recognised consequence of oropharyngeal dysphagia. It is distinct from aspiration pneumonitis which is an acute lung injury occurring after inhaling a large volume of regurgitated gastric contents [7]. The degree of aspiration that can be tolerated before developing aspiration pneumonia varies between individuals. A landmark study by Susan Langmore [8] identified the risk factors for developing aspiration pneumonia as dependence for oral feeding, dependence for oral care, number of decayed teeth, number of medications, current smoking, tube feeding and reduced mobility. These factors contrast with the risk factors for aspiration which include decreased consciousness, compromised airway defence mechanisms, dysphagia, gastroesophageal reflux disease and recurrent vomiting [7]. Aspiration is more likely to lead to pneumonia if the aspirated material is pathogenic to the lungs or the host resistance is compromised [8]. These factors occur more commonly in the elderly, those with reduced physical activity, multiple comorbidities, malnutrition, decreased salivary clearance, poor oral hygiene impaired cough reflex and poor immune defence [7].

Aspiration of solid food can cause mechanical obstruction, resulting in acute respiratory distress or asphyxia [7]. The degree of pulmonary distress will depend upon the size of the aspirated material and its location within the airway [7]. It can result in a granulomatous inflammatory reaction with localised bronchial stenosis in addition to mechanical obstruction. Aspiration may be an underappreciated cause of bronchiolitis [7]. Other consequences of oropharyngeal dysphagia include malnutrition and dehydration. Malnutrition can increase susceptibility to infection and the likelihood of developing aspiration pneumonia.

## Assessment of Oropharyngeal Dysphagia

The role of the SLP is to assess the oral and pharyngeal phases of the swallow, provide differential diagnosis and design the treatment program [2]. In certain diseases immediate referral for SLP assessment is warranted. For example, dysphagia assessment within 24-h of acute stroke will decrease the incidence of aspiration pneumonia [9]. Indicators for SLP referral include the presence of diseases known to result in dysphagia and the presence of signs and symptoms of dysphagia such as coughing and choking on food, hyposensitive cough, difficulty managing saliva and delayed swallow.

## Screening Tests for Aspiration

Screening tests for aspiration are designed to identify patients who are at risk of dysphagia and indicate referral to SLP [10]. Screening is less comprehensive than a formal clinical assessment of oropharyngeal dysphagia and can be conducted by a range of professionals within the multidisciplinary team. Used well they can reduce the risk of pneumonia in specific patient populations. The potential problem with screening tests is that they rely on the patient to have an intact cough reflex. Absence of cough when swallowing water during the screening test, is often presumed to indicate no aspiration. However the absence of cough may be due to a hyposensitive cough whereby the patient has failed to cough in response to aspiration. This is known as silent aspiration and can be difficult to appreciate if the cough is absent. Identifying aspiration requires a comprehensive swallowing assessment and should not be based solely on a sip or water swallow test.

## Clinical Assessment of Oropharyngeal Dysphagia

Formal clinical assessment of oropharyngeal dysphagia conducted by SLP involves a thorough case history including previous medical and surgical history and current medications, symptoms and eating behaviour. The assessment involves observation of respiratory status including $SpO_2$ level if available, respiratory rate and signs of breathing difficulty. Judgement of alertness, attention, level of distraction, cognition, and language are required as they impact on patient safety, cognitive function during eating and impact on the rehabilitation process. The clinical assessment involves comprehensive evaluation of the oral cavity, dentition, and motor and sensory functions of cranial nerves V, VII, IX, X and XII. Assessment of airway protection includes cough, phonation and hyolaryngeal excursion during dry swallow and the ability to manage secretions. Reflexive swallowing is tested using a range of food and fluid consistencies and sizes to examine the oral and pharyngeal phases of swallowing including mastication, oral transfer, airway protection and aspiration risk.

Oropharyngeal dysphagia needs to be differentially diagnosed from other disease that can mimic oropharyngeal dysfunction. For example, oesophageal dysphagia may result in referred laryngeal and pharyngeal symptoms. Some patients may complain of periodic choking episodes, yet on careful questioning, these episodes consist of a sensation of laryngeal closure while food is still in the oral cavity. This phenomenon is not pure choking and may be more consistent with Vocal Cord Dysfunction and laryngeal hypersensitivity than oropharyngeal dysphagia. Making these distinctions for the patient can avoid unnecessary investigations and treatments, and reduce anxiety around the condition.

## Instrumental Assessment of Oropharyngeal Dysphagia

Instrumental assessment of oropharyngeal dysphagia can be used to complement the clinical assessment. Video Fluoroscopic Swallow Study (VFSS) is a dynamic radiological examination of the oral, pharyngeal and sometimes oesophageal phases of the swallow. A range of food and fluid textures and bolus sizes may be trialled along with therapeutic swallowing manoeuvres. The VFSS provides an objective evaluation of normal and abnormal swallow physiology and identifies the reason for aspiration, and pharyngeal pooling and other abnormalities. However there are limitations of VFSS including radiation exposure, inability to examine swallow function representative of an actual meal and the effect of the contrast medium on food and fluid consistency [11].

As the name suggests, the Fibreoptic Endoscopic Evaluation of Swallowing (FEES) involves transnasal insertion of a flexible fiberoptic endoscope into the hypopharynx to enable direct observation of the pharyngeal and laryngeal structures before and during deglutition. This test provides objective feedback about the pharyngeal phase of the swallow including saliva management. It is more portable than VFSS and as there is no radiation exposure hence the examination can be repeated and last as long as clinically necessary [12]. The disadvantages of FEES include discomfort, gagging, vasovagal syncope, epistaxis, mucosal perforation [12] and inability to examine the oral phase of the swallow. Furthermore, topical anaesthetics, if used, will reduce pharyngeal sensation which may influence the study result.

## Treatment of Oropharyngeal Dysphagia

The primary goal of SLP management of the patient with oropharyngeal dysphagia is to minimise aspiration and prevent the development or exacerbation of aspiration pneumonia, while maximising nutrition and hydration [13]. Swallowing and coughing are the two reflexes responsible for airway protection. Pitts argues that they occur in response to aspiration as 'meta-behaviours' and that both are required to protect the airway from aspiration [14]. It then follows that both cough and swallowing need to be considered during intervention for oropharyngeal dysphagia.

The SLP role in the management of oropharyngeal dysphagia is summarised in Table 27.1. The SLP will often determine whether or not the patient is safe for oral intake and if so the most appropriate food and fluid textures to prevent aspiration.

| **Table 27.1** Summary of speech-language pathology intervention strategies for oropharyngeal dysphagia | Determine whether the patient is safe for oral intake |
|---|---|
| | Recommend the safest food and fluid consistencies |
| | Implement transitional feeding |
| | Prescribe therapeutic exercise programs and swallow manoeuvres |
| | Identify safe swallowing strategies for the individual patient |
| | Recommend optimal posture for swallowing |

The options are broadly classified as full oral, texture modified or non-oral. Enteral feeding may be required for patients who are not safe for oral intake and the decision around this is made in collaboration with the multidisciplinary team. Texture modified food and fluids may be beneficial for patients who are unsafe on particular consistencies as they reduce the need for chewing and coordinated bolus manipulation. Reduced viscosity of these texture modified foods may slow oral and pharyngeal transit thus giving the individual time to protect their airway prior to transit.

The SLP may also prescribe therapeutic dysphagia exercise programs in order to strengthen oropharyngeal musculature, improve coordination of the swallow and compensate for oral and pharyngeal deficits [15]. These exercises are designed to improve pharyngeal transit and reduce aspiration. For example, the supraglottic swallow technique involves voluntarily closure of the vocal folds before swallowing therefore improving the duration and timing of airway protection. It may also increase tongue strength during the swallow [16]. Many dysphagia therapy exercises and techniques require intact cognition and careful concentration before every mouthful, and if this is lacking supervision during meals may be required.

## Aspiration and Quality of Life

Although aspiration is serious, there are circumstances where minimising aspiration needs to be balanced with quality of life in the treatment process. This is particularly pertinent in individuals with chronic or progressive conditions. The decision making regarding non-oral feeding or restricting food and fluid textures can be complex particularly when the perspectives of the patient, family and multidisciplinary team members differ. There can be different opinions about whether the patient is aspirating, the likelihood of improvement, the potential consequences of aspiration, and the patient and family's willingness to accept these consequences. If aspiration is acute or exacerbated by an acute illness a more restrictive treatment option may be indicated in the short term. In chronic dysphagia, restrictive treatment options such as texture modified diets or non-oral feeding may be less acceptable to patients, families and their doctors. Furthermore, prolonged restrictionin cases of chronic aspiration where negative consequences are predicted, decisions regarding feeding and nutritional options are often made by the multidisciplinary team including patient and family rather than by the SLP in isolation. The range of treatment options including predicted risks and benefits need to be outlined to the patient and family. Although the goal is to prevent aspiration there can be negative consequences of the treatments used to prevent aspiration. Tube feeding has risks including the risk of insertion, tube displacement, infection and aspiration of refluxed feeds. In elderly individuals, tube feeding does not reduce morbidity and actually increases the risk of aspiration pneumonia, partly through aspiration of bacteria laden saliva and refluxed tube feeds [17, 18]. Texture modified diets and thickened fluids can contribute to malnutrition and dehydration if intake is inadequate [19].

The Frazier water protocol [20] is used in some settings. It allows for the free consumption of water between meals in patients with good oral hygiene, mobility and respiratory status even if they are known to be aspirating thin fluids. Strict oral hygiene before and after each meal is required to reduce aspiration of bacteria along with saliva. The rationale for this protocol is that although aspiration will occur, it will occur with an inert liquid in the presence of a clean oral cavity thus reducing the chance of bacteria and large food particles being aspirated. It therefore improves quality of life while minimising the risk of developing aspiration pneumonia.

## Laryngeal Hyper-Responsiveness Syndrome

In contrast to dysphagia which results in reduced airway protection, laryngeal hyper-responsiveness involves increased or excessive airway protection. Laryngeal hypersensitivity is a common underlying feature of several laryngeal conditions including chronic refractory cough, paradoxical vocal fold movement (PVFM) and some forms of muscle tension dysphonia. Due to the clinical overlap between these conditions they will be referred to as laryngeal hyper-responsiveness syndromes in this chapter.

Chronic refractory cough is defined as a cough that has lasted for longer than eight weeks and is refractory to medical management based on the anatomic diagnostic protocol.

PVFM, also known as Vocal Cord Dysfunction, is a disorder whereby the vocal folds adduct involuntarily and episodically during inspiration leading to symptoms of inspiratory dyspnoea, stridor, throat tightness, dysphonia and cough. There is no standardised definition of PVFM and no agreement on exact diagnostic criteria. Chronic refractory cough and PVFM may occur in isolation or the two conditions can co-occur.

Laryngeal hyper-responsiveness syndromes have reduced thresholds for triggering protective airway responses. Therefore laryngeal closure and cough become heightened and are triggered by low levels of innocuous stimuli such as talking or cold air. This is evidenced by increased cough reflex sensitivity in both chronic refractory cough and PVFM whereby cough is triggered by low levels of capsaicin [21, 22].

The mechanism for laryngeal hyper-responsiveness was hypothesised as a reaction to central nervous system changes resulting in hyperexcitability of the sensory motor pathways [23]. Causative factors include emotional distress, habitual postural muscle patterns, gastroesophageal reflux and post viral illness [23]. These factors can lead to chronic laryngeal motor stimulation and increased sensory irritation whereby neural plasticity alters the central neural control of the laryngeal structures. Laryngeal hyper-responsiveness syndromes are often the result of maladaptive compensatory mechanisms whereby the patient perceives an urge to cough, coughs in response to that urge and subsequently the threshold for triggering the cough is lowered [23].

The consequences of laryngeal hyper-responsiveness are rarely life threatening but can cause significant patient distress and have an enormous impact on quality of life [24]. There is an increased incidence of dysphonia in patients with laryngeal hyper-responsiveness syndrome [25] which contributes to the morbidity of the condition.

Reflux and lung disease may also affect phonation and contribute to the development or exacerbation of voice disorders. A voice disorder is defined as a deviation in pitch, quality and loudness compared to those of a similar age, gender, cultural background and geographic location [26]. Voice disorders can result from organic laryngeal conditions, neurological disease, respiratory disease, psychological conditions and habitual environmental factors. They can have a significant impact on quality of life, particularly for individuals who rely on their voice vocationally. Numerous mechanisms can underlie dysphonia, however the key mechanisms described here will include reduced lung capacity, reflux laryngitis and laryngeal hypersensitivity.

Conditions such as asthma and chronic obstructive pulmonary disease that result in airway obstruction may also result in dysphonia. Respiratory function is essential for phonation. The most efficient phonation occurs at mid-air pressure levels and mid lung volume levels of air [27]. The passive forces of expiration are generally sufficient for speech [27] but additional power can be supplied by active exhalation. The respiratory airstream needs to overcome the resistance of the approximated vocal folds to promote abduction and subsequent vocal fold vibration [26]. If lung capacity is reduced it may be difficult to create adequate phonation threshold pressure in order to set the vocal folds into oscillation.

Dysphonia in asthma may be the result of impaired respiratory function or vocal fold changes caused by cough or inhaled corticosteroids [28]. Dysphonia in chronic obstructive pulmonary disease is related to the degree of airway obstruction, weakness and inadequate volume due to impaired respiratory function [28]. Insufficient subglottic pressure may be generated leading to reduced vocal fold closure and breathy vocal quality. Some individuals may compensate for poor respiratory support by taking more frequent breaths during speech. Others may utilise excess laryngeal effort to compensate for impaired respiratory function which leads to deterioration in voice quality and increased laryngeal trauma.

Reflux laryngitis is the term used to describe an inflammatory condition of the vocal folds resulting from refluxate reaching the level of the posterior vocal folds region causing tissue irritation and occasionally oedema and ulceration [26]. Key symptoms are rough vocal quality, vocal fatigue, globus sensation and throat clearing. While laryngopharyngeal reflux is recognised in voice disorders it is thought to be less significant as a cause for cough [29].

## SLP Assessment of Laryngeal Hyper-Responsiveness Syndromes

Referral to SLP for management of laryngeal hyper-responsiveness syndromes usually occurs following comprehensive medical management. Serious medical disease, such as lung pathology and asthma, needs to be excluded prior to commencing behavioural intervention. In short, we do not want to suppress cough in a patient with a compromised airway. SLP's typically deal with the subset of chronic cough that is refractory to medical treatment rather than all cases of chronic cough [30]. However, there are currently no guidelines around the degree of medical assessment and treatment that is needed prior to SLP intervention for cough. For example, diagnostic options for gastroesophageal reflux disease include 24-h ambulatory pH monitoring, gastroscopy, oesophagoscopy and empiric trials of proton pump inhibitors, however the extent to which these options should be trialled before referral to SLP is unclear. The relationship between gastroesophageal reflux and PVFM requires further research and the benefits of treating asymptomatic GERD in patients with VCD are unknown.

SLP assessment of laryngeal hypersensitivity syndrome involves case history in order to determine the nature, severity and characteristics of the patient symptoms, and the associated environmental and medical factors. In many cases symptoms are triggered by non-tussive stimuli, subthreshold tussive stimuli, abnormal laryngeal sensation or by talking. Patient rated symptom scales can be used to quantify the patient perception of symptoms. They include the Leicester Cough Questionnaire [31], Newcastle Laryngeal Hypersensitivity Questionnaire [32], Cough Severity Index [33], Dyspnoea Severity Index [34], the Symptom Frequency and Severity Scale [35], the Voice Handicap Index [36] and the Reflux Symptom Index [37]. These scales all have different purposes and the choice of scale(s) is often determined by the syndrome indicated in the case history. Interestingly, laryngeal sensation is significantly worse in patients with laryngeal hyperresponsiveness syndromes compared to healthy controls ($p < 0.001$) but with no significant difference between patients with these various laryngeal syndromes ($p = 0.951$) [22, 32] (Fig. 27.2).

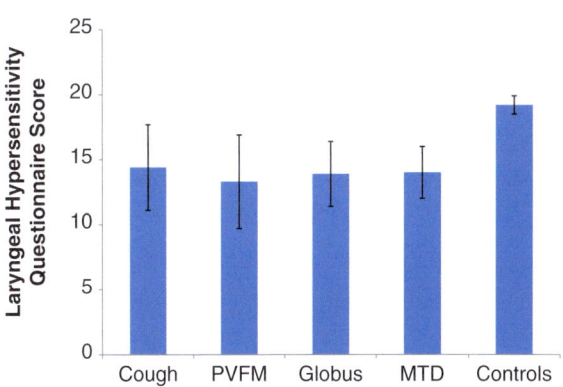

**Fig. 27.2** Comparison of laryngeal hypersensitivity questionnaire scores between patients with chronic cough, paradoxical vocal fold movement, globus pharyngeus, muscle tension dysphonia and healthy controls. The cut-off for normal function is 17.1

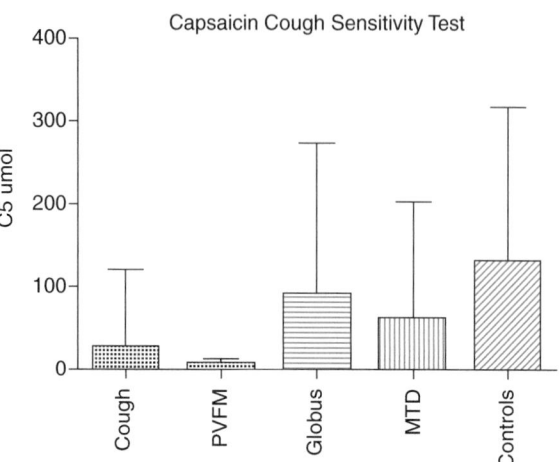

**Fig. 27.3** Comparison of capsaicin cough reflex sensitivity results between patients with chronic refractory cough, paradoxical vocal fold movement (PVFM), globus pharyngeus, muscle tension dysphonia (MTD) and healthy controls [22]

Following case history and symptom ratings, vocal hygiene factors including hydration and phonotraumatic behaviours are addressed as these can contribute to laryngeal irritation and exacerbate symptoms. Clinical assessment of oromusculature, cough, breathing and phonation is then conducted. Voice assessment tasks extend the voice to the limits of duration, pitch and loudness and can subsequently trigger cough to a greater extent than typical conversation. Instrumental assessment including acoustic voice analysis, electroglottography, nasendoscopy, hypertonic saline challenge and capsaicin cough sensitivity testing are also beneficial. The emotional impact of symptoms may need to be explored in some patients.

Cough reflex sensitivity testing determines the threshold for cough, but more importantly provides the opportunity to observe the patient's cough behaviour when exposed to tussive stimuli. For example, do they attempt to suppress a cough or do they cough at the first sign of an urge to cough? Interestingly, cough reflex sensitivity was significantly lower in patients with the laryngeal hyper-responsiveness syndromes compared to healthy controls ($p < 0.001$) [22] (Fig. 27.3).

## SLP Treatment of Laryngeal Hypers-Responsiveness Syndromes

SLP treatment for laryngeal hyper-responsiveness syndromes is distinct from medical management and has an emphasis on behavioural management of symptoms. Behaviour change is a critical component of most areas of SLP practice. Treatment aims to control functions typically considered outside of an individual's control such as swallowing, phonation, cough and breathing.

SLP treatment for laryngeal hyper-responsiveness syndromes involves four components: education, symptom control techniques, reducing laryngeal irritation and psychoeducational counselling [38–40]. Education facilitates the understanding of the rationale for therapy. It includes the reason for cough or laryngeal symptoms, the capacity for voluntary control of these symptoms, and the difference between essential cough where coughing is required to expectorate a foreign body or excess phlegm, and unnecessary cough that occurs in response to irritation.

There are a range of symptom control techniques which can be used to control cough and involuntary laryngeal closure. The choice of technique depends upon the specific symptoms and individual ability of the patient. The exercises are initially taught in the clinical setting during asymptomatic periods and then are gradually utilised outside the clinical setting to prevent or interrupt the symptoms occurring. The exercises must be practiced extensively with multiple repetitions in order for them to become automatic. Attention must be paid to ensure that the techniques are performed accurately. The treatment technique used for dysphonia will vary according to the underlying pathology but generally aims to achieve more efficient phonation in order to normalise pitch, loudness, quality and ease of phonation.

Laryngeal irritation is addressed by improving surface and systemic hydration, which is often reduced in patients with laryngeal hyper-responsiveness syndromes, and through reducing exposure to laryngeal irritants. Laryngeal irritants include inhaled or ingested substances such as fumes, smoke, alcohol and caffeine. Triggers are identified and avoided in the short term where practical. Once the patient has adequate control over their symptoms exposure to the triggers is gradually reintroduced. Phonotraumatic behaviours such as hard glottal attacks, excessive phonation or prolonged phonation at suboptimal pitch and loudness can exacerbate laryngeal irritation.

While it is beyond the scope of SLP practice to diagnose reflux, SLP are well placed to facilitate behaviour change in relation to reflux management. Lifestyle strategies for reflux such as smoking cessation, diet modification, weight loss and elevating the head of the bed [41] are important in reducing laryngeal irritation [42, 43]. Although most patients have received advice about lifestyle management options by their medical practitioner, it is our clinical experience that few patients have implemented these strategies. Furthermore, the SLP may have a role in reinforcing the adherence to the medical management of reflux. Some patients who are prescribed Proton Pump Inhibitors for cough cease taking it early either because they do not get classic reflux symptoms or because there is not an immediate response to the medication.

### Conclusion

Disorders resulting from reflux, aspiration and lung disease may affect a variety of laryngeal functions including cough, breathing, phonation and swallowing. These conditions may result in hypo or hyper laryngeal sensitivity which subsequently manifest as laryngeal dysfunction. The SLP has an important role in identifying the underlying behaviour, improving voluntary control of laryngeal behaviour, improving airway protection and preventing aspiration pneumonia.

## References

1. Steidl E, Ribeiro CS, Gonçalves BF, Fernandes N, Antunes V, Mancopes R. Relationship between dysphagia and exacerbations in chronic obstructive pulmonary disease: a literature review. Int Arch Otorhinolaryngol. 2015;19(1):74–9.
2. Groher M, Crary M. Dysphagia: clinical management in adults and children. St. Louis: Mosby Elsevier; 2010.
3. Addington WR, Stephens R, Widdicombe J, Rekab K. Effect of stroke location on the laryngeal cough reflex and pneumonia risk. Cough. 2005;1(1):4.
4. Addington WR, Stephens RE, Gilliland KA. Assessing the laryngeal cough reflex and the risk of developing pneumonia after stroke: an interhospital comparison. Stroke. 1999;30(6):1203–7.
5. Ward K, Seymour J, Steier J, Jolley CJ, Polkey MI, Kalra L, et al. Acute ischaemic hemispheric stroke is associated with impairment of reflex in addition to voluntary cough. Eur Respir J. 2010;36(6):1383–90.
6. Hu X, Yi ES, Ryu JH. Aspiration-related deaths in 57 consecutive patients: autopsy study. PLoS One. 2014;9(7):e103795.
7. Hu X, Lee JS, Pianosi PT, Ryu JH. Aspiration-related pulmonary syndromes. Chest. 2015;147(3):815–23.
8. Langmore SE, Terpenning MS, Schork A, Chen Y, Murray JT, Lopatin D, et al. Predictors of aspiration pneumonia: how important is dysphagia? Dysphagia. 1998;13(2):69–81.
9. Hinchey JA, Shephard T, Furie K, Smith D, Wang D, Tonn S. Formal dysphagia screening protocols prevent pneumonia. Stroke. 2005;36(9):1972–6.
10. Logemann JA, Veis S, Colangelo L. A screening procedure for oropharyngeal dysphagia. Dysphagia. 1999;14(1):44–51.
11. American Speech-Language-Hearing Association. Guidelines for speech-language pathologists performing videofluoroscopic swallowing studies [Guidelines]. 2004 [cited 2015 1/5/2015]. Available from http://www.asha.org/policy/GL2004-00050/.
12. Nacci A, Ursino F, La Vela R, Matteucci F, Mallardi V, Fattori B. Fiberoptic endoscopic evaluation of swallowing (FEES): proposal for informed consent. Acta Otorhinolaryngol Ital. 2008;28(4):206–11.
13. Sura L, Madhavan A, Carnaby G, Crary MA. Dysphagia in the elderly: management and nutritional considerations. Clin Interv Aging. 2012;7:287–98.
14. Pitts T, Rose MJ, Mortensen AN, Poliacek I, Sapienza CM, Lindsey BG, et al. Coordination of cough and swallow: a meta-behavioral response to aspiration. Respir Physiol Neurobiol. 2013;189(3):543–51.
15. Langmore SE, Pisegna JM. Efficacy of exercises to rehabilitate dysphagia: a critique of the literature. Int J Speech Lang Pathol. 2015;17(3):222–9.
16. Fujiwara S, Ono T, Minagi Y, Fujiu-Kurachi M, Hori K, Maeda Y, et al. Effect of supraglottic and super-supraglottic swallows on tongue pressure production against hard palate. Dysphagia. 2014;29(6):655–62.
17. Langmore SE, Skarupski KA, Park PS, Fries BE. Predictors of aspiration pneumonia in nursing home residents. Dysphagia. 2002;17(4):298–307.
18. Langdon PC, Lee AH, Binns CW. High incidence of respiratory infections in 'nil by mouth' tube-fed acute ischemic stroke patients. Neuroepidemiology. 2009;32(2):107–13.
19. McGrail A, Kelchner L. Barriers to oral fluid intake: beyond thickened liquids. J Neurosci Nurs. 2015;47(1):58–63.
20. Panther K. The Frazier free water protocol. Perspect Swallowing Swallowing Disord (Dysphagia). 2005;14:4–9.
21. Ryan N, Gibson P. Cough reflex hypersensitivity and upper airway hyperresponsiveness in vocal cord dysfunction with chronic cough. Respirology. 2006;11(Suppl 2):A48.
22. Vertigan AE, Bone SL, Gibson PG. Laryngeal sensory dysfunction in laryngeal hypersensitivity syndrome. Respirology. 2013;18(6):948–56.
23. Morrison M, Rammage L, Emami A. The irritable larynx syndrome. J Voice. 1999;13(3):447–55.

24. Dicpinigaitis PV, Tso R, Banauch G. Prevalence of depressive symptoms among patients with chronic cough. Chest. 2006;130(6):1839–43.
25. Vertigan AE, Theodoros DG, Winkworth AL, Gibson PG. Perceptual voice characteristics in chronic cough and paradoxical vocal fold movement. Folia Phoniatr Logop. 2007;59(5):256–67.
26. Stemple J, Glaze L, Klaben B. Clinical voice pathology: theory and management. 4th ed. Brisbane: Plural Publishing; 2010.
27. Boone D, McFarlane S, VonBerg S, Zraick R. The voice and voice therapy. 8th ed. Sydney: Allyn & Bacon; 2009.
28. Verdolini K, Rosen C, Branski R. Classification manual for voice disorders-I. Mahwah: Lawrence Erlbaum Associates; 2006.
29. Birring S. Controversies in the evaluation and management of chronic cough. Am J Respir Crit Care Med. 2011;183(6):708–15.
30. Gibson PG, Chang AB, Glasgow NJ, Holmes PW, Katelaris P, Kemp AS, et al. CICADA: cough in children and adults: diagnosis and assessment. Australian cough guidelines summary statement. Med J Aust. 2010;192(5):265–71.
31. Birring S, Prudon B, Carr A, Singh S, Morgan M, Pavord I. Development of a symptom specific health status measure for patients with chronic cough: Leicester Cough Questionnaire. Thorax. 2003;58:339–43.
32. Vertigan A, Bone S, Gibson PG. Development and validation of the Newcastle laryngeal hypersensitivity questionnaire. Cough. 2014;10(1):1.
33. Shembel AC, Rosen CA, Zullo TG, Gartner-Schmidt JL. Development and validation of the cough severity index: a severity index for chronic cough related to the upper airway. Laryngoscope. 2013;123(8):1931–6.
34. Gartner-Schmidt J, Shembel AC, Zullo T, Rosen CA. Development and validation of the dyspnea index (DI): a severity index for upper airway-related dyspnea. J Voice. 2014;28(6):775–82.
35. Vertigan A, Theodoros D, Gibson P, Winkworth A. Voice and upper airway symptoms in people with chronic cough and paradoxical vocal fold movement. J Voice. 2007;21(3):361–83.
36. Jacobson H, Johnson A, Grywalski C, Silbergleit A, Jacobson G, Benninger M. The voice handicap index (VHI): development and validation. Am J Speech Lang Pathol. 1997;6:66–70.
37. Belafsky PC, Postma GN, Koufman JA. Validity and reliability of the reflux symptom index (RSI). J Voice. 2002;16(2):274–7.
38. Vertigan A, Theodoros D, Gibson PG, Winkworth A. Efficacy of Speech pathology management for chronic cough: a randomised placebo controllled trial of treatment efficacy. Thorax. 2006;61(12):1065–9.
39. Vertigan A, Theodoros D, Winkworth A, Gibson P. Chronic cough: a tutorial for speech language pathologists. J Med Speech Lang Pathol. 2007;15:189–206.
40. Mathers-Schmidt B. Paradoxical vocal fold motion: a tutorial on a complex disorder and the Speech-Language pathologists role. Am J Speech Lang Pathol. 2001;10:111–25.
41. Kaltenbach T, Crockett S, Gerson LB. Are lifestyle measures effective in patients with gastroesophageal reflux disease? An evidence-based approach. Arch Intern Med. 2006;166(9):965–71.
42. Ness-Jensen E, Hveem K, El-Serag H, Lagergren J. Lifestyle intervention in gastroesophageal reflux disease. Clin Gastroenterol Hepatol. 2015;6(15):00635–7.
43. Haruma K, Kinoshita Y, Sakamoto S, Sanada K, Hiroi S, Miwa H. Lifestyle factors and efficacy of lifestyle interventions in gastroesophageal reflux disease patients with functional dyspepsia: primary care perspectives from the LEGEND study. Intern Med. 2015;54(7):695–701.

# Anti Reflux Surgery

## 28

Zainab Rai, Alyn H. Morice, and Peter Sedman

## Introduction

Surgery may be necessary to control gross reflux disease, particularly when anatomical abnormalities underlie the pathophysiology. Treatment is generally less successful when directed at isolated airway reflux and aspiration since the refluxate consists mainly of a gaseous mist which even the tightest 'wrap' will not be able to control. When successful however, repeated admissions for recurrent aspiration can be abruptly terminated.

**Case Report Via Email**
19th August 2015
   Dear Professor Morice,
   I just read an article about you on the internet and thought you might be interested in my story.
   I cannot remember the exact year but about 13 years ago I came to see you at Castle Hill about my chronic asthma, for the past 20 years before I had been in and out of hospital every week with bad asthma attacks and had got to the stage when I could barely walk down the street and had a nebuliser at home which I used a lot.
   After I came to see you and you suggested I had a laprascopic nissen fundoplication to help my asthma I was booked in to have it and then the week before I had my worst asthma attack and was in ICU on a life support machine for a week then in hospital for a month afterwards, when I had recovered enough I then had the operation you suggested.

---

Z. Rai · P. Sedman
Hull and East Yorkshire Hospitals NHS Trust, Hull, UK
e-mail: zainab.rai@nhs.net; peter.sedman@hey.nhs.uk

A. H. Morice (✉)
HYMS, University of Hull, Hull, UK
e-mail: a.h.morice@hull.ac.uk

I wanted you to know that since I had the operation I have not had a single asthma attack nor any symptoms, I have gone from being on constant steroids and nebulisers and in and out of hospital to living a normal life, I use no medication at all except for serotide (sic) 250 morning and night.

Your suggestion of the operation was a life saver for me and my life has been totally changed, I would be interested to know if you have the time to tell me how the operation worked so dramatically to end my asthma symptoms as I have asked various GPs and they don't have an answer.

Yours sincerely,

## Anatomy of the Oesophagus

The human oesophagus is approximately 25 cm long (10 in.) and starts in the neck at the lower border of the cricoid cartilage, at the level of the sixth vertebra. It travels through the mediastinum to end in the abdomen at the cardiac orifice of the stomach [1].

Structurally, the oesophagus comprises of 4 distinct layers; the outer connective tissue layer known as the areolar tissue, followed by the muscular layer which contains longitudinal muscle fibres and internal circular fibres. The oesophageal musculature is striated in the upper third and smooth in the lower two thirds. Below the muscular layer lies the submucosal layer containing mucus glands, followed finally by the mucosal layer consisting of stratified epithelium which in health makes an abrupt change to columnar epithelium marking the end of the oesophagus and the start of the stomach [2].

Anatomically, the oesophagus can be thought of in two distinct parts; cervical and thoracic. The cervical oesophagus starts in the neck and deviates slightly to the left. Its anterior relations include the trachea and thyroid gland. Posteriorly lie the sixth and seventh vertebrae and the pre vertebral muscles covered by the pre vertebral fascia. On either side, the cervical oesophagus is related to the common carotid artery and recurrent laryngeal nerve. Additionally on the left side, the subclavian artery and terminal part of the thoracic duct lie in close proximity.

The thoracic oesophagus traverses both the superior and posterior mediastinum. It returns to the midline at the level of the fifth thoracic vertebra before reaching the oesophageal opening at T10 in the diaphragm. Anteriorly, the thoracic oesophagus is crossed by the trachea, pericardium (which acts to separate the oesophagus from the left atrium) and the left bronchus which causes a slight constriction. Posteriorly, lie several structures including the thoracic vertebrae, the thoracic duct, azygos vein and tributaries and the descending aorta. On the left side, the thoracic oesophagus is related to the left subclavian artery, the terminal part of the aortic arch, the left recurrent laryngeal nerve, thoracic duct and left pleura. On the right side the azygos vein and right pleura form key relations [1].

The oesophageal nerve plexus consists of fibres from the vagus nerve (parasympathetic contribution) and visceral branches of the sympathetic nerve.

The vagus delivers two types of fibres to the plexus; the pre-ganglionic cholinergic parasympathetic fibres and afferent fibres. The pre-ganglionic fibres have cell bodies located in the dorsal motor nucleus of the vagus and synapse within the walls of the oesophagus in on the terminal ganglia. The afferent fibres from the vagus nerve are involved in autonomic reflexes. Ultimately, the two vagi nerves reform to make the vagal trunks with the left vagus forming the anterior trunk and the right forming the posterior trunk.

The second set of fibres are contributed by the sympathetic trunk and also deliver two distinct type of neurons; the sympathetic post-ganglionic fibres and afferent fibres which are primarily involved in relaying pain sensation [3].

## The Oesophagus and Reflux

Human beings as bi-pedal creatures are particularly at risk of gaseous airway reflux due to the evolutionary changes to the upper gastro-intestinal tract. In other mammals, the oesophagus lies horizontally with the stomach at the distal end positioned at a right angle, so that food boluses 'drop' into the stomach. In humans, the oesophagus is straightened and thus the anatomical barrier created by the right angle drop is obliterated. There is some compensation by the diaphragmatic crura through which the human oesophagus traverses, however the diaphragm is a mobile structure and therefore the risk of airway reflux is increased during episodes of phonation and in particular laughing, during which the intra-abdominal pressure fluctuates. An additional evolutionary change that serves to increase the risk of airway reflux in humans is the separation of the soft palate from the epiglottis and arytenoids which acts to permanently expand the oropharynx therefore making the transit of material from the stomach and oral cavity easy [4].

## Lower Oesophageal Sphincter

In the human oesophagus there is no distinct anatomical sphincter at the lower end of the oesophagus, none the less a sphincter mechanism exists as evidenced by the fact that generally, bending or lying flat does not cause a reflux.

The lower oesophageal sphincter is a complicated system. There are 5 key features that contribute to the sphincter effect at the lower oesophagus [5]:

1. A high pressure zone at the terminal oesophagus. This is physiological and can be easily demonstrated by oesophageal manometry.
2. The densely packed mucosal folds at the cardiac orifice effectively 'plugging' the oesophagus
3. The diaphragmatic crural sling which pinches the oesophagus
4. The oblique angle at which the oesophagus enters the stomach which acts to create a valve-like effect
5. The intra-abdominal positive pressure acting on the terminal part of the oesophagus that lies in the abdomen [6].

## Surgery and the Oesophagus

Surgical intervention in reflux disease is crucially dependant on the pathological process leading to the reflux. The pathology is basically of two types. Firstly there is a disorder of the lower oesophageal sphincter such as laxity or frequent transient openings [7]. Secondly there may be a disorder of the motility of the oesophagus leading to poor clearance of gastro-oesophageal reflux or oesophago-pharyngeal reflux [8, 9]. Currently this latter pathological process is not amenable to surgical intervention, although in future methods of exciting oesophageal peristalsis through electrical stimulation may be developed. The problem with oesophageal dysmotility is that ineffective peristaltic waves maybe further inhibited by any correction of lower oesophageal sphincter anatomy and the patient may experience an increase in symptoms coupled with gas bloat. Thus it is crucial that before any surgery is contemplated the precise pathophysiological mechanisms are elucidated. The development of high resolution oesophageal manometry has greatly helped this area and the high quality images now coupled with impedance measurements greatly enhances the ability to predict surgical outcomes (see Chap. 10). We undertake multi-disciplinary team meetings where surgical, gastroenterological and respiratory opinions are combined in the full evaluation of the patient.

## Surgical Techniques to Improve Lower Oesophageal Sphincter Tone

The advent of laparoscopic fundoplication has revolutionised surgical management of reflux disease. Whilst there is much controversy as to the precise technique leading to the 'wrap' there is little evidence in randomised control trials of the superiority of one technique over another. Individual centres through the familiarity with their preferred technique advocate full or partial 'wrap' and perhaps expertise and frequent experience are more important than the technique itself [10].

The most commonly used method of fundoplication is Nissen's fundoplication and it is briefly described below (see Fig. 28.1).

The first Nissen's fundoplication was carried out in 1955 by Dr. Rudolp Nissen to treat severe oesophagitis, however it wasn't until the 1970s that [11] the procedure gained popularity and today is considered to be the gold standard in the surgical management of airway reflux disease, gastro-oesophageal reflux disease and surgical repair of hiatus hernia.

The surgery involves plicating or 'wrapping' the gastric fundus around the lower oesophagus thus mechanically reinforcing the lower oesophageal sphincter. The 'wrapped' fundus is then sutured in place. There are several different degrees of plication that can be performed; similarly a wrap can be made both anteriorly and posteriorly.

Although the initial Nissen's fundoplication was an open procedure, over the last 4 decades a laparoscopic approach to this procedure has gained favour and is now the synonymous with Nissen's. The technique described in this chapter is a laparoscopic 360° anterior wrap.

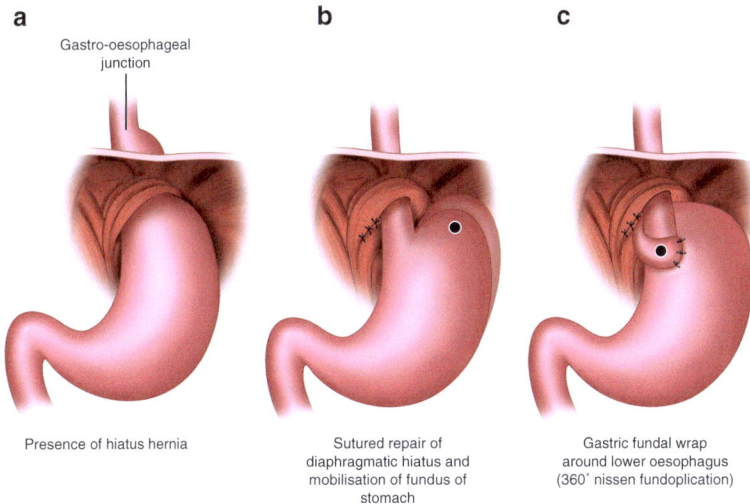

**Fig. 28.1** Schematic diagram of Nissen fundoplication—after a drawing by Mr P Sedman

A number of varying methods may be employed for port placements and these depend largely on individual surgeon's preference. Most surgeons will place of a total of 5 ports for a Nissen's fundoplication. These include; a supra-umbilical port, which serves as the camera port, a subcostal port in the right mid-clavicular line. An atraumatic liver retractor is inserted through this port to lift up the left hemiliver thereby exposing the hiatus. Retraction of the hemiliver may be facilitated either by an assistant of by a self-retraining apparatus. Another 2 port sites are created subcostally, one to the right of the midline and the other to the left of the midline. Instruments through these ports are used to carry out dissection during the procedure. A final port site is fashioned in the left midclavicular line, subcostally. This port is used for additional instruments that may be needed during the procedure [12].

Once the hiatus is exposed, the lesser omentum is opened preserving the hepatic branch of the anterior vagus nerve. Dissection is then carried out towards the diaphragm bilaterally so that the crura are exposed. Using blunt dissection the oesophagus is separated from the diaphragmatic crura. Once the oesophagus has thus been separated circumferentially, a nylon tape is inserted through the left sub-costal, midclavicular port and the oesophagus is circled. By retracting the nylon tape anteriorly, the posterior hiatus of the oesophagus is revealed. Using precise dissection the posterior aspect of the oesophagus is mobilised.

In the traditional Nissen's, a bougie is inserted into the oesophagus prior to the wrap to ensure that the patency of the oesophagus is not compromised. There are a number of alternative methods that can be employed intra-operatively to reduce the risk of post-operative dysphagia. The exact technique depends on individual surgeons preferences, and may include the insertion of an intra-oesophageal bougie or the free movement of a 10 mm instrument or bougie passed adjacent to the oesophagus [13].

With the aid of atraumatic Babcock graspers, the fundus of the stomach is wrapped around the lower oesophagus such that the anterior and posterior walls of the stomach are meet anteriorly. This is then secured with interrupted sutures. A few of these sutures should contain the oesophageal wall to stop post-operative sliding of the cardia of the stomach.

The final stage of the procedure involves a thorough examination of the abdomen to ensure good haemostasis. The port are subsequently removed under direct vision and fascia closed with non-absorbable sutures. The skin may be closed with absorbable sutures or glue.

Complications of this operation are of two main types. Initially many patients describe dysphagia or food sticking. This usually resolves over a couple of months but can be intractable and the fundoplication may need to be reversed. Secondly, the objective of the procedure is to prevent reflux and whilst this is highly effective against liquid acid reflux which can be a major cause aspiration, it is less effective against gaseous airway reflux, since no matter how tight the wrap, sufficient lumen is required to allow the food to transit and thus gas may leak back. The two consequences of this is that success against symptoms such as cough, which is caused by the particulate matter in the gaseous reflux are successfully treated in approximately two thirds of cases and the other third may suffer the consequences of gaseous bloat adding additional abdominal symptoms to those from the upper airway. Because of this morbidity our view is that the surgical option should only be considered when there is failure of medical treatment and the patient is suffering from intolerable symptoms or is in danger of potentially fatal aspiration.

## References

1. Drake RL, Vogl W, Tibbitts AW. Gray's anatomy for students. Philadelphia: Elsevier/Churchill Livingston; 2005.
2. Patti MG, Gantert W, Way LW. Surgery of the esophagus. Anatomy and physiology. Surg Clin North Am. 1997;77:959–70.
3. Woodland P, Sifrim D, Krarup AL, Brock C, Frokjaer JB, Lottrup C, Drewes AM, Swanstrom LL, Farmer AD. The neurophysiology of the esophagus. Ann N Y Acad Sci. 2013;1300:53–70.
4. Laitman JT, Reidenberg JS. The human aerodigestive tract and gastroesophageal reflux: an evolutionary perspective. Am J Med. 1997;103:2S–8S.
5. Boyce HW. The normal anatomy around the oesophagogastric junction: an endoscopic view. Best Pract Res Clin Gastroenterol. 2008;22:553–67.
6. Dent J. Approaches to driving the evolving understanding of lower oesophageal sphincter mechanical function. J Smooth Muscle Res. 2007;43:1–14.
7. Allen CJ, Newhouse MT. Gastroesophageal reflux and chronic respiratory disease. Am Rev Respir Dis. 1984;129:645–7.
8. Fouad YM, Katz PO, Hatlebakk JG, Castell DO. Ineffective esophageal motility: the most common motility abnormality in patients with GERD-associated respiratory symptoms [see comments]. Am J Gastroenterol. 1999;94:1464–7.
9. Kastelik JA, Aziz I, Thompson R, Redington AE, Ojoo J, Buckton GK, Smith CM, Dakkak M, Morice AH. Gastroesophageal dysmotility as a cause of chronic persistent cough. Am J Respir Crit Care Med. 2001;163:A60.

10. Andolfi C, Plana A, Furno S, Fisichella PM. Paraesophageal hernia and reflux prevention: is one fundoplication better than the other? World J Surg. 2017;41:2573.
11. Cooper JD, Jeejeebhoy KN. Gastroesophageal reflux: medical and surgical management. Ann Thorac Surg. 1981;31:577–93.
12. DeMeester TR, Bonavina L, Albertucci M. Nissen fundoplication for gastroesophageal reflux disease. Evaluation of primary repair in 100 consecutive patients. Ann Surg. 1986;204:9–20.
13. Mathavan VK, Yuh JN, Marks JM. Long-term evaluation of patients undergoing laparoscopic antireflux surgery without bougie placement. J Laparoendosc Adv Surg Tech A. 2009;19:7–12.

# Index

**A**
Acid secretion, 33
Acid suppression
  in cystic fibrosis, 322
  extra-digestive GERD
    effectiveness and failure, 279
    management, 278–281
  geographical variations, 269
  medical management, 270
  proton pump inhibitors
    efficacy of, 272–274
    extra-digestive GERD, 277–278
    maintenance, 274–276
    safety concerns, 281–285
Acute aspiration model, 149
Acute respiratory failure, 236
$\beta_2$ Agonists, 334–336
Airflow obstruction, 138
Airway disease
  asthma, 61
  COPD, 60–61
  cystic fibrosis, 61–63
  prokinectics, 297
  reflux inhibitors, 295
Airway hyper-responsiveness (AHR), 138
Airway reflux, 49
  characteristics, 82
  combine questionnaires, 86
  HARQ, 85–86
  PRSQ, 84–85
  RSI, 83
  SERQ, 83–84
Alcohol consumption, 17
Alveolar macrophages (AMs), 151
American College of Gastroenterology
      guidelines, 155
American Society for Parenteral and Enteral
      Nutrition (A.S.P.E.N.), 230

$\gamma$-aminobutyric acid (GABA), 294
Animal models, 42
Antacid PPI therapy, 155–157
Anti-cholinergics, 337
Antisecretory drugs, 272
Arbaclofen placarbil, 294
Aspartate proteases, 31
Aspiration, 55, 263
  cystic fibrosis, 189
  contribution of, 238
  pneumonia, 261, 345
    treatment, 263
  tracheal cuff shape, 240
  VAEs, 236
Association of Gastrointestinal Physiologists
      Guidelines, 120
Asthma, 42, 61, 307–308
  antacid PPI therapy, 155–157
  aspiration markers, 150
  causes, 142, 144–145
  diagnosis, 3
  flatulent, 4
  life-style modifications, 157
  multiple inflammatory stimuli, 138
  non-eosinophilic forms, 141
  obesity, 154
  obstructive sleep apnea, 152–154
  principal, 138
  therapy, 138
  triggers, 6
Azithromycin, 305, 306, 319–321
  in cystic fibrosis, 323–324

**B**
Baclofen, 294
Barium esophagram, 106
Bernoulli's Principle, 144

Bile acids, 34, 42, 45, 151
   aspriation of, 191
   concentration, 189, 190
   in saliva, 189
Boyle's Law, 144
British Thoracic Society, 3
Bronchial responsiveness
   aforementioned study, 74
   negative mechanistic study, 74
   treatment of GERD, 75
Bronchiectasis, 314–316
   aetiology, 175–178
   bacteriology of, 178–179
   description, 175
   effect of treatment, 182
   *Helicobacter pylori*, 180–181
   high-resolution computed tomography, 177
   investigation, 181
   quality of life and, 181
Bronchiolitis obliterans, macrolide, 308–314
Bronchiolitis obliterans syndrome (BOS), 64, 213, 217
Bronchodilators
   anti-cholinergics, 337
   $\beta_2$ agonists, 334–336
   nebulised recombinant human DNase, 338
   theophyllines, 336–337

**C**
*Cacochymia*, 4
Caffeine, 35
Capsaicin, 35
Capsaicin inhalation cough challenge, 73
Cell models, 43–48
Cervical oesophagus, 358
Chenodeoxycholic acid (CDCA), 45
Cholecystokinin, 141
Chronic allograft rejection, 220
Chronic aspiration, 149
Chronic cough, 59, 154, 206, 210
   end-stage lung disease, 214
   reflux, 101
Chronic obstructive pulmonary disease (COPD), 42, 60–61
   azithromycin, 319–321
   cigarette smoking, 317
   clarithromycin, 319
   clinical course, 316
   definition, 165
   exacerbations, 165
   erythromycin, 318
   gastroesophageal reflux disease
      epidemiology and prevalence, 166
      exacerbations, 168–169
      implications, 170

   outcomes, 170
   potential mechanisms, 167–168
   prevalent, 317
Chronic refractory cough, 349
Chyle, 6
Chyme, 30
Cilostazol, 264
Cisapride, 297
Citric acid, 73
Clarithromycin, 305, 306, 319
Cochrane Database Systematic Review, 230
Comprehensive Reflux Symptom Scale (CReSS), 86
Concomitant pulmonary disease, 213
Continuous maintenance therapy, 276
Continuous positive airway pressure (CPAP), 152
Conventional oesophageal manometry, 116
COPD, *see* Chronic obstructive pulmonary disease (COPD)
*COPDGene*, 169
Copenhagen City Heart study, 171
Cough, 128, 131
   detection, 127–128
   events, 129–131
   frequency, 128
   GERD-associated, 208
   limitations of current methodology, 126
   mechanism, 122
   monitoring
      anti-tussive medications, 131
      relationship between type and site of GOR, 128
   reflex
      depression, 263
      sensitivity testing, 72, 73, 352
   severity, 126–127
   sound, 127, 131
Cough reflex sensitivity
   capsaicin inhalation cough challenge, 73
   citric acid, 73
   clinical trial, 72
   preclinical study, 72
Cough-specific Quality of Life Questionnaire (CQLQ), 127
Cystic fibrosis (CF), 61–63
   acid suppression, 322
   airway inflammation, 188
   autosomal recessive multisystem disorder, 322
   azithromycin, 323–324
   bile acids, 191
   characteristics, 188
   lung disease, 322
   lung function, 190
   prevalence, 188, 322

reflux mechanisms, 189
treatment, 191, 192

### D
Depression, of cough reflex, 263
Diagnostic confusion, 3
Dietary intake, 35–36
Distal esophageal reflux, 145
Distal intestinal obstruction syndrome (DIOS), 188
Dopaminergic pathway, 295
Duodenogastric reflux, 34
Dyspepsia, 7
Dysphagia, in elderly, 262
Dysphonia, 4, 350

### E
End-stage lung disease (ESLD)
    development, 214
    reflux prevalence in patients, 215
Erythromycin, 304–306, 318
Esophagopharyngeal reflux, 108
Exocrine secretions, 32
Extra-digestive GERD, 277, 278
Extra-esophageal reflux (EER), 241
Extra-esophageal syndromes, 140

### F
Fibreoptic endoscopic evaluation of swallowing (FEES), 347
Flatulent asthma, 5
Flexible bronchoscopy, 238
Fractalkine, 43

### G
Gamma scintigraphy, 108
Gastric fluid, 149
Gastric microbiome, 33–34
Gastric mucus, 32
Gastric secretion
    aspartate proteases, 31
    control, 32–33
    endocrine cells, 30
    glands, 30
    hydrogen ions, 31
    mucin, 32
    stomach acid, 31
Gastro oesophageal reflux (GOR), 55
Gastroesophageal reflux disease (GERD), 93, 246–252
    acid suppression, 23–24
    anti-reflux surgery, 20–21

chronic cough
    barium swallow, 208
    clinical presentation, 206
    epidemiology, 206
    24-H oesophageal pH monitoring, 209
    management, 208
    mechanisms, 207–208
    multichannel intraluminal impedance, 209
    oesophageal manometry, 208
    pathophysiology, 207
    treatment, 209
classical symptoms, 81
clinical conditions, 9
cough, 125
definition, 9, 81
diagnosis, 10, 12–13
    barium swallow, 16
    oesophageal manometry, 16
    pH-impedance monitoring, 14–16
    proton pump inhibitor trial, 13–14
    scintigraphy, 16
    tests, 12, 105
    UGIE, 14
endoluminal therapy, 20
epidemiology, 10–12, 140, 166
exacerbations, 168
*Helicobacter pylori*, 24
implications, 170
lifestyle modification, 17
manifestations, 81
medical therapy
    acid neutralization, 17–19
    barrier forming agents, 19
    mucosal protective, 20
    prokinetic agents, 20
    selective serotonin reuptake inhibitors, 20
    tricyclic antidepressants, 20
outcomes, 170
pathophysiology, 293
pediatrics, 246
    endoscopy and biopsies, 249
    esophageal pH monitor, 248
    history and physical examination, 247
    lifestyle changes, 251
    multiple intraluminal impedance, 248
    non-pharmacologic treatment, 250
    pathophysiology, 246
    pharmacologic treatment, 251
    prevalence, 246
    surgical treatment, 252
potential mechanisms, 167
prevalence, 11, 166
surgery, 157–158
symptoms, 9, 15, 71, 205
therapy, 17

Gastrointestinal (GI) motility disorders, 228
Gastrointestinal tract, 249
Gastro-oesophageal pressure gradients (GOPG), 119
Global Initiative for Chronic Obstructive Lung Disease (GOLD), 165
GERD, *see* Gastroesophageal reflux disease (GERD)

## H

Haematoxylin, 42
*Helicobacter pylori* (HP), 24, 33
    bronchiectasis, 180–181
Hiatal hernias (HH), 177
High resolution oesophageal manometry (HRM)
    catheters, 117
    fundamental advantage, 117
    perform, 120
    physiological measurement, developments, 121
    technical theory, 117
    trace, 122
High-resolution computed tomography (HRCT), 177, 197
Histamine2 (H2) antagonists, 251
Hospital-acquired pneumonia (HAP), 8
Hull airways reflux questionnaire (HARQ), 85–86, 181
Human gastric juice, 94
Humid, *see* Flatulent asthma

## I

Idiopathic pulmonary fibrosis (IPF), 49, 57
    aetiology, 215
    acute exacerbations, 198
    anti-acid medications, 200
    asymptomatic GERD, 198
    cause and effect, 197
    clinical features, 195
    contradictions, 217
    development, 216
    evaluate GER in, 196
    incidence and prevalence, 195
    lifestyle modifications, 199
    natural history, 198
    non-acid reflux, 198
    pathogenesis, 196
    progression, 199
    proton pump inhibitors, 200
Ilaprazole, 23

Intensive care unit (ICU)
    aspiration, 229
    critically-ill patients, 228
    gastric *vs.* post-pyloric, 230
    GI motility disorders, 228
    stress ulcer prophylaxis, 228–229
    ventilator-associated pneumonia, 230–231
Intragastric imaging, 32
IPF, *see* Idiopathic pulmonary fibrosis (IPF)
Itopride, 297

## L

Lansoprazole, 170
Laparoscopic fundoplication, 360
Laryngeal hyper-responsiveness syndrome
    assessment, 351
    causative factors, 349
    conditions, 350
    consequences, 350
    feature, 349
    management, 351
    mechanism, 349
    treatment, 352–353
    triggering protective airway responses, 349
Laryngitis, 350
Laryngopharyngeal reflux (LPR), 61, 99, 280
Leicester Cough Monitor (LCM), 127
Leicester Cough Questionnaire (LCQ), 126–127
Lesogaberan, 294
Lipid laden alveolar macrophages (LLM), 189, 238, 239
Lower oesophageal sphincter, 359
Lung allograft dsyfunction, 217–220
Lung disease, 350
    antibacterial effect, 306–307
    with GOR
        airway disease, 60–64
        parenchymal disease, 57–60
    immunomodulatory effect, 307
    NTM, 179–180
    prokinetic effect, 305–306
Lung Sound Monitoring Device, 130
Lung transplantation, 64

## M

Macro-aspiration, 236
Macrolide, 303
    antibiotics, 170
    history of, 304

in lung disease
    antibacterial effect, 306–307
    immunemodulatory effect, 307
    prokinetic effect, 305–306
in respiratory disease
    asthma, 307
    bronchiectasis, 314–316
    bronchiolitis obliterans, 308–314
Magnetic resonance imaging (MRI), 110–111
Mechanical ventilation, 236
Metabotropic glutamate receptor 5 (mGluR5), 295
Microaspiration, 59, 122, 237
Microbiome, 65
Mixed disciplinary team (MDT), 64
Morbid obesity, 21
Mucin, 32
Multiple Intraluminal Impedance (MII), 248
Mycobacterium avium complex (MAC), 179

## N
NCFB, *see* Non-cystic fibrosis bronchiectasis (NCFB)
Nebulised recombinant human DNase (rhDNase), 338
Nissen's fundoplication, 360
Nitric oxide, 34
Non-acid reflux, 49
Non-alloimmune injury, 64
Non-cardiac chest pain (NCCP), 278
Non-cystic fibrosis bronchiectasis (NCFB), 63
Non-erosive reflux disease (NERD), 273
Non-gastric secretions, 34

## O
Obesity, 17
Obstructive sleep apnea (OSA), 153
Oesophageal dysmotility, 122
Oesophageal hypersensitivity, 23
Oesophageal manometry, cough, 126
Oesophagus
    anatomy, 358–359
    dysmotility, 360
    in humans, 359
Omeprazole+succinic acid, 23
Oral care, 263
Oropharyngeal dysphagia, 344
    aspiration, 345, 348
    assessment, 346
    clinical assessment, 346
    consequences, 345
    instrumental assessment, 347
    oral and pharyngeal phases, 344
    quality of life, 348
    respiratory disease, 345
    screening test, 346
    solid food, 345
    swallowing, 344
    treatment, 347

## P
Par Vagum, 6
Parenchymal disease, 58
Pediatrics, in GERD
    diagnosis, 247–249
    pathophysiology, 246
    prevalence, 246
    treatment, 250–253
Pepsin, 31, 238
    analysis, 96–98
    asthma and GERD, 151
    concentration, 99
    detection, 95
    history, 93–94
    identification, 95
    nomenclature, 94
    predictive power, 239
    structure, 94
Pepsinogen secretion, 33
Peptest, 98
Pharyngeal reflux symptom questionnaire (PRSQ), 84–85
pH-impedance monitoring
    indication, 15
    wireless pH, 16
Pneumonia, 345
    in elderly, 261
    treatment, 263
Pressure sensitivity, 115
Prokinetics, 295
Proton pump inhibitors (PPI), 240
    consumption, 19
    cystic fibrosis, 191
    discontinuation, 23
    efficacy, 18
    ineffectuality, 19
    infants, 251
    IPF, 200
    trial, 13–14
Pulmonary aspiration, 237
Pulmonary micro-aspiration, 168
Pulmonary scintigraphy, 189

**R**
Rabeprazole, 23
Rat gastroduodenal reflux models, 41
Reflux, 4
　anatomy, 92
　animal models, 41–42
　aspiration, 149–150
　biomarkers, 249
　cell models, 43–48
　diagnostic tests, 95
　human study, 49–51
　MRI imaging technique, 110–111
　neural mechanisms, 60
　nuclear medicine, 108–110
　oesophagitis, 35
　peptest, 98
　prevalence, 93
　surgical intervention, 360
　treatment, 357
　in upper airway, 146–148
　X-ray, 106–108
Reflux symptom index (RSI), 83
Refluxate
　chemical composition, 30, 36
　in lung, 49
　lung aspiration, 109
　saliva secretion, 34
　short-chain fatty acids, 34
　tissues to, 30
Respiration, 262
　bronchiectasis, 314–316
　bronchiolitis obliterans, 308–314

**S**
Saliva, 34
Salivary amylase, 238
Salivary pepsin, 98
Smoking, 17
Society of Critical Care Medicine (SCCM), 230
Speech-language pathologists (SLP)
　laryngeal conditions, 344
　laryngeal hyper-responsiveness syndrome
　　assessment, 351
　　causative factors, 349
　　conditions, 350
　　consequences, 350
　　feature, 349
　　management, 351
　　mechanism, 349
　　treatment, 352–353

　　triggering protective airway
　　　responses, 349
　oropharyngeal dysphagia
　　aspiration, 345, 348
　　assessment, 346
　　clinical assessment, 346
　　consequences, 345
　　instrumental assessment, 347
　　oral and pharyngeal phases, 344
　　quality of life, 348
　　respiratory disease, 345
　　screening test, 346
　　solid food, 345
　　swallowing, 344
　　treatment, 347
S-Tenatoprazole, 23
Stretta, 20
Sucralfate, 20
Supine anteroposterior esophagram, 107
Supraoesophageal reflux questionnaire
　(SERQ), 83–84
Surgical fundoplication, 66
Swallowing, 262
Symptom Association Probability (SAP)
　Index, 125, 130

**T**
Tenatoprazole, 23
Theophyllines, 336–337
Thoracic oesophagus, 358
Transepithelial resistance (TER), 45
Transient lower oesophageal sphincter
　relaxation (TLOSR), 117, 294

**U**
Upper aerodigestive tract, 34
Upper gastrointestinal contrast
　radiography, 249
Upper gastrointestinal endoscopy (UGIE),
　14, 249

**V**
Ventilator associated events (VAEs), 236
Ventilator-associated pneumonia (VAP),
　230–231, 236
VitaloJak monitor, 127
Vocal cord dysfunction, 349
Vonoprazan, 23

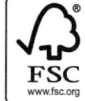

MIX
Papier aus verantwortungsvollen Quellen
Paper from responsible sources
FSC® C105338

If you have any concerns about our products,
you can contact us on
**ProductSafety@springernature.com**

In case Publisher is established outside the EU,
the EU authorized representative is:
**Springer Nature Customer Service Center GmbH**
**Europaplatz 3, 69115 Heidelberg, Germany**

Printed by Libri Plureos GmbH
in Hamburg, Germany